Essentials of Medical Terminology

Second Edition

To my loving parents,
Bill and Renee Ozorio,

and to my brothers,
Michael, Stephen, and Timothy

Essentials of Medical Terminology

Second Edition

Juanita Davies, B.Sc. HRA

DELMAR
™
THOMSON LEARNING

Australia Canada Mexico Singapore Spain United Kingdom United States

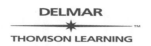

DELMAR

THOMSON LEARNING

Essentials of Medical Terminology, 2nd Edition
by Juanita Davies, B.Sc. HRA

Health Care Publishing Director:
William Brottmiller

Executive Editor:
Cathy L. Esperti

Acquisitions Editor:
Sherry Gomoll

Editorial Assistant:
Jennifer Conklin

Executive Marketing Manager:
Dawn F. Gerrain

Channel Manager:
Jennifer McAvey

Technology Project Manager:
Laurie Davis

Technology Project Specialist:
Joe Saba

Art/Design Coordinator:
Robert Plante

Cover Design:
SchoolhouseGraphics.com

Project Editor:
David Buddle

Production Coordinator:
Anne Sherman

For permission to use material from this text or product, contact us by
Tel   (800) 730-2214
Fax   (800) 730-2215
www.thomsonrights.com

Library of Congress Cataloging-in-Publication Data
Davies, Juanita J.
   Essentials of medical terminology / Juanita J. Davies. — 2nd ed.
      p. cm.
   Includes index.
   ISBN 0-7668-3110-8
   1. Medicine—Terminology   I. Title.
R123 .D28 2001
610'.1'4—dc21
                                                    2001037125

NOTICE TO THE READER

Contents

Preface

Who This Book Is For

Essentials of Medical Terminology, second edition, is designed specifically for students taking a one-semester medical terminology course. Every word of the text has been written with the goal of making it possible for a wide range of students to acquire a basic medical terminology vocabulary in 15 to 16 weeks. The exercises and Instructor's Manual are practical, straightforward, and extensive enough that most instructors will not need to supplement them. Answers to exercises are provided to enable students to take responsibility for monitoring their own learning. The Instructor's Manual makes it possible for the text to be used in a variety of learning modes and environments.

Strategy for Learning

Students should master Chapter 1 before moving on to other chapters. It describes a simple method of analyzing medical terms that has proved effective for my own students over the years. Chapters 2, 3, and 4 introduce standard roots, suffixes, and prefixes. They should also be learned before other chapters. The remaining chapters teach the terms associated with each body system in a variety of sequences to suit your needs. They contain just enough anatomy and physiology to make the chapters interesting and the terms easily understandable, but not so much that the student gets bogged down.

Part of completing a chapter is doing the exercises in the text as well as on the CD-ROM. Students should also take personal responsibility for studying the terminology tables and self-testing for mastery. Because the tables are the heart of the text, they are designed to make learning and remembering the terms as easy as possible. Terms are chunked in association with common word elements. Tables are placed where it makes the most sense from a learning perspective. Explanatory notes are used when extra information will enhance the learning experience.

Essentials of Medical Terminology, second edition, is a useful and effective learning tool. The chapter pedagogical elements include:

- **Chapter Organization**—an outline of all major chapter headings.
- **Chapter Objectives**—an outline of key content covered in the chapter. These objectives, along with the workbook and practice software exercises, may be used to test students' understanding of the chapter content.
- **Introduction**—a brief paragraph describing the main chapter content.
- **Anatomy and Physiology Coverage**—terminology introduced in the context of the basic anatomy and physiology of each body system to give students a reference point—something to "hang their hat on" when studying medical terms.

- **Term Analysis and Definition Section**—word elements (root, suffixes, or prefixes) are introduced and then followed by several examples of terms using the particular word element. This clustering or "chunking" of new terms makes retention easier.
- **Review of Terms**—a comprehensive review at the end of each chapter includes terms categorized into the following groups: anatomy and physiology, pathology, diagnosis, and clinical and surgical procedures. It is a perfect summary to help reinforce words learned throughout the chapter.
- **Abbreviations**—the most common abbreviations and definitions for the topic of each chapter are listed.
- **Putting It All Together**—extensive exercises that include short-answer, matching, building medical words, spelling, identification, and defining exercises.

New to This Edition

SPECIAL FEATURES

- Appendixes B, **Word Element to Definition**, and C, **Definition to Word Element**, have been added to facilitate quick translation.
- The definitions of new suffixes, roots, and prefixes have been added to each chapter, highlighting new word elements for the student to study.
- Memory keys have been reformatted to highlight different ideas within each key.
- Chapters have been reorganized to cluster related systems.
- New illustrations have been added to facilitate student learning.
- Illustrations are in four colors to enhance the visibility of anatomical structures.

CHANGES TO THE CHAPTERS

Chapter 7, The Skeletal System—Student learning is enhanced by the addition of new information about joints as well as a new table summarizing the location of skeletal structures.

Chapter 10, The Eyes and Ears—Student learning is enhanced by the addition of new information on cataracts and deafness.

Chapter 12, The Cardiovascular System—Student learning is enhanced by the expansion of information relating to the pulse.

Chapter 13, Blood and the Immune and Lymphatic Systems—The text is updated by the addition of information relating to antibody-antigen reaction.

Chapter 14, The Respiratory System—Because the condition is increasingly prevalent, information relating to bronchial asthma has been added.

Chapter 15, The Digestive System—Sections on types of teeth and types of hernias have been added.

Chapter 17, The Female Reproductive System and Obstetrics—The chapter has been expanded to include new information on the placenta, human chorionic gonadotrophic hormone, amniocentesis, and chorionic villus sampling.

Features of the Book

SOFTWARE
A free Student Practice CD-ROM is packaged with the textbook to help students maximize learning. The CD-ROM's appealing exercises and games will help students remember even the most difficult terms. See the Student Practice CD-ROM for more details.

READABILITY
Much attention has been paid to maintaining a reading level suitable for intended students.

MEMORY KEYS
Memory keys are used throughout the text to emphasize and encapsulate basic concepts. This feature not only facilitates learning but also makes review and study easier.

PHONETIC PRONUNCIATION
All of the important terms are followed by easy-to-read, phonetic pronunciations.

ILLUSTRATIONS
Many illustrations have been included to give this text the visual enhancements needed to help students learn medical terminology. Illustrations have also been placed in the analysis tables to provide instant visualization.

Instructor's Manual

An *Instructor's Manual* has been created to assist with lesson preparation and student performance assessment. The *Instructor's Manual* includes:

- Developing a Medical Terminology Course—includes two sample syllabi (15-week and 10-week courses), as well as grading policy ideas and test and quiz suggestions
- Chapter tests for each of the 17 chapters of the textbook
- Midterm exam
- Final exam
- Word element quizzes for each of the body system chapters

About the Author

Juanita Davies has taught anatomy and medical terminology since 1973. She has also written extensively on the subject of medical terminology. Her early work includes *A Programmed Learning Approach to Medical Terminology* and a computerized testbank containing 15,000 questions that students have been using since 1985. Her first book with Delmar, *Modern Medical Language*, is a combination of anatomy and medical terminology. Her third book, *A Quick Reference to Medical Terminology*, is currently in production.

Acknowledgments

Special thanks to Cathy Esperti, Executive Editor, whose timely and knowledgeable advice greatly improved the quality of this text. Thank you also to the production and editorial staff for their suggestions and support in completing this project.

And to my husband, Jim, thank you for taking time out of your busy schedule to proof-read the final manuscript. Your assistance was invaluable.

Reviewers

Special appreciation goes to the following reviewers for their insights, comments, suggestions, and attention to detail, which were very important in guiding the development of this textbook.

Jean Fisher, MBA, MS, RRT
Director of Clinical Education, Assistant Professor
University of Charleston
Charleston, WV

Robert Formanek, MT (ASCP), CMA
Instructor
Gateway Technical College
Elkhorn, WI

Paulette Nitkiewicz, BSN, RN, CMA
Program Director, Instructor
Laurel Business Institute
Uniontown, PA

Sylvia Nobles, CRNP, MSN
Director, Instructor
Trenholm State Technical College
Montgomery, AL

How to Use the Student Practice CD-ROM

The Student Practice CD-ROM packaged with this text has been specifically designed to accompany *Essentials of Medical Terminology*, second edition, to help you learn even the toughest medical terms. By using these exercises and games, you'll challenge yourself and other students and make your study of medical terms more effective.

This software can be used for practice, review, or self-testing, or it can be used with the timed Speed Test to see how quickly you can answer the questions. The software will track your correct and incorrect answers and can print out a report of how you've done. The software includes more than 800 questions covering 17 chapters. The exercises and activities include:

- **Application Exercises**—multiple choice, fill-in, and labeling
- **Game Activities**—crossword puzzles, hangman, concentration, tic-tac-toe, and a board game

Getting started is easy. Follow the simple directions in the book to install the program on your computer. Then take advantage of the features. If you get stuck, press F1 for on-line help covering all parts of the software.

System Requirements

- Microsoft® Windows® 95 or better
- 486 MHz CPU (Pentium recommended)
- 16 MB or more of RAM
- Double-spin CD-ROM drive
- 10 MB or more free hard drive space
- 256-color display or better

Setup Instructions

1. Insert disk into CD-ROM player.
2. From the Start Menu, choose **RUN**.
3. In the **Open** text box, enter **d:setup.exe** then click the **OK** button. (Substitute the letter of your **CD-ROM** drive for **d:**.)
4. Follow the installation prompts from there.

Basic Medical Terminology

C H A P T E R

1

Learning Medical Terms

CHAPTER OBJECTIVES

On completion of this chapter, you will be able to do the following:

1. Pronounce medical terms
2. Define parts that make up medical terms
3. Analyze component parts of medical terms
4. Identify words with no prefixes or roots
5. Understand when a combining vowel is used or not used
6. Distinguish between a combining vowel and a combining form
7. Pluralize medical terms

INTRODUCTION

Medical terminology is used to describe such things as parts of the body, locations in the body, bodily functions, diseases, surgical and clinical procedures, measurements, medical instruments, and many others. Each medical term describes in a single word something that would otherwise require several words to express. For example, the term *appendicitis* is a short form of saying "inflammation of the appendix."

Medical terminology is most easily learned by using an organized approach called **term analysis**, which is what this chapter is about. When you have mastered term analysis, you will be ready to learn the meanings of the most common parts of medical terms, which are the subjects of Chapters 2, 3, and 4. All of the remaining chapters deal with medical terminology used in relation to the various systems of the human body.

At various places in the book, you will find short summaries of information called **memory keys**. Their purpose is to make study and review easier. They are also a useful way for you to check your understanding of key concepts as you read through the text. There are also lots of exercises at the end of each chapter, which allow you to test yourself to ensure that you have learned the essentials.

At the end of Chapters 6 through 17, there is a review of the terms pertinent to the body system being studied. The medical terms have been grouped into specialties; that is, all the anatomical terms are grouped together, all the pathologic terms are grouped together, and all the diagnostic and surgical terms are grouped together. As a review, the student can define the term in the space provided.

1.1   Pronunciation Guide

It is very important that you know how to pronounce the medical terms you learn. If you cannot pronounce a term, it will be difficult for you to remember how to spell it, and accurate spelling is very important. However, the proper pronunciation of a medical term is not always obvious. Therefore, all difficult terms in their first appearance in this book are typed in bold print and are followed by a common pronunciation. Many terms have more than one accepted pronunciation, so do not be surprised if from time to time your instructor prefers a pronunciation different from the one given in this book. In these cases, simply strike out the pronunciation given here, and replace it with the version your instructor prefers.

The system of pronunciation in this book is quite simple. Each term is respelled using combinations of letters that are commonly known to have a particular sound. For instance, *tion* will be written as *shun*. When the letters *a* and *u* are to be pronounced as they are in the word *acute*, they will be rewritten as *ah* and *you*, respectively. The long *a* sound as in the word *pain* is written as *ay*. The long *i* sound is written as *igh* or *eye*. Long *e* is written as *ee*. Short *e* is *eh* when it stands alone as a syllable, and otherwise is just *e*. Long *o* is written as *oh*. The syllables of the respelled term are separated by hyphens (-). The most strongly emphasized syllable is written in bold type with capital letters (e.g., **BOLD**). Any syllable with secondary emphasis is written in bold but without capitals (e.g., **bold**). To help you put this all together, here are a few examples:

Syllable	Pronunciation	Example
tion	shun	regurgitation (ree-**gur**-jih-**TAY**-shun)
short a sound	ah	acute (ah-**KYOUT**)
short e sound	eh	hematemesis (**hee**-mah-**TEM**-eh-sis)
short i sound	ih	adipose (**AD**-ih-pohs)
long a sound	ay	pain (payn)
long e sound	ee	ileitis (**ill**-ee-**EYE**-tis)
long i sound	igh or eye	rhinitis (rye-**NIGH**-tis) ileitis (**ill**-ee-**EYE**-tis)
long o sound	oh	anorexia (**an**-oh-**RECK**-see-ah)
long u sound	you	acute (ah-**KYOUT**)

1.2   The Parts of Medical Terms

Medical terms are made up of the following word elements: **prefixes**, **roots**, and **suffixes**. Not all terms have all three parts, but let's start by looking at an example that does.

periarthritis (**per**-ee-ar-**THRIGH**-tis)

peri-   prefix
arthr   root
-itis   suffix

The first part is the prefix. Whenever a prefix stands alone in this book, it is followed by a hyphen (for example, the prefix in the above example, if standing alone, would be written as peri-). You will learn all the common prefixes in Chapter 4. The root in the example (**arthr**) is in the middle, in bold type. In this book, all roots are in bold type, so that you can easily identify them. You will get an introduction to the common roots in Chapter 2. The last part of our example is the suffix. Whenever a suffix stands alone in this book, it is preceded by a hyphen (e.g., -itis). Suffixes are dealt with in Chapter 3. When you learn the common prefixes, roots, and suffixes, you will be able to understand the meaning of terms you have not seen before by simply analyzing the term using the method described in the next section.

Memory Key   The parts of medical terms are prefixes, roots, and suffixes.

1.3   How to Analyze Medical Terms

When you analyze a term, always start with the suffix. Look again at the example in section 1.2. The suffix is -itis, which means "inflammation." Now look at the prefix, peri-. It means "around." By combining these two, you know that the term refers to "inflammation around something." Now look at the middle of the term. It is the root "**arthr**," meaning joint. Putting it all together, we learn that peri**arthr**itis means inflammation around a joint. It is important that you fully understand the proper procedure for analyzing terms.

Memory Key	To analyze a term, always start with the suffix. Then go to the beginning of the word; it will be either a prefix or a root. If there is an additional part in that term, it will be a root.

1.4   Terms with No Prefix

Some terms have no prefix. An example is

arthritis (ar-**THRIGH**-tis)

-itis   suffix meaning "inflammation"
arthr   root meaning "joint"

The meaning of the complete medical term, reading from the suffix to the beginning of the word, is "inflammation of a joint."

Table 1-1 gives additional examples of terms with no prefix.

TABLE 1-1

EXAMPLES OF TERMS WITH NO PREFIX

Term	Definition
gastritis (gas-**TRY**-tis)	inflammation of the stomach
hepatitis (**hep**-ah-**TYE**-tis)	inflammation of the liver
carditis (kar-**DYE**-tis)	inflammation of the heart
adenitis (**ad**-eh-**NIGH**-tis)	inflammation of a gland
cardiology (**kar**-dee-**OL**-oh-jee)	study of the heart
gastrology (gas-**TROL**-oh-jee)	study of the stomach
hepatology (**hep**-ah-**TOL**-oh-jee)	study of the liver

| Memory Key | Some terms have a suffix and a root, with no prefix. |

1.5   Terms with No Root

Some terms consist of a prefix and suffix, with no root at all. An example is

neoplasm (**NEE**-oh-plazm)

neo-   prefix meaning "new"
-plasm   suffix meaning "growth"

The meaning of the complete term is "new growth."

1.6   Terms with Two Roots

Some terms have two roots followed by a suffix. Examples are

osteoarthritis (oss-tee-oh-ar-**THRIGH**-tis)

-itis   suffix meaning "inflammation"
-oste/o   root meaning "bone"
arthr   root meaning "joint"

The meaning of the complete term is inflammation of the bone and joint.

gastroenteritis (**gas**-troh-en-ter-**EYE**-tis)

-itis   suffix meaning "inflammation"
gastr/o   root meaning "stomach"
enter/o   root meaning "intestine"

The meaning of the complete term is "inflammation of the stomach and intestine."

When two roots are combined, there will be an additional vowel placed between them to make pronunciation easier. This is called a **combining vowel**, which is discussed in the next section.

| Memory Key | When a term has two roots, they are joined with a combining vowel and are followed by a suffix. |

1.7   The Combining Vowel

A combining vowel is a vowel, usually *o*, that combines two roots or a root and a suffix. Using the example *osteoarthritis*, you can see that the vowel *o* joins the two roots *oste* and *arthr*. The *o* in this case is a combining vowel. Its only purpose is to aid pronunciation. Similarly, in *gastroenteritis*, the combining vowel *o* joins the two roots *gastr* and *entr*.

In the above examples, a combining vowel is used between two roots, as in osteoarthritis and gastroenteritis. But when a root is followed by a suffix, a combining vowel is used *only when the suffix begins with a consonant.* In Table 1-1, the term *cardiology* uses the combining vowel *o* between the root and suffix because the suffix -logy begins with a consonant.

> **cardi**ology (**kar**-dee-**OL**-oh-jee)
>
> -logy   suffix meaning "the study of"
> **cardi**   root meaning "heart"
> /o   combining vowel

In the example *gastritis*, there is no combining vowel between the word root **gastr** and the suffix -itis because the suffix starts with a vowel.

> **gastr**itis (gas-**TRY**-tis)
>
> -itis   suffix meaning "inflammation"
> **gastr**   root meaning "stomach"

Although *o* is by far the most common combining vowel, occasionally *e* or *i* is used. An example using *e* is **chol**elith (**KOH**-lee-lith), meaning "gallstones," and an example using *i* is **dent**iform (**DEN**-tih-form), meaning "shaped like a tooth."

> **chol**elith (**KOH**-lee-lith)
>
> -lith   suffix meaning "stone"
> **chol**   root meaning "gall"
> /e   combining vowel

> **dent**iform (**DEN**-tih-form)
>
> -form   suffix meani ng "shape"
> **dent**   root meaning "tooth"
> /i   combining vowel

Note that in the examples *cholelith* and *dentiform*, the combining vowel is used because the suffix starts with a consonant. Rare exceptions to this rule are the terms *biliary* (**BILL**-ee-air-ee), which means "pertaining to the bile ducts," and *angiitis* (an-jee-**EYE**-tis), which refers to inflammation of a blood vessel. Angiitis is also frequently written angitis (an-**JEYE**-tis).

Table 1-2 provides examples of when a combining vowel is used and not used.

TABLE 1-2

PROPER USE OF A COMBINING VOWEL

Term	Explanation
gastritis (gas-**TRY**-tis)	no combining vowel is used because the suffix -itis starts with a vowel
gastrology (gas-**TROL**-oh-jee)	the combining vowel is used because the suffix -logy starts with a consonant

continued on page 9

Table 1-2 *continued from page 8*

Term	Explanation
cephalgia (seh-**FAL**-jee-ah)	no combining vowel is used because the suffix -algia starts with a vowel
hepatopathy (**hep**-ah-**TOP**-ah-thee)	the combining vowel is used because the suffix -pathy starts with a consonant

Memory Key A combining vowel is used between two roots. Between a root and a suffix, the combining vowel is used when the suffix begins with a consonant.

1.8 The Combining Form

You have already learned what a combining vowel is. The **combining form** is the name given to a root that is followed by a combining vowel. For example, the root **arthr**, written in its combining form, is

arthr/o

Notice that in many of the above examples, the root is separated from the combining vowel by a slash (/). This indicates that the *o* may or may not be used in a medical word. Other examples of combining forms are provided in Table 1-3. Note that the combining form is often easier to pronounce than the root alone.

Memory Key The combining form is the root plus the combining vowel.

TABLE 1-3

ADDITIONAL EXAMPLES OF COMBINING FORMS

Combining Form	Root	Meaning
gastr/o	**gastr**	stomach
hepat/o	**hepat**	liver
aden/o	**aden**	gland
cardi/o	**cardi**	heart

1.9   Plurals

Plurals are formed in various ways, depending on which letters are at the end of a term. To form the plural of singular terms ending in *is*, change the *i* to an *e*, as shown in the following examples:

Singular	Plural
diagnosis (**dye**-ag-**NOH**-sis)	diagnoses (**dye**-ag-**NOH**-seez)
pelvis (**PEL**-vis)	pelves (**PEL**-veez)
neurosis (new-**ROH**-sis)	neuroses (new-**ROH**-seez)

To form the plural of many singular words ending in *us*, change the *us* to an *i*, as shown in the following examples:

Singular	Plural
bronchus (**BRONG**-kus)	bronchi (**BRONG**-kye)
bacillus (bah-**SILL**-us)	bacilli (bah-**SILL**-eye)
calculus (**KAL**-kyou-lus)	calculi (**KAL**-kyou-lye)
embolus (**EM**-boh-lus)	emboli (**EM**-boh-lye)

There are a few exceptions. For example, the plural of *virus* (**VYE**-rus) is *viruses* (**VYE**-rus-ez), and the plural of *sinus* (**SIGH**-nus) is *sinuses* (**SIGH**-nus-ez).

The plural of singular words ending in *a* is formed by adding an *e* to the word, as shown in the following examples. Modifiers in Latin must agree with the noun. For example, the plural of *vena cava* is *venae cavae*.

Singular	Plural
sclera (**SKLEHR**-ah)	sclerae (**SKLEHR**-ee)
scapula (**SKAP**-you-lah)	scapulae (**SKAP**-you-lee)
vena cava (**VEE**-nah **CAV**-ah)	venae cavae (**VEE**-nee **CAV**-ee)

Singular terms ending in *um* are pluralized by changing the *um* to an *a*, as shown in the following examples:

Singular	Plural
acetabulum (**ass**-eh-**TAB**-you-lum)	acetabula (**ass**-eh-**TAB**-you-lah)
capitulum (ka-**PIT**-you-lum)	capitula (ka-**PIT**-you-lah)
septum (**SEP**-tum)	septa (**SEP**-tah)
diverticulum (**dye**-ver-**TICK**-you-lum)	diverticula (**dye**-ver-**TICK**-you-lah)

To form the plural of singular words ending in *ix* or *ex*, change the ending to *ices*, as shown in the following examples:

Singular	Plural
calix (**KAY**-licks)	calices (**KAY**-lih-seez)
cervix (**SER**-vicks)	cervices (**SER**-vih-seez)
index (**IN**-decks)	indices (**IN**-dih-seez)
varix (**VAR**-icks)	varices (**VAR**-ih-seez)

Singular words ending in *oma* are made plural by the addition of a *ta* or *s*, as shown in the following examples:

Singular	Plural
adenoma (**ad**-eh-**NOH**-mah)	**aden**omata or **aden**omas (**ad**-eh-no-**MA**-tah) (**ad**-eh-**NOH**-mahz)
carcinoma (**kar**-sih-**NOH**-mah)	**carcin**omata or **carcin**omas (**kar**-sin-oh-**MA**-tah) (**kar**-sin-**OH**-mahz)
fibroma (figh-**BROH**-mah)	**fibr**omata or **fibr**omas (figh-broh-**MA**-tah) (figh-**BROH**-mahz)

To form the plural of singular words ending in *nx*, change the *x* to *g* and add *es*, as shown in the following examples:

Singular	Plural
larynx (**LAR**-inks)	**laryn**ges (**LAR**-in-jeez)
phalanx (**FAH**-lanks)	**phalan**ges (fah-**LAN**-jeez)

To form the plural of singular words ending in *on*, change the *on* to an *a* or simply add an *s*, as shown in the following example:

Singular	Plural
ganglion (**GANG**-glee-on)	**gangli**a or **gangli**ons (**GANG**-glee-ah) (**GANG**-glee-onz)

To form the plural of singular words ending in *ax*, change the *ax* to *aces*, as shown in the following example:

Singular	Plural
thorax (**THOH**-racks)	**thor**aces (**THOH**-rah-sees)

Memory Key	Remember the following rules:		
	is→es	um→a	nx→nges
	us→i	ix→ices	on→a, or simply add an *s*
	a→ae	oma→omata; omas	ax→aces

1.10   Putting It All Together

Exercise 1-1   FILL IN THE BLANKS

1. The three parts of a medical term are the _____ , _____ , and

_____ .

2. The component part usually found at the end of a medical word is the _____ .

3. When you analyze a medical term you start with the _____ , and then define the

_____ .

4. The root in periarthritis is _____ .

5. The difference between the combining form and combining vowel is _____

_____ .

Exercise 1-2   TRUE OR FALSE

1. The term *carditis* has no prefix.   T   F

2. An example of a word with no root is *gastrology*.   T   F

3. In the term *hepatopathy*, the combining vowel is used because
   the suffix starts with a consonant.   T   F

4. A combining vowel is not used between two roots.   T   F

5. The prefix peri- means "around."   T   F

Exercise 1-3   SINGULARS AND PLURALS

Give the plural for the following singular forms.

Singular   **Plural**

1. thorax   _____

2. neurosis   _____

3. ganglion   _____

4. virus   _____

5. phalanx   _____

6. fibroma   _____

7. varix   _____

8. diverticulum   _____

9. scapula   _____

10. embolus   _____

Give the singular for the following plural forms.

Plural   **Singular**

1. larynges   _____

2. carcinomas   _____

3. calices   _____

4. acetabula   _____

5. sclerae   _____

6. bronchi   _____

7. diagnoses   _____

8. sinuses   _____

9. septa   _____

10. indices   _____

Roots of Each Body System

2

CHAPTER ORGANIZATION

This chapter will help you learn basic anatomical roots. It is divided into the following sections:

CHAPTER OBJECTIVES

On completion of this chapter, you will be able to do the following:

1. Define *anatomy* and *physiology*
2. Describe the levels of organization into which the body is arranged
3. Name the body systems
4. Define and spell common anatomical roots

INTRODUCTION

This chapter starts by introducing you to some basic concepts related to the study of the human body. It will prepare you for learning the roots you need to know for this and the following chapters on suffixes and prefixes.

The roots in this chapter are grouped according to body systems. You will find it much easier to remember each root if you associate it with a mental picture of the organs it refers to. The roots you will encounter in this chapter will give you a foundation, a base for building medical terms found in Chapters 3 and 4. Additional roots pertinent to each body system can be found in Chapters 6 through 17. Note that the roots in the tables of this chapter are expressed in their combining forms, as described in Chapter 1.

2.1   Anatomy and Physiology

Two terms you will encounter often in this text are *anatomy* and *physiology*. Anatomy is the study of the parts of the body. The names and locations of the muscles of the body exemplify anatomy. Physiology is the study of how the body parts work. Gas exchange at the alveolar-capillary membrane is an example of physiology.

Memory Key	Anatomy is the study of structure. Physiology is the study of function.

2.2   Levels of Organization

All life consists of microscopic living structures called *cells*, which perform various functions in the body. Regardless of their function, all cells are similar—though not identical—in structure. They have an outer membrane and various internal structures that absorb nutrients, create protein, fight bacteria, excrete wastes, and store various products created within the cell. In other words, the cell is a structural and functional unit despite its size. Cells make up the cellular level, which is the first level of organization of the body. The next level is called *tissue*. Cells combine to make tissues such as muscle and bone. Tissues combine to make up *organs*, such as the heart and liver. Related organs make up *organ systems*, such as the cardiovascular and skeletal systems. All of the organ systems go together to form the human body. To summarize, the various levels of organization of the body are cells, tissues, organs, organ systems, and the entire body (the organism). Figure 2-1 illustrates these levels of organization. Later in this chapter, all of the individual organ systems are illustrated.

Memory Key	The levels of organization of the body, from smallest to largest, are cells, tissues, organs, systems, organism.

2.3   Organ Systems

Twelve organ systems (often called body systems) make up the human body. These systems work together to perform all the necessary functions of life. The following figures illustrate all of these systems. Included with each figure is a list of the common anatomical roots of each system.

Memory Key There are 12 organ (body) systems: integumentary, skeletal, muscular, digestive, nervous, endocrine, eyes and ears, cardiovascular, lymphatic and immune, respiratory, urinary, and reproductive.

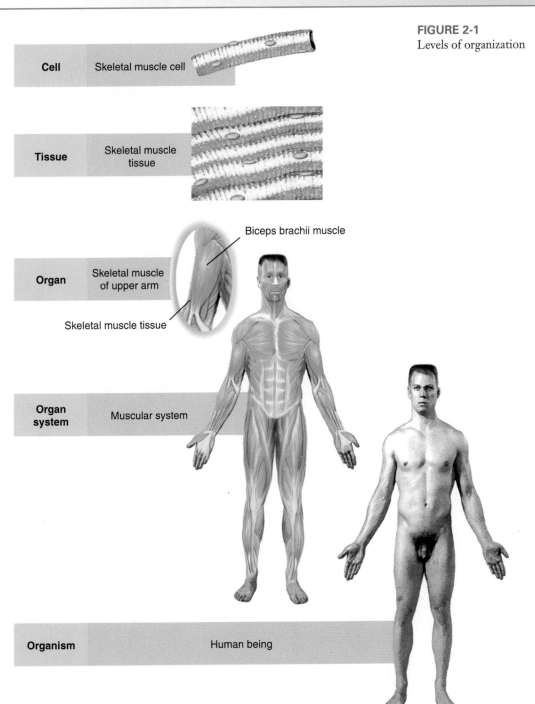

FIGURE 2-1
Levels of organization

Cell   Skeletal muscle cell

Tissue   Skeletal muscle tissue

Biceps brachii muscle

Organ   Skeletal muscle of upper arm

Skeletal muscle tissue

Organ system   Muscular system

Organism   Human being

2.4   Common Anatomical Roots

BODY AS A WHOLE

Root	Meaning
adip/o; lip/o; steat/o	fat
axill/o	armpit
bi/o	life
cephal/o	head
cervic/o	neck
cyt/o	cell
hist/o; histi/o	tissue
path/o	disease
viscer/o	internal organs

FIGURE 2-2
Integumentary system: skin and accessory organs such as hair, nails, sweat glands, oil glands

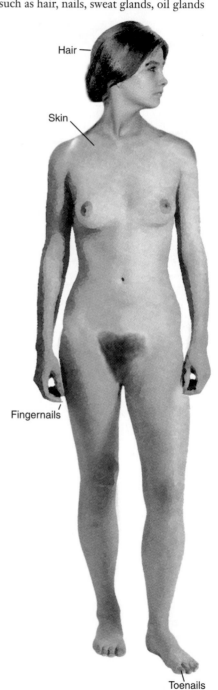

Hair

Skin

Fingernails

Toenails

SKIN (INTEGUMENTARY SYSTEM)

Root	Meaning
cili/o; pil/o	hair
derm/o; dermat/o; cutane/o	skin
onych/o; ungu/o	nail

SKELETAL SYSTEM

Root	Meaning
arthr/o	joint
chondr/o	cartilage
crani/o	skull
cost/o	rib
myel/o	bone marrow (also means spinal cord)
oste/o	bone
pelv/o	pelvis
spin/o	spine; spinal (vertebral) column; backbone
vertebr/o; spondyl/o	vertebra

FIGURE 2-3
Skeletal system: bones, cartilage, joints

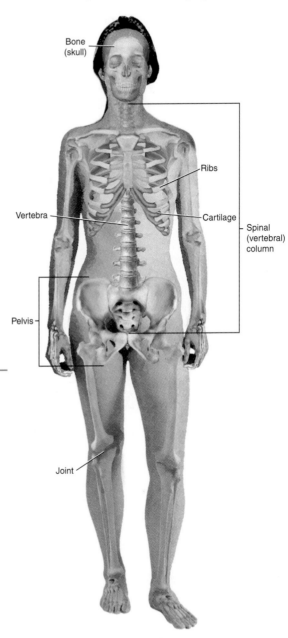

Bone (skull)

Ribs

Vertebra

Cartilage

Spinal (vertebral) column

Pelvis

Joint

MUSCULAR SYSTEM

Root	Meaning
my/o; muscul/o	muscle
tend/o; tendin/o	tendon

FIGURE 2-4
Muscular system: muscles and tendons

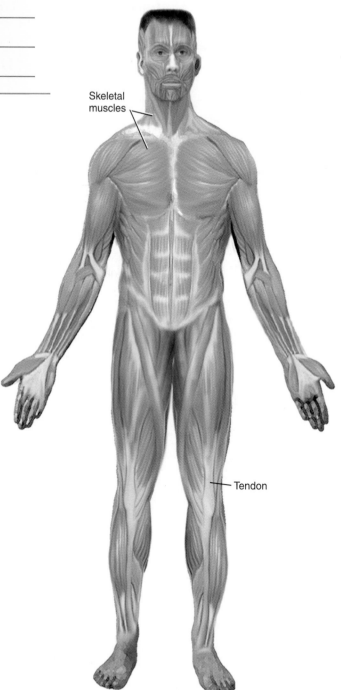

Skeletal muscles

Tendon

NERVOUS SYSTEM; EYES, EARS

Root	Meaning
blephar/o	eyelid
cerebr/o; encephal/o	brain
myel/o	spinal cord (also means bone marrow)
neur/o	nerve
ophthalm/o; ocul/o	eye
ot/o	ear

FIGURE 2-5
Nervous system and organs of special sense: brain, spinal cord, nerves, eyes, ears

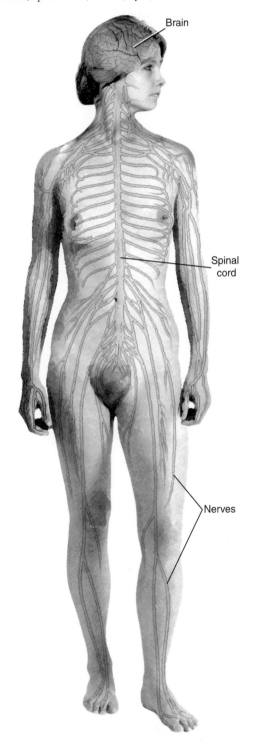

ENDOCRINE SYSTEM

Root	Meaning
aden/o	gland
adren/o	adrenal gland
parathyroid/o	parathyroid gland
pituitar/o	pituitary gland
thyroid/o	thyroid gland

FIGURE 2-6

Endocrine system: pituitary, thyroid, parathyroid, adrenal, and pineal glands; thymus, portions of the hypothalamus and the pancreas; ovaries; testes. Also included are hormonal secretions from each gland.

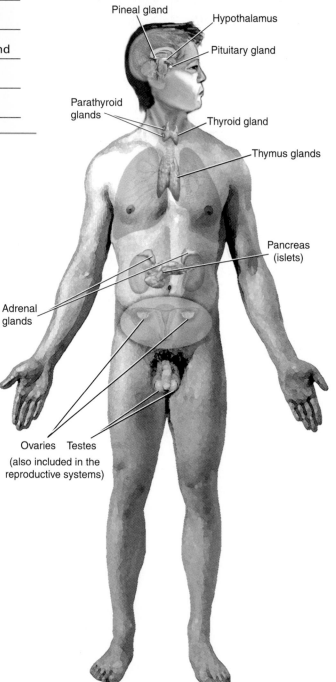

Pineal gland
Hypothalamus
Pituitary gland
Parathyroid glands
Thyroid gland
Thymus glands
Pancreas (islets)
Adrenal glands
Ovaries   Testes
(also included in the reproductive systems)

CIRCULATORY SYSTEM

Root	Meaning
angi/o; vascul/o; vas/o	vessel
arteri/o	artery
cardi/o	heart
hem/o; hemat/o	blood
ven/o; phleb/o	vein

FIGURE 2-7
Circulatory system: heart, arteries, veins, capillaries, blood

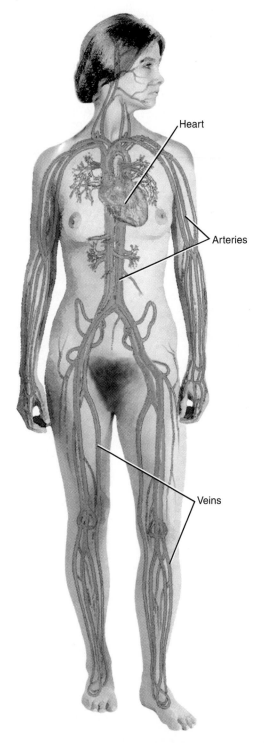

Heart

Arteries

Veins

LYMPHATIC AND IMMUNE SYSTEMS

Root	Meaning
adenoid/o	adenoids
lymph/o	lymph (clear, watery fluid)
lymphaden/o	lymph glands; lymph nodes
lymphangi/o	lymph vessels
splen/o	spleen
tonsill/o	tonsils

FIGURE 2-8

Lymphatic and immune systems: thymus, bone marrow, spleen, tonsils, lymph nodes, lymph capillaries, lymph vessels, lymphocytes, lymph

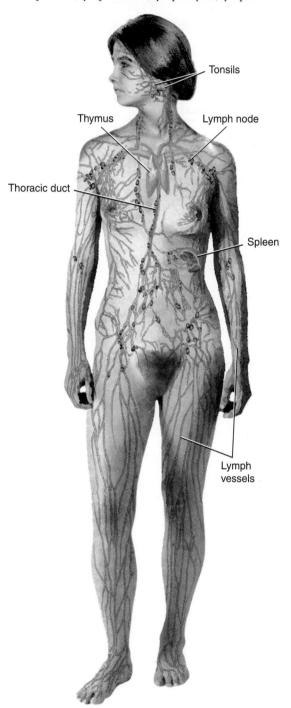

Tonsils

Thymus

Lymph node

Thoracic duct

Spleen

Lymph vessels

RESPIRATORY SYSTEM

Root	Meaning
alveol/o	air sac; alveolus
bronch/o; bronchi/o	bronchus
bronchiol/o	small bronchial tubes
laryng/o	voice box; larynx
nas/o; rhin/o	nose
pharyng/o	throat; pharynx
phren/o	diaphragm
pneum/o; pneumon/o; pulmon/o	lungs
thorac/o	chest
trache/o	windpipe; trachea

FIGURE 2-9
Respiratory system: lungs, nasal cavity, pharynx, larynx, trachea, bronchi, bronchioles

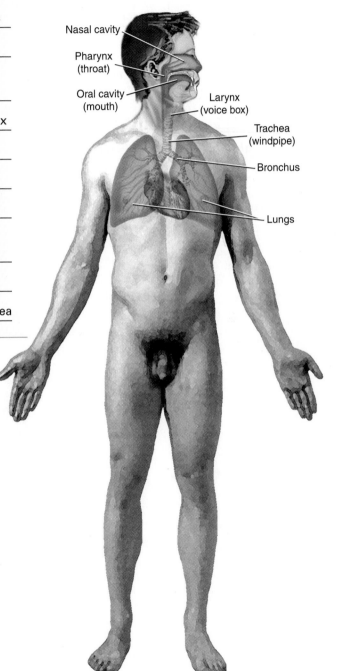

DIGESTIVE SYSTEM

Root	Meaning
abdomin/o	abdomen
cheil/o	lips
col/o	large intestine; colon
enter/o	small intestine
esophag/o	esophagus
gastr/o	stomach
gloss/o; lingu/o	tongue
hepat/o	liver
or/o; stomat/o	mouth
pharyng/o	throat; pharynx (also part of the respiratory system)
rect/o	rectum

FIGURE 2-10
Digestive system: mouth, pharynx, esophagus, stomach, small intestine, large intestine, salivary glands, pancreas, gallbladder, liver

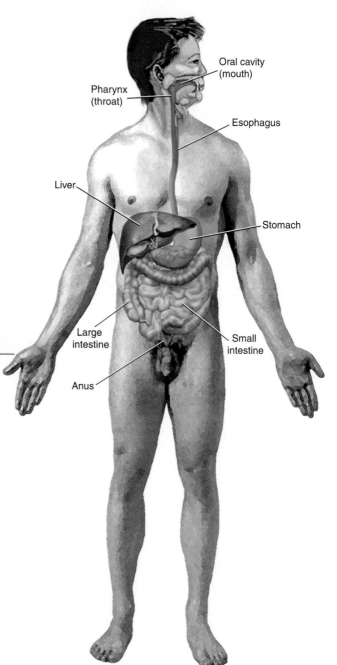

URINARY SYSTEM

Root	Meaning
cyst/o	bladder
ren/o; nephr/o	kidneys
ureter/o	ureters
urethr/o	urethra

FIGURE 2-11
Urinary system: kidneys, ureters, urinary bladder, urethra

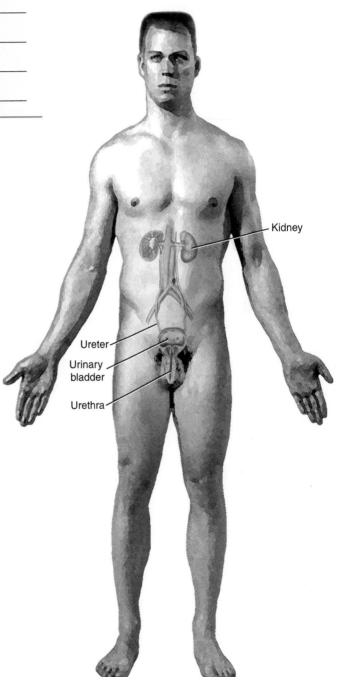

Kidney

Ureter

Urinary bladder

Urethra

MALE REPRODUCTIVE SYSTEM

Root	Meaning
epididym/o	epididymis
orchid/o; test/o; testicul/o	testicle; testis
phall/o	penis
prostat/o	prostate gland
vas/o	ductus (vas) deferens

FIGURE 2-12
Male reproductive system: testes, epididymides, ductus deferens, ejaculatory ducts, penis, seminal vesicles, prostate gland

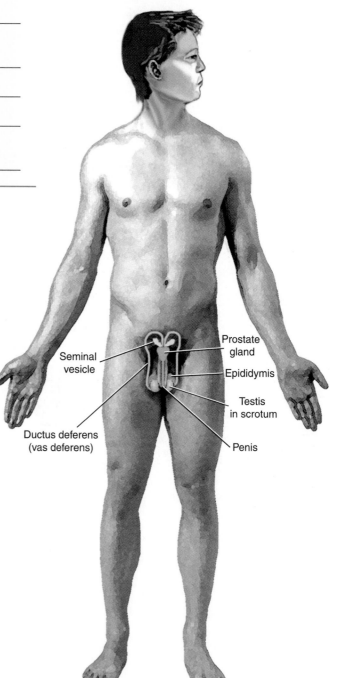

FEMALE REPRODUCTIVE SYSTEM

Root	Meaning
colp/o; vagin/o	vagina
gynec/o	female
mast/o; mamm/o	breast
oophor/o; ovari/o	ovary
salping/o	fallopian tubes; uterine tubes
uter/o; hyster/o; metr/o	uterus
vulv/o	vulva; external genitalia

FIGURE 2-13
Female reproductive system: ovaries, uterine tubes, uterus, vagina, external genitalia, mammary glands

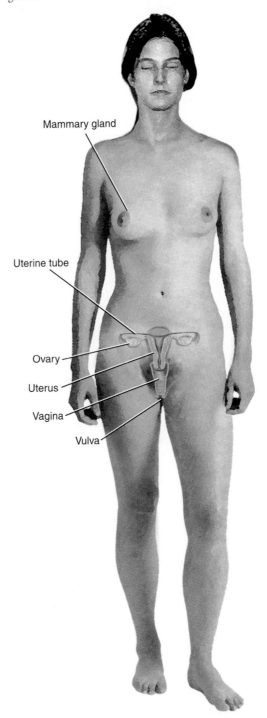

Mammary gland

Uterine tube

Ovary

Uterus

Vagina

Vulva

2.5   Putting It All Together

DEFINITIONS

Give the meaning of the following combining forms.

1. arthr/o _____

2. ot/o _____

3. cyst/o _____

4. rect/o _____

5. encephal/o _____

6. gastr/o _____

7. bronchi/o; bronch/o _____

8. angi/o _____

9. hemat/o _____

10. steat/o _____

11. oste/o _____

12. cardi/o _____

13. nephr/o _____

14. cyt/o _____

15. blephar/o _____

16. cili/o _____

17. rhin/o _____

18. splen/o _____

19. arteri/o _____

20. path/o _____

21. neur/o _____

22. abdomin/o _____

23. tonsill/o _____

24. myel/o _____

25. bi/o _____

26. trache/o _____

27. ophthalm/o _____

28. hepat/o   _____

29. viscer/o   _____

30. cephal/o   _____

Exercise 2-2   ROOTS

Give the root for the medical term for each of the following.

1. armpit   _____

2. head   _____

3. nail   _____

4. cartilage   _____

5. skull   _____

6. tendon   _____

7. eye   _____

8. small intestine   _____

9. colon   _____

10. tongue   _____

11. ductus deferens   _____

12. thyroid gland   _____

13. vein   _____

14. lung   _____

15. chest   _____

16. lymph vessels   _____

17. external genitalia   _____

18. testicle   _____

19. epididymis   _____

20. ovary   _____

Exercise 2-3   SHORT ANSWER

1. Define _anatomy_ and _physiology_. _____

2. Name 12 body systems and at least two organs in each. _____

_____

_____

_____

_____

_____

_____

_____

_____

_____

_____

_____

C H A P T E R

Suffixes

3

CHAPTER ORGANIZATION

This chapter will help you learn about medical suffixes. It is divided into the following sections:

CHAPTER OBJECTIVES

On completion of this chapter, you will be able to do the following:

1. Spell and give the meaning for suffixes
2. Distinguish suffixes that signify pathologic conditions from those that signify diagnostic and surgical procedures
3. Identify suffixes used to convert medical nouns to adjectives
4. Define, spell, and pronounce the medical terms that use the suffixes in this chapter

INTRODUCTION

You learned in Chapter 1 that suffixes are the first things to look at when analyzing a term. The most common ones are grouped into four sections in this chapter. In each section, you will find the suffix definition first, then examples of terms using the suffix. Each example is accompanied by a pronunciation guide and a definition. Make sure you know the pronunciation first. Then work to remember the meaning.

You may find that in this and other chapters, memory aids are useful. Many students realize that remembering suffix, prefix, and root meanings is aided by associating them with a particular visualization or other sensory association. For example, the first suffix, -algia, means "pain." It may be best remembered by recalling a particular pain you have experienced and associating it with the suffix. Similarly, you might remember the second suffix, -cele, by imagining a huge hernia coming out of your intestine when you say the suffix to yourself. The more outrageous the imagined association, the more likely you are to remember.

3.1   Additional Word Elements

Use these additional word elements when studying the medical terms in this chapter.

Root	Meaning
acr/o	top; extremities
carcin/o	cancer
don/o	donates
glyc/o	sugar
pharmac/o	drug
physi/o	nature
practition/o	practice
sect/o	cut

3.2 Suffixes Used to Indicate Pathologic Conditions

Pathology means the study of disease processes. The suffixes below describe disease, symptoms, or abnormalities.

	-algia	pain
Term	**Term Analysis**	**Definition**
cephalalgia (sef-**AL**-jee-ah)	**cephal/o** = head	headache
arthralgia (ar-**THRAL**-jee-ah)	**arthr/o** = joint	joint pain
otalgia (oh-**TAL**-gee-ah)	**ot/o** = ear	earache
	-cele	**hernia (protrusion or displacement of an organ through a structure that normally contains it)**
cystocele (**SIS**-toh-seel)	**cyst/o** = bladder	hernia of the urinary bladder; protrusion of the bladder onto the vaginal walls (see Figure 3-1)

FIGURE 3-1
Cystocele

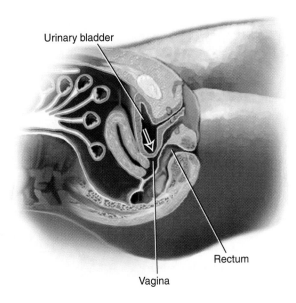

Urinary bladder

Rectum

Vagina

FIGURE 3-2
Rectocele

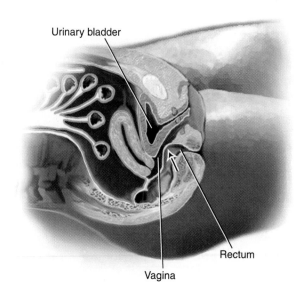

Urinary bladder

Rectum

Vagina

Term	Term Analysis	Definition
rectocele (**RECK**-toh-seel)	**rect/o** = rectum	hernia of the rectum; protrusion of the rectum onto the vaginal wall (see Figure 3-2)
encephalocele (en-**SEF**-ah-loh-**seel**)	**encephal/o** = brain	hernia of the brain
	-dynia	**pain**
gastrodynia (**gas**-troh-**DIN**-ee-ah)	**gastr/o** = stomach	stomach pain
mastodynia (**mas**-toh-**DIN**-ee-ah)	**mast/o** = breast	breast pain
	-emesis	**vomiting**
hematemesis (**hee**-mah-**TEM**-eh-sis)	**hemat/o** = blood	vomiting of blood
	-emia	**blood condition**
glycemia (glye-**SEE**-mee-ah)	**glyc/o** = sugar	sugar in the blood

	-ia	state of; condition
Term	**Term Analysis**	**Definition**
pneumonia (new-**MOH**-nee-ah)	**pneumon/o** = lung	condition of the lung (most commonly known as an inflammation of the lung)

	-itis	**inflammation (the redness, swelling, heat, and pain that occurs when the body protects itself from injury)**
enteritis (**en**-ter-**EYE**-tis)	**enter/o** = small intestine	inflamed small intestine
stomatitis (sto-mah-**TYE**-tis)	**stomat/o** = mouth	inflamed mouth
spondylitis (**spon**-dih-**LYE**-tis)	**spondyl/o** = vertebra	inflamed vertebra

Memory Key Inflammation has two *ms*; inflamed has only one *m*.

	-lysis	**destruction; separation; breakdown**
hemolysis (hee-**MO**-lih-sis)	**hem/o** = blood	breakdown of blood

Memory Key To remember the meaning of -lysis, think of the word *analysis*, meaning to "break down or separate into parts."

	-malacia	softening
cerebromalacia (**ser**-eh-broh-mah-**LAY**-shee-ah)	**cerebr/o** = brain	softening of the brain
chondromalacia (**kon**-droh-mah-**LAY**-shee-ah)	**chondr/o** = cartilage	softening of cartilage

	-megaly	enlargement
Term	**Term Analysis**	**Definition**
visceromegaly (**VIS**-er-oh-**meg**-ah-lee)	**viscer/o** = internal organs	enlargement of the internal organs
	-oma	**tumor; mass**
lipoma (lih-**POH**-mah)	**lip/o** = fat	tumor containing fat
myoma (my-**OH**-mah)	**my/o** = muscle	tumor of muscle
	-osis	**abnormal condition**
nephrosis (neh-**FROH**-sis)	**nephr/o** = kidney	abnormal condition of the kidney
	-pathy	**disease process**
ureteropathy (you-**ree**-ter-**OP**-pah-thee)	**ureter/o** = ureter (a tube leading from each kidney to the bladder for the passage of urine)	disease process of the ureter
	-penia	**decrease, deficiency**
cytopenia (**sigh**-toh-**PEE**-nee-ah)	**cyt/o** = cell	deficiency of cells
	-phobia	**irrational fear**
acrophobia (**ack**-roh-**FOH**-bee-ah)	**acr/o** = top, extremities	fear of heights

FIGURE 3-3
Blepharoptosis

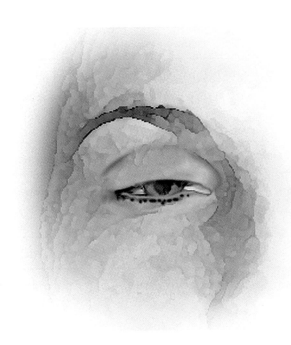

	-ptosis	**downward displacement; drooping; prolapse; sagging**
Term	**Term Analysis**	**Definition**
blepharoptosis (**blef**-ah-rop-**TOH**-sis)	**blephar/o** = eyelid	drooping eyelid (see Figure 3-3)
nephroptosis (**nef**-rop-**TOH**-sis)	**nephr/o** = kidney	drooping kidney
	-ptysis	**spitting**
hemoptysis (he-**MOP**-tih-sis)	**hem/o** = blood	spitting up of blood
	-rrhage; rrhagia	**bursting forth**
hemorrhage (**HEM**-or-idj)	**hem/o** = blood	bursting forth of blood; bleeding
gastrorrhagia (**gas**-troh-**RAY**-jee-ah)	**gastr/o** = stomach	bleeding from the stomach

	-rrhea	flow; discharge
Term	**Term Analysis**	**Definition**
otorrhea (**oh**-toh-**REE**-ah)	**ot/o** = ear	discharge from the ear
	-rrhexis	rupture
splenorrhexis (**splee**-nor-**ECKS**-sis)	**splen/o** = spleen	ruptured spleen
	-sclerosis	hardening
arteriosclerosis (ar-**tee**-ree-oh-skleh-**ROH**-sis)	**arteri/o** = artery	hardening of the arteries
	-spasm	sudden, involuntary contraction
blepharospasm (**BLEF**-ah-roh-spazm)	**blephar/o** = eyelid	sudden, involuntary contraction of the eyelid
	-stenosis	narrowing; stricture
phlebostenosis (**fleb**-oh-steh-**NOH**-sis)	**phleb/o** = vein	narrowing of a vein
	-y	process
neuropathy (new-**ROP**-ah-thee)	**neur/o** = nerve **path/o** = disease	disease process of the nerve

3.3   Suffixes Used to Indicate Diagnostic and Surgical Procedures

Diagnosis of pathologic conditions involves using many different standard procedures, depending on the symptoms displayed by the patient. If the diagnosis indicates that surgery is required, then the appropriate surgical procedures will be recommended. Common suffixes associated with diagnostic and surgical procedures are listed next.

	-centesis	surgical puncture to remove fluid
Term	**Term Analysis**	**Definition**
abdominocentesis (ab-**dom**-ih-noh-sen-**TEE**-sis)	**abdomin/o** = abdomen	surgical puncture to remove fluid from the abdomen
thoracocentesis (**thoh**-rah-koh-sen-**TEE**-sis)	**thorac/o** = chest	surgical puncture of the chest wall to remove excess fluid from around the lungs
	-desis	surgical binding; surgical fusion
arthrodesis (ar-throh-**DEE**-sis)	**arthr/o** = joint	surgical fusion of a joint
	-ectomy	excision; surgical removal
oophorectomy (oh-**of**-oh-**RECK**-toh-mee)	**oophor/o** = ovary	excision of the ovary
tonsillectomy (**ton**-sih-**LECK**-toh-me)	**tonsill/o** = tonsils	excision of the tonsils
	-graphy	process of recording; producing images
mammography (mam-**OG**-rah-fee)	**mamm/o** = breast	producing images of the breast (by the use of x-rays) (see Figure 3-4)
myelography (**my**-eh-**LOG**-rah-**FEE**)	**myel/o** = spinal cord	producing images of the spinal cord (by the use of x-rays)
computed **tomo**graphy (CT) (toh-**MOG**-rah-fee)	**tom/o** = to cut	x-ray beam rotates around the patient detailing the structure at various depths. The information is computer analyzed and converted to a picture of the body part. Common body parts studied in this fashion include the abdomen, kidneys, brain, and chest.

FIGURE 3-4
Mammography

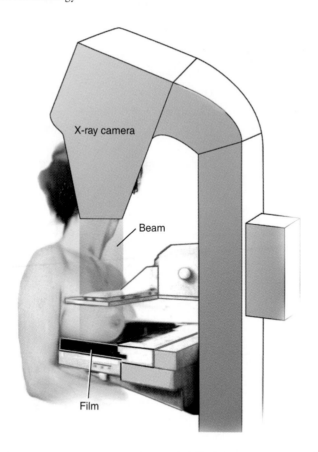

X-ray camera

Beam

Film

	-gram	record; writing
Term	**Term Analysis**	**Definition**
lymphangiogram (lim-**FAN**-jee-oh-**gram**)	**lymphangi/o** = lymph vessel	record of the lymph vessel (by the use of x-rays)
	-graph	**instrument used to record**
cardiograph (**KAR**-dee-oh-graf)	**cardi/o** = heart	instrument used to record heart activity
	-metry	**to measure; measurement**
pelvimetry (pel-**VIM**-eh-tree)	**pelv/i** = pelvis	measurement of the pelvis. *NOTE:* A pelvimetry is performed to confirm the size of the maternal pelvis in situations in which the pelvis is thought to be too small for the delivery of the baby.

	-meter	**instrument used to measure**
Term	**Term Analysis**	**Definition**
craniometer (**kray**-nee-**OM**-eh-ter)	**crani/o** = skull	instrument used to measure the skull

	-opsy	**to view**
biopsy (**BYE**-op-see)	**bi/o** = life	a procedure involving the removal of a piece of living tissue, which is then microscopically examined for any abnormalities

	-pexy	**surgical fixation**
nephropexy (**NEF**-roh-**peck**-see)	**nephr/o** = kidney	surgical fixation of the kidney

	-plasty	**surgical reconstruction; surgical repair**
orchidoplasty (**OR**-kid-oh-**plas**-tee)	**orchid/o** = testicle	surgical reconstruction of the testicle

	-rrhaphy	**suture; sew**
colporrhaphy (kol-**POR**-ah-fee)	**colp/o** = vagina	suturing of the vagina

	-scope	**instrument used to visually examine (a body cavity or organ)**
bronchoscope (**BRONG**-koh-skope)	**bronch/o** = bronchus	instrument used to visually examine the interior of the bronchus (for examples of endoscopes, see Figure 4-1)

	-scopy	process of visually examining (a body cavity or organ)
Term	**Term Analysis**	**Definition**
bronchoscopy (brong-**KOS**-koh-pee)	**bronch/o** = bronchus	process of visually examining the bronchus (remember that -y means "process")

Memory Key | The suffix *-y* means "process."

	-stasis	stoppage; stopping; controlling
hemostasis (**he**-moh-**STAY**-sis)	**hem/o** = blood	stoppage of blood
	-stomy	new opening
tracheostomy (**tray**-kee-**OS**-toh-mee)	**trache/o** = trachea; windpipe	new opening into the trachea
	-tome	instrument used to cut
myotome (**MY**-oh-tohm)	**my/o** = muscle	instrument used to cut muscle
	-tomy	process of cutting; incision
tenotomy (teh-**NOT**-oh-mee)	**ten/o** = tendon	process of cutting a tendon

3.4   General Suffixes

The following is a list of general suffixes you need to know to understand a great number of medical terms:

	-cyte	cell
Term	**Term Analysis**	**Definition**
adipocyte (**AD**-ih-poh-**sight**)	**adip/o** = fat	fat cell

Term	Term Analysis	Definition
histiocyte (**HISS**-tee-oh-**sight**)	**histi/o** = tissue	tissue cell
	-er; -or; -ician; -logist; -ist	**specialist; one who specializes; specialist in the study of**
practitioner (prack-**TISH**-un-er)	**practition/o** = practice	one who has obtained the proper requirements to work in a specific field of study
organ donor (**DOH**-nor)	**don/o** = donate	one who donates organ tissue to be used in another body
physician (fih-**ZIH**-shun)	**physi/o** = nature	specialist in the study of medicine who has graduated from a recognized school of medicine and is licensed by the appropriate authority to practice
neurologist (new-**ROL**-oh-jist)	**neur/o** = nerve	specialist in the study of the nervous system and its disorders
pharmacist (**FARM**-ah-sist)	**pharmac/o** = drug	specialist licensed to prepare and dispense drugs
	-ion	**process**
section (**SECK**-shun)	**sect/o** = to cut	process of cutting
	-logy	**study of; process of study**
hepatology (hep-ah-**TOL**-oh-jee)	**hepat/o** = liver	study of the liver
physiology (fiz-ee-**OL**-oh-jee)	**physi/o** = nature	study of function (the study of how a structure functions)
	-plasia	**formation; development**
chondroplasia (kon-droh-**PLAY**-zee-ah)	**chondr/o** = cartilage	formation of cartilage

	-poiesis	production; manufacture; formation
Term	**Term Analysis**	**Definition**
hematopoiesis (**he**-mah-toh-poi-**EE**-sis)	**hemat/o** = blood	production of blood
	-trophic; -trophy	**development; growth; nutrition**
thyrotrophic hormone (**thigh**-roh-**TROH**-fick)	**thyr/o** = thyroid gland	a substance having an influence on the thyroid gland

3.5   Adjectival Suffixes

Adjectival suffixes describe special qualities or relationships.

	-genic	**produced by; producing**
Term	**Term Analysis**	**Definition**
carcinogenic (**kar**-sih-noh-**JEN**-ick)	**carcin/o** = cancer	producing cancer (agent that produces cancer)
	-oid	**resembling**
osteoid (**OS**-tee-oyd)	**oste/o** = bone	resembling bone
	-ole; -ule	**small**
bronchiole (**BRONG**-kee-ohl)	**bronchi/o** = bronchus	small bronchus
venule (**VEN**-youl)	**ven/o** = vein	small vein
	-ac; -al; -ary; -eal; -ic; -ous	**pertaining to**
cardiac (**KAR**-dee-ack)	**cardi/o** = heart	pertaining to the heart

Term	Term Analysis	Definition
renal (**REE**-nal)	**ren/o** = kidney	pertaining to the kidney
mammary (**MAM**-ah-ree)	**mamm/o** = breast	pertaining to the breast
pharyngeal (**far-IN**-jee-al)	**pharyng/o** = throat; pharynx	pertaining to the throat
gastric (**GAS**-trik)	**gastr/o** = stomach	pertaining to the stomach
venous (**VEE**-nus)	**ven/o** = vein	pertaining to a vein

NOTE: Although there are some exceptions, the suffixes meaning "pertaining to" are not generally interchangeable with a given root. For example, one can create the adjectives *renal* and *cardiac*, but not renac, renar, renary, cardiar, cardieal, cardious, or cardiose.

3.6   Putting It All Together

Exercise 3-1   DEFINING SUFFIXES

Define the following suffixes.

Suffixes indicating pathologic conditions:

1. -algia _____

2. -dynia _____

3. -emesis _____

4. -osis _____

5. -cele _____

6. -malacia _____

7. -oma _____

8. -penia _____

9. -emia _____

10. -ptosis _____

11. -rrhage _____

12. -rrhexis _____

13. -stenosis _____

Suffixes indicating diagnostic and surgical procedures:

14. -ectomy _____

15. -gram _____

16. -graph _____

17. -opsy _____

18. -plasty _____

19. -scope _____

20. -stasis _____

21. -tome _____

General suffixes:

22. -cyte _____

23. -ist _____

24. -ion _____

25. -logy _____

26. -poiesis _____

Adjectival suffixes:

27. -genic _____

28. -oid _____

29. -ole _____

30. -ac; -al; -ary; -eal; -ic; -ous _____

Exercise 3-2   IDENTIFYING SUFFIXES

Give the suffix for the following:

1. hernia _____

2. instrument used to measure _____

3. blood condition _____

4. inflammation _____

5. destruction _____

6. enlargement _____

7. abnormal condition _____

8. irrational fear _____

9. drooping _____

10. spitting _____

11. flow, discharge _____

12. hardening _____

13. process _____

14. surgical fusion _____

15. process of recording _____

16. to measure _____

17. surgical fixation _____

18. suture _____

19. process of visually examining
    (a body cavity or organ) _____

20. stopping _____

21. instrument used to cut _____

22. cell _____

23. study of _____

24. formation _____

25. resembling _____

Exercise 3-3   IDENTIFYING SUFFIXES MEANING "PERTAINING TO"

Place a check mark beside each suffix that means "pertaining to."

1. -al _____

2. -ous _____

3. -eal _____

4. -oma _____

5. -ary _____

6. -ule _____

7. -ic _____

8. -ole _____

9. -ac _____

10. -oid _____

Exercise 3-4	IDENTIFYING SUFFIXES INDICATING A DIAGNOSTIC OR SURGICAL PROCEDURE

Place a check mark beside the suffix indicating a diagnostic or surgical procedure.

1. -sclerosis _____

2. -ectomy _____

3. -plasia _____

4. -stomy _____

5. -cyte _____

6. -pexy _____

7. -rrhaphy _____

8. -rrhexis _____

9. -rrhagia _____

10. -penia _____

Exercise 3-5	DEFINITIONS

Define the following terms.

1. mastodynia _____

2. hematemesis _____

3. enteritis _____

4. cerebromalacia _____

5. nephrosis _____

6. blepharoptosis _____

7. otorrhea _____

8. phlebostenosis _____

9. mammography _____

10. orchidoplasty _____

11. tenotomy _____

12. bronchoscopy _____

13. histiocyte _____

14. pharmacist _____

15. chondroplasia _____

Exercise 3-6   USING ADJECTIVAL SUFFIXES

Complete the medical word by using the correct adjectival suffix to indicate "pertaining to."

Example: cardi**ac**. -ac is the adjectival suffix.

1. ren/   _____

2. mamm/   _____

3. pharyng/   _____

4. gastr/   _____

5. ven/   _____

Exercise 3-7   SPELLING

Place a check mark beside the terms that are spelled incorrectly. Correct the misspelled words.

1. ophorectomy   _____

2. inflamation   _____

3. cephalgia   _____

4. pelvmetry   _____

5. hemolysis   _____

6. spleenorrhexis   _____

7. physiology   _____

8. orchidoplaste   _____

9. hemostasis   _____

10. practitionar   _____

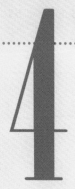

C H A P T E R

Prefixes

CHAPTER ORGANIZATION

This chapter has been designed to help you learn about medical prefixes. It is divided into the following sections:

CHAPTER OBJECTIVES

On completion of this chapter, you will be able to do the following:

1. Give meanings for prefixes
2. Distinguish prefixes that signify direction and position from those that signify negation or number
3. Identify prefixes that have the same meaning
4. Identify prefixes that are opposite in meaning
5. Define, spell, and pronounce medical terms that use the prefixes in this chapter

INTRODUCTION

Prefixes tell us how, why, where, when, how much, how many, what position, and what direction. This chapter introduces you to the most common prefixes but starts by listing new roots, suffixes, and their meanings used in this chapter. The remaining sections display the prefix and its meaning first, followed by examples of terms using the prefix. As in Chapter 3, learn pronunciation first, then the meaning.

4.1   Additional Word Elements

Use these additional word elements when studying the medical terms in this chapter.

Root	Meaning
cellul/o	cell
cis/o	to cut
comat/o	deep sleep
digest/o	digestion
duct/o	to draw
later/o	side; lateral
nat/o	birth
sept/o	infection
son/o	sound

Suffix	Meaning
-aise	ease
-ar	pertaining to
-cuspid	projection; cusps
-drome	to run
-form	shape; form

continued on page 54

continued from page 53

Suffix	Meaning
-genous	produced by
-gnosis	knowledge
-mortem	death
-plasm	development; formation
-tropia	turning
-version	turning; tilting

4.2   Prefixes Referring to Direction and Position

The prefixes below tell us which direction, where, when, and how much.

	ab-	away from
Term	**Term Analysis**	**Definition**
abduction (ab-**DUCK**-shun)	-ion = process **duct/o** = to draw	process of drawing away from (see Figure 8-3B)

	ad-	toward
adduction (ah-**DUCK**-shun)	-ion = process **duct/o** = to draw	process of drawing toward (see Figure 8-3B)

Memory Key | The prefix ad- means "to draw toward." Remember this example: when you add something, you bring it toward you.

	ante-	before
antenatal (an-tee-**NAY**-tal)	-al = pertaining to **nat/o** = birth	pertaining to before birth

Memory Key The prefix ante- means "before." Both the prefix and its meaning contain the letter *e*, making them easy to remember. Compare with anti- (against) in section 4.3.

	circum-	around
Term	**Term Analysis**	**Definition**
circum**duct**ion (**ser**-kum-**DUCK**-shun)	-ion = process **duct/o** = to draw	process of drawing a part in a circular motion (see Figure 8-3E)
	dia-	**through; complete**
diameter (dye-**AM**-eh-ter)	-meter = measurement	measurement from edge to edge of a circle
diagnosis (**dye**-ag-**NOH**-sis)	-gnosis = knowledge	one disease is differentiated from another disease after complete knowledge is obtained of the disease through a study of the signs and symptoms, and laboratory, x-ray, and other diagnostic procedures
	ecto-	**outside**
ectogenous (eck-**TOJ**-eh-nus)	-genous = produced by; produced from	produced from the outside; infection that originates from the outside
	endo-	**within**
endoscope (**EN**-doh-skohp)	-scope = instrument used to visually examine a body cavity or organ	instrument used to visually examine a body cavity or organ. *NOTE:* Endoscopes are named after the organ being examined. For example, in Figure 4-1, a gastroscope, laparoscope, and a colonoscope are used to visualize the stomach, abdominal cavity, and colon, respectively.

FIGURE 4-1

Endoscopes: (A) gastroscope, (B) laparoscope, (C) colonoscope

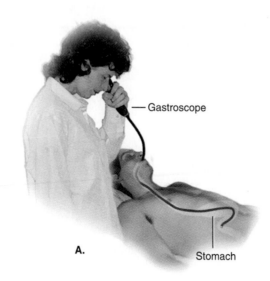

Gastroscope

Stomach

A.

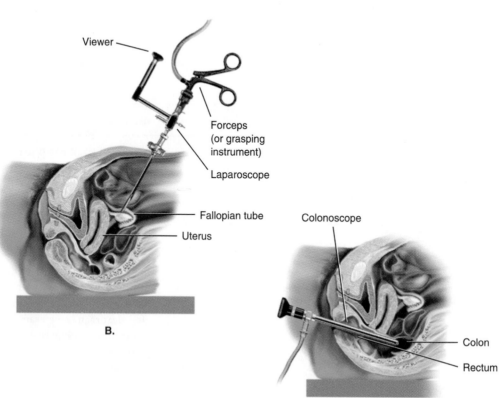

Viewer

Forceps
(or grasping
instrument)

Laparoscope

Fallopian tube

Uterus

B.

Colonoscope

Colon

Rectum

C.

	epi-	**upon; on; above**
Term	**Term Analysis**	**Definition**
epigastric (ep-ih-**GAS**-trick)	-ic = pertaining to **gastr/o** = stomach	pertaining to upon the stomach

	e-; ex-; exo-; extra-	**out; outward; outside**
eversion (ee-**VER**-zhun)	-version = process of turning	process of turning out, as in the turning of the sole of the foot outward (see Figure 4-2)
excision (eck-**SIH**-zhun)	-ion = process **cis/o** = cut	process of cutting out
extraocular (**ecks**-trah-**OCK**-you-lar)	-ar = pertaining to **ocul/o** = eye	pertaining to outside the eye

Memory Key   Ex- means "out," as in exit.

FIGURE 4-2
Inversion and eversion

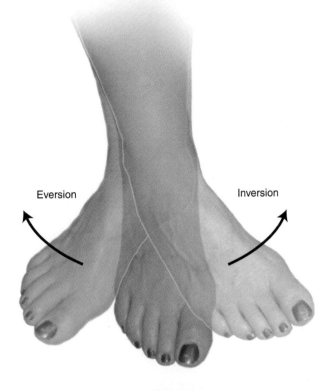

Eversion   Inversion

	hyper-	**excessive; above**
Term	**Term Analysis**	**Definition**
hyperplasia (**high**-per-**PLAY**-see-ah)	-plasia = formation; development	excessive formation
	hypo-	**below; under; deficient**
hypo**gastr**ic (high-poh-**GAS**-trick)	-ic = pertaining to **gastr/o** = stomach	pertaining to below the stomach
	in-	**in; into**
in**cis**ion (in-**SIH**-zhun)	-ion = process **cis/o** = to cut	process of cutting into. *NOTE:* Types of incisions include (A) McBurney, over the appendix; (B) Pfannenstiel, a curved lower abdominal incision; (C) subcostal, below the ribs; (D) suprapubic, above the pubic area; (E) transverse, a horizontal incision; (F) midline or epigastric, vertical incision at the midline; (G) paramedian, vertical incision near the midline; and (H) umbilical cord incision, through the umbilicus for scopic surgery (see Figure 4-3)
inversion (in-**VER**-zhun)	-version = process of turning	process of turning in as in the turning of the sole of the foot inward (see Figure 4-2)
	infra-	**below; beneath**
infra**costal** (in-frah-**KOS**-tal)	-al = pertaining to **cost/o** = rib	pertaining to below the ribs
	inter-	**between**
inter**cellul**ar (**in**-ter-**SEL**-you-lar)	-ar = pertaining to **cellul/o** = cell	pertaining to between the cells

FIGURE 4-3
Types of abdominal incisions

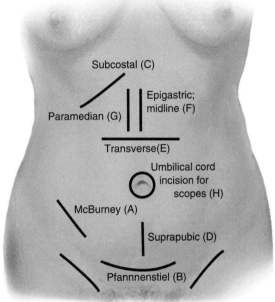

	intra-	within
Term	**Term Analysis**	**Definition**
intracranial (**in**-trah-**KRAY**-nee-al)	-al = pertaining to **crani/o** = skull	pertaining to within the skull
	meta-	**beyond**
metaplasia (met-ah-**PLAY**-zha)	-plasia = formation; development	change in formation
metastasis (meh-**TAS**-tah-sis)	-stasis = stopping; controlling	the uncontrolled spread of cancerous cells from one organ to another. *NOTE:* A malignant tumor will undergo metastasis.
	para-	**beside; near**
paranasal (**par**-ah-**NAY**-sal)	-al = pertaining to **nas/o** = nose	pertaining to near the nose

	per-	through
Term	**Term Analysis**	**Definition**
percutaneous (per-kyou-TAY-nee-us)	-ous = pertaining to cutane/o = skin	pertaining to through the skin
	peri-	around
perineuritis (per-ih-nyou-RYE-tis)	-itis = inflammation neur/o = nerve	inflammation around a nerve
	post-	after
postmortem (pohst-MOR-tehm)	-mortem = death	after death
	pre-	before; in front of
prenatal (pre-NAY-tal)	-al = pertaining to nat/o = birth	pertaining to before birth; referring to the fetus
	pro-	before
prodrome (proh-drohm)	-drome = to run	symptom or symptoms occurring before the onset of disease. For example, chest pain, tiredness, and shortness of breath are prodromal symptoms of a heart attack.
prognosis (pragh-NOH-sis)	-gnosis = knowledge	prediction or forecast of the outcome of the disease
	retro-	back; behind
retroversion (ret-roh-VER-zhun)	-version = process of turning	backward turning or tipping of an organ
	sub-	under; below
subcutaneous (sub-kyou-TAY-nee-us)	-ous = pertaining to cutane/o = skin	pertaining to under the skin. For example, subcutaneous fat (see Figure 4-4)

FIGURE 4-4
Skin and subcutaneous fat

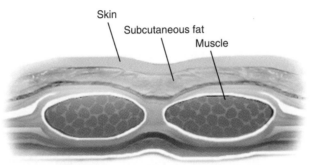

Skin

Subcutaneous fat

Muscle

Term	Term Analysis	Definition
sublingual (sub-**LING**-gwahl)	-al = pertaining to **lingu/o** = tongue	pertaining to under the tongue
	supra-	**above**
suprarenal (**soo**-prah-**REE**-nal)	-al = pertaining to **ren/o** = kidney	pertaining to above the kidney
	trans-	**across**
transection (tran-**SECK**-shun)	-ion = process **sect/o** = cut	process of cutting across (see Figure 4-5)

FIGURE 4-5
Transection

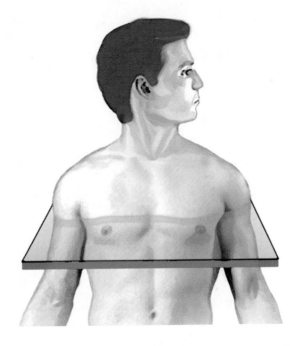

	ultra-	beyond
ultra**sono**graphy (**ul**-trah-son-**OG**-rah-fee)	-graphy = process of recording **son/o** = sound	process of recording an image of internal structures by using high-frequency sound waves. Also known as ultrasound (see Figure 4-6)

FIGURE 4-6
Ultrasonography.
(A) Ultrasonography is often used to monitor fetal development during pregnancy.
(B) Fetal ultrasound

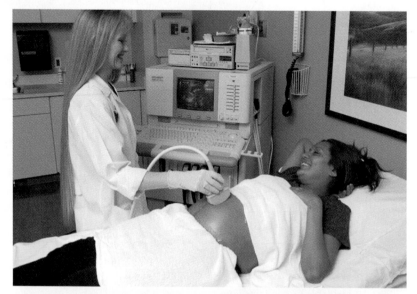

A.

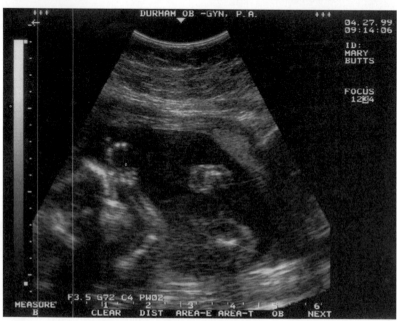

B.

4.3   Negative Prefixes

The prefixes below mean against, not, or lacking.

	anti-	against
Term	**Term Analysis**	**Definition**
anti**biotic** (**an**-tih-bye-**OT**-ick)	-tic = pertaining to **bi/o** = life	drug used to kill harmful bacteria

> **Memory Key**   The prefix anti- means "against." Both the prefix and its meaning contain the letter *i*, making them easy to remember. Compare with ante- (before) in section 4.2.

	a-; an-	no; not; lack of
a**septic** (ay-**SEHP**-tick)	-ic = pertaining to **sept/o** = infection	free from infectious material
anemia (ah-**NEE**-me-ah)	-emia = blood condition	lack of red blood cells (RBCs); lack of hemoglobin (Hgb)

	contra-	against; opposite
contra**lateral** (**kon**-trah-**LAH**-ter-al)	-al = pertaining to **later/o** = side	pertaining to the opposite side

	in-	not
in**digest**ible (**in**-dih-**JES**-tih-bl)	-ible = able to be; tending to **digest/o** = digestion	not capable of being digested

> **Memory Key**   The prefix in- becomes ir- before *r*, and im- before *m* and *p*.

4.4 Prefixes Referring to Numbers

The prefixes below tell us how many.

	bi-; di-	**two**
Term	**Term Analysis**	**Definition**
bilateral (bye-**LAT**-er-al)	-al = pertaining to later/o = side	pertaining to two sides

Memory Key	A bicycle has two wheels.

dissection (dye-**SECK**-shun)	-ion = pertaining to sect/o = to cut	to cut into two pieces

	hemi-; semi-	**half**
hemigastrectomy (**hem**-ee-gas-**TRECK**-toh-mee)	-ectomy = excision gastr/o = stomach	excision of half the stomach
semicomatose (**sem**-ee-**KOH**-mah-tohs)	semi- = half comat/o = deep sleep	state of unconsciousness from which the patient may be aroused

	mono-; uni-	**one**
monocyte (**MON**-oh-sight)	-cyte = cell	blood cell with a single nucleus
unilateral (**you**-nih-**LAT**-er-al)	-al = pertaining to later/o = side	pertaining to one side

	multi-; poly-	**many**
multiform (**MUL**-tih-form)	-form = shape; form	having many shapes
polyadenoma (**pol**-ih-**ad**-eh-**NOH**-mah)	-oma = tumor aden/o = gland	tumor of many glands

	quadri-	four
Term	**Term Analysis**	**Definition**
quadrilateral (kwad-rih-**LAT**-er-al)	-al = pertaining to later/o = side	pertaining to four sides

	tri-	three
tricuspid (try-**KUS**-pid)	-cuspid = projection; cusp	three cusps or projections. *NOTE:* The tricuspids or molars are teeth with three projections for grinding and cutting food.

Memory Key   A trio is a group of three.

4.5   Miscellaneous Prefixes

The prefixes below tell us various qualities.

	ana-	apart; up
Term	**Term Analysis**	**Definition**
anatomy (ah-**NAT**-oh-mee)	-tomy = process of cutting; to cut	the study of the structure of the body. *NOTE:* This term is derived from the fact that, to study structure, one must cut up or dissect the body.

	auto-	self
autopsy (**AW**-top-see)	-opsy = to view	internal and external examination of the body after death to determine the cause of death. Also called necropsy or postmortem examination

	brady-	slow
bradycardia (brad-ee-**KAR**-dee-ah)	-ia = state of; condition cardi/o = heart	pertaining to a slow heartbeat

	dys-	bad; abnormal; difficult; painful
Term	**Term Analysis**	**Definition**
dysplasia (dis-**PLAY**-see-ah)	-plasia = development; formation	abnormal development
	macro-	**large**
macro**cephal**ia (**mack**-roh-seh-**FAY**-lee-ah)	-ia = state of; condition **cephal/o** = head	excessively large head
	mal-	**bad**
malaise (mah-**LAYZ**)	-aise = ease	a feeling of uneasiness or discomfort. A sign of illness
	micro-	**small**
microscope (**MYE**-kroh-skohp)	-scope = instrument used to visually examine	instrument used to visually examine very small objects
	neo-	**new**
neoplasm (**NEE**-oh-plazm)	-plasm = development; formation	new formation of tissue such as an abnormal growth or tumor
	pan-	**all**
pan**hyster**ectomy (**pan**-hiss-ter-**ECK**-toh-mee)	-ectomy = excision; surgical removal **hyster/o** = uterus	excision of all the uterus
	syn-; sym-	**together; with; joined**
syn**arthr**otic (**sin**-ar-**THRAH**-tick)	-tic = pertaining to **arthr/o** = joint	a type of joint in which the bones are joined
symmetry (**SIM**-eh-tree)	-metry = process of measuring	like parts on opposite sides of the body are similar in form, size, and position

Memory Key	syn- becomes sym- before *m*, *b*, and *p*.

	tachy-	fast; rapid
Term	**Term Analysis**	**Definition**
tachy**cardi**a (**tack**-ee-**KAR**-dee-ah)	-ia = condition **cardi/o** = heart	pertaining to fast heartbeat

4.6   Summary of Prefixes That Have the Same Meaning

Some prefixes mean the same thing. For example, epi-, hyper-, and supra- all mean "above." Below is a list of such prefixes:

Meaning	Prefix
above	epi-; hyper-; supra-
against	anti-; contra-
around	circum-; peri-
bad	dys-; mal-
before	ante-; pre-; pro-
below	hypo-; infra-; sub-
outside	e-; ex-; extra
within	endo-; intra-

4.7   Summary of Prefixes That Have the Opposite Meaning

Some prefixes mean exactly the opposite of each other. For example, ab- means "away from" and ad- means "toward." Below is a list of opposite prefixes:

Meaning	Prefix
away from	ab-
toward	ad-
before	ante-; pre-; pro-
after	post-
outside	ecto-; ex-; extra-; e-
within; inward	endo-; in-; intra-
above	epi-; hyper-; supra-
below	hypo-; infra-; sub-
fast	tachy-
slow	brady-
excessive	hyper-
deficient	hypo-
large	macro-
small	micro-
apart	ana-
together; with; joined	syn-

4.8   Putting It All Together

Exercise 4-1   DEFINING PREFIXES

Underline, then define, the prefix in each word.

1. circumduction _____

2. epigastric _____

3. hyperplasia _____

4. infracostal _____

5. metastasis _____

6. postmortem _____

7. retroversion _____

8. transection _____

9. contralateral _____

10. hemigastrectomy _____

11. tricuspid   _____

12. macrocephalia   _____

13. neoplasm   _____

14. synarthrotic   _____

15. tachycardia   _____

Exercise 4-2   MATCHING

Match the word in Column A with its meaning in Column B.

Column A	Column B
_____ 1. ectogenous	A. study of structure
_____ 2. incision	B. slow breathing
_____ 3. dysplasia	C. lack of red blood cells
_____ 4. bilateral	D. produced from the outside
_____ 5. anatomy	E. pertaining to between the cells
_____ 6. perineuritis	F. abnormal development
_____ 7. anemia	G. a feeling of uneasiness or discomfort
_____ 8. intercellular	H. pertaining to two sides
_____ 9. bradypnea	I. inflammation around the nerve
_____ 10. malaise	J. process of cutting

Exercise 4-3   OPPOSITES

Write the prefix that is opposite in meaning to each of the following.

1. ab-   _____

2. ante-   _____

3. hyper-   _____

4. endo-   _____

5. brady-   _____

6. micro-   _____

7. syn-   _____

8. epi-   _____

Exercise 4-4   COMPLETION

Complete the word by placing the correct prefix in the blank provided. Definitions are given in the right-hand column.

Example: ***per*** cutaneous   through the skin

1. _____-duction   process of drawing away from

2. _____-natal   before birth; referring to the fetus

3. _____-cision   process of cutting out

4. _____-cision   process of cutting into

5. _____-drome   a symptom occurring before the onset of disease

6. _____-section   process of cutting across

7. _____-digestible   not digestible

8. _____-lateral   pertaining to one side

9. _____-adenoma   tumor of many glands

10. _____-cardia   fast heartbeat

Exercise 4-5   IDENTIFYING PREFIXES WITH THE SAME MEANING

Write the prefixes that mean:

1. bad   _____

2. below   _____

3. above   _____

4. against   _____

5. before   _____

6. around   _____

PART II

Body Systems

C H A P T E R

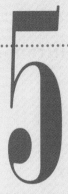

Body Organization

CHAPTER ORGANIZATION

This chapter will help you learn basic anatomy. It is divided into the following sections:

CHAPTER OBJECTIVES

On completion of this chapter, you will be able to do the following:

1. Name the cavities of the body and their organs
2. Define anatomical position
3. List and define correct terminology used for direction and abdominopelvic regions and quadrants
4. Locate the body cavities and abdominopelvic regions and quadrants
5. Analyze, define, spell, and pronounce medical terms found in this chapter
6. Define abbreviations common to body organization

INTRODUCTION

This chapter will teach you the common medical terms related to the organization of the body in its various cavities. You will also learn the terms used to describe the positions of the body and the placement of various body parts.

5.1   Cavities and the Arrangement of Body Parts

The body consists of a number of cavities, just as a backpack is divided into different pouches. The two main body cavities are the **dorsal** (**DOOR**-sal), or back, cavity and the **ventral** (**VEN**-tral), or front, cavity. Each is subdivided into smaller cavities. The dorsal cavity contains the **cranial cavity** (**KRAY**-nee-al) and **spinal cavity** (**SPY**-nal). As the names imply, the cranial cavity contains the brain, and the spinal cavity contains the spine. The ventral cavity contains the **thoracic** (thoh-**RAS**-ick), **abdominal** (ab-**DOM**-ih-nal), and **pelvic** (**PEL**-vick) cavities.

The **diaphragm** (**DYE**-ah-fram), the major respiratory muscle, separates the thoracic cavity from the abdominal cavity. The abdominal cavity contains such digestive organs as the stomach, large and small intestines, pancreas, gallbladder, and liver. It also contains the spleen, kidneys, and ureters.

The **pelvic cavity** contains reproductive and urinary organs (excluding the kidneys and ureters). The abdominal and pelvic cavities are frequently referred to as one cavity, called the **abdominopelvic cavity** (ab-**dom**-ih-noh-**PEL**-vick). The body cavities are illustrated in Figure 5-1.

Memory Key	• Major cavities are the dorsal and ventral. • Subdivisions of the dorsal cavity are the cranial and spinal cavities. • Subdivisions of the ventral cavity are the thoracic, abdominal, and pelvic cavities.

5.2   Directional Terminology

ANATOMICAL POSITION

Just as we need directional terms (east, west, etc.) to describe the world we live in, we need directional terms to describe locations in the body. However, the body can be upright, lying down, and facing different directions. This situation creates a problem in trying to describe location, and it is for this reason that the concept of a standard **anatomical position** was developed (see Figure 5-2A). In the anatomical position, the body is standing erect, arms by the side, with head, palms, and feet facing forward. All directional terms assume that the body is in this position. One must constantly keep the anatomical position in mind when using directional terms.

Memory Key	The anatomical position: standing erect, arms at side, with head, palms, and feet facing forward.

FIGURE 5-1
Body cavities

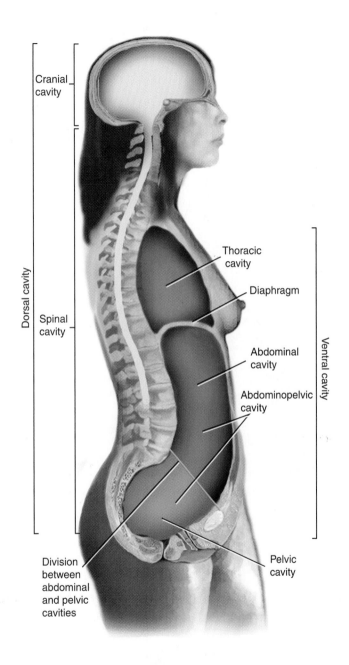

FIGURE 5-2

Directional terms relating to the anatomical position: (A) anatomical position, (B) lateral view of the body, (C) directional terms deep and superficial, (D) supine, (E) prone, (F) dorsum and plantar

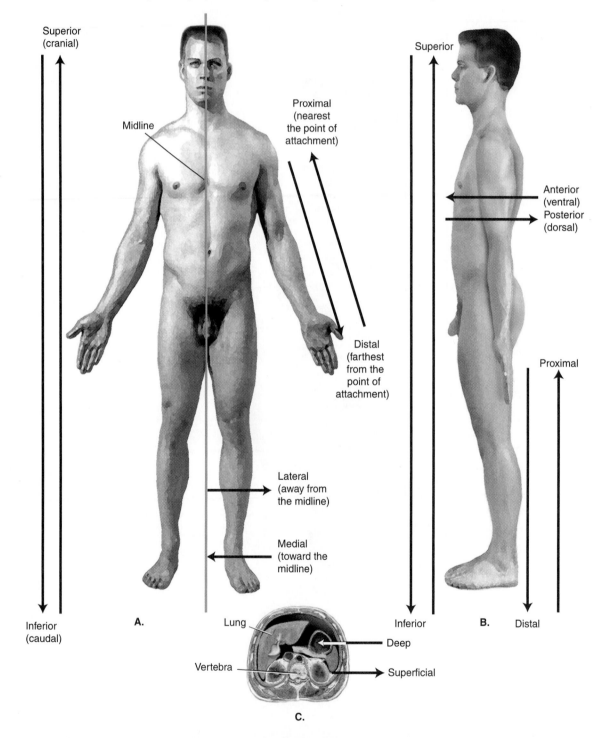

FIGURE 5-2 *continued*

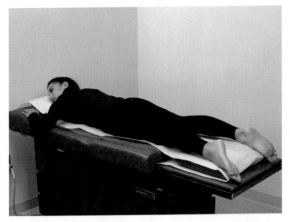

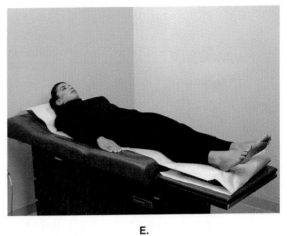

D.

E.

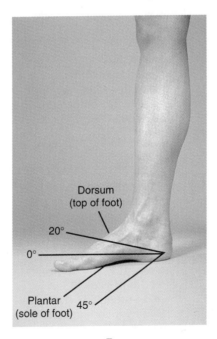

F.

DIRECTIONAL TERMS

Directional terms are required for describing the position of body parts, particularly in relation to each other. Table 5-1 lists the directional terms and provides examples of their use. Figure 5-2 illustrates the use of the terms.

TABLE 5-1

DIRECTIONAL TERMINOLOGY

Directional Term	Definition	Example
superior or cranial	above; toward the head	The head is superior to the neck. Cranial nerves originate in the head.
inferior or caudal	below; toward the lower end of the body or tail	The neck is inferior to the head. Caudal anesthesia is injected in the lower spine
anterior or ventral	front surface of the body; belly side of the body	The thoracic cavity is anterior to the spinal cavity.
posterior or dorsal	back surface of the body	The spinal cavity is posterior to the thoracic cavity.
medial	toward the midline (The midline is an imaginary line drawn down the center of the body from the top of the head to the feet.)	The big toe is medial to the small toe.
lateral	away from the midline	The small toe is lateral to the big toe.
proximal	nearest the point of attachment to the trunk. (*NOTE:* This definition is used primarily to describe directions on the arms and legs.)	The elbow is proximal to the wrist, and the wrist is proximal to the fingers.
	toward the point of origin. (*NOTE:* This definition is used primarily to describe directions pertaining to the digestive tract, with the mouth as the point of origin.)	The stomach is proximal to the intestines.
distal	farthest from the point of attachment to the trunk; farthest from the point of origin	The knee is distal to the hip, and the ankle is distal to the knee. The intestines are distal to the stomach, and the stomach is distal to the throat.

continued on page 79

Table 5-1 *continued from page 78*

Directional Term	Definition	Example
superficial	near the surface of the body	The skin is superficial to underlying organs.
deep	away from the surface of the body	Muscles are deep to the skin.
supine	lying on the back, face up. (*NOTE:* In relation to the arms, *supine* means the palms are facing toward the front.)	During an operation, the patient may be placed in the supine position.
prone	lying on the abdomen, face down. (*NOTE:* In relation to the arms, *prone* means the palms are facing toward the back.)	During an operation, the patient may be placed in the prone position.
plantar	sole of the foot	Plantar warts are on the sole of the foot.
dorsum	upper portion of the foot	The dorsum of the foot is the top portion.
peripheral	away from the center	Peripheral nerves are the nerves away from the brain and spinal cord. Peripheral blood vessels are in the extremities.

Memory Key To remember the term *supine*, notice that supine has "up" as part of the word.

ABDOMINOPELVIC REGIONS AND QUADRANTS

The abdominopelvic area of the body has been divided into regions and quadrants for purposes of describing areas of pain and the location of organs within the abdominopelvic cavity. There are nine abdominal regions and four quadrants. Figure 5-3 illustrates the regions. Figure 5-4 illustrates the quadrants.

FIGURE 5-3
Abdominopelvic regions

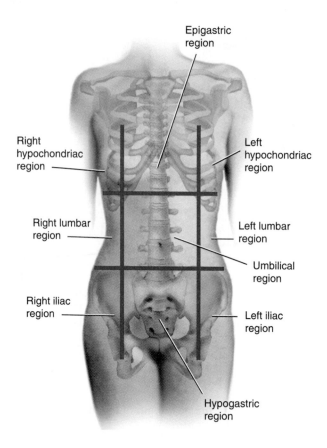

Epigastric region

Right hypochondriac region

Left hypochondriac region

Right lumbar region

Left lumbar region

Umbilical region

Right iliac region

Left iliac region

Hypogastric region

FIGURE 5-4
Abdominopelvic quadrants

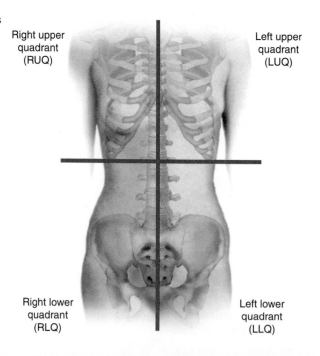

Right upper quadrant (RUQ)

Left upper quadrant (LUQ)

Right lower quadrant (RLQ)

Left lower quadrant (LLQ)

5.3   Additional Word Elements

Use these additional word elements when studying the medical terms in this chapter.

Root	Meaning
anter/o	front
caud/o	tail
dors/o	back
infer/o	inferior
inguin/o	groin
phren/o	diaphragm
poster/o	posterior
proxim/o	near
super/o	superior
ventr/o	front

5.4   Term Analysis and Definition

	gastr/o	stomach
Term	**Term Analysis**	**Definition**
epigastric (ep-ih-**GAS**-trick)	-ic = pertaining to epi- = upon; above	pertaining to upon the stomach. Refers to an abdominal region
hypogastric (**high**-poh-**GAS**-trick)	-ic = pertaining to hypo- = below; deficient	pertaining to below the stomach. Refers to an abdominal region
	ili/o	hip
iliac (**ILL**-ee-ack)	-ac = pertaining to	pertaining to the hip

SUFFIXES

	-al	pertaining to
Term	**Term Analysis**	**Definition**
caudal (**KAW**-dal)	**caud/o** = tail	pertaining to the tail; toward the tail (see Figure 5-2A)
cranial (**KRAY**-nee-al)	**crani/o** = skull	pertaining to the skull (see Figure 5-2A)
dorsal (**DOOR**-sal)	**dors/o** = back	pertaining to the back (see Figure 5-2B)
inguinal (**ING**-gwih-nal)	**inguin/o** = groin	pertaining to the groin
medial (**MEE**-dee-al)	**medi/o** = middle	pertaining to the middle (see Figure 5-2A)
proximal (**PROCK**-sih-mal)	**proxim/o** = near; close	pertaining to that which is near a point of reference (see Figure 5-2A)
spinal (**SPYE**-nal)	**spin/o** = spine; spinal column; backbone	pertaining to the spine
ventral (**VEN**-tral)	**ventr/o** = front	pertaining to the front
visceral (**VIS**-er-al)	**viscer/o** = internal organ	pertaining to the internal organs

	-ic	pertaining to
pelvic (**PEL**-vick)	**pelv/o** = pelvic	pertaining to the pelvis
phrenic (**FREN**-ick)	**phren/o** = diaphragm	pertaining to the diaphragm
thoracic (thoh-**RAS**-ick)	**thorac/o** = chest; thorax	pertaining to the chest

	-ior	pertaining to
anterior (an-**TEER**-ee-or)	**anter/o** = front	pertaining to the front of the body or organ (see Figure 5-2B)
inferior (in-**FEER**-ee-or)	**infer/o** = below; downward	pertaining to below or in a downward position; a structure below another structure (see Figure 5-2B)

Term	Term Analysis	Definition
posterior (pos-**TEER**-ee-or)	**poster/o** = back	pertaining to the back of the body or an organ (see Figure 5-2B)
superior (soo-**PEER**-ee-or)	**super/o** = above; toward the head	pertaining to a structure or organ situated either above another or toward the head (see Figure 5-2B)

5.5   Abbreviations

Abbreviation	Meaning
LLQ	left lower quadrant
LUQ	left upper quadrant
RLQ	right lower quadrant
RUQ	right upper quadrant

5.6   Putting It All Together

Exercise 5-1   TRUE OR FALSE

1. The diaphragm is a muscle.	T	F
2. The liver is located in the pelvic cavity.	T	F
3. The abdominal cavity is inferior to the thoracic cavity.	T	F
4. The big toe is lateral to the small toe.	T	F
5. The wrist is proximal to the elbow.	T	F
6. Prone is lying on the back, face up.	T	F
7. The left iliac region is in the left lower quadrant.	T	F
8. *Supine* refers to the palms facing toward the back.	T	F
9. *Dorsum* may refer to the back portion of a structure.	T	F
10. The right hypochondriac region of the abdomen is in the RUQ.	T	F

Exercise 5-2   MATCHING

Match each directional term in Column A with its meaning in Column B.

	Column A	**Column B**
_____	1. superior	A. away from the midline
_____	2. superficial	B. toward the midline
_____	3. peripheral	C. near or toward the surface of the body
_____	4. lateral	D. away from the center
_____	5. proximal	E. farthest away from the point of attachment to the trunk
_____	6. caudal	F. above
_____	7. medial	G. nearest the point of attachment to the trunk
_____	8. distal	H. toward the tail

Exercise 5-3   DEFINITIONS

Underline the root or combining form, then define the medical word.

1. hypogastric _____

2. iliac   _____

3. dorsal   _____

4. inguinal   _____

5. visceral   _____

6. cranial   _____

7. phrenic   _____

8. anterior   _____

9. superior   _____

10. thoracic   _____

11. caudal   _____

6

The Skin
(Integumentary System)

CHAPTER ORGANIZATION

This chapter will help you understand the skin (the integumentary system). It is divided into the following sections:

CHAPTER OBJECTIVES

On completion of this chapter, you will be able to do the following:

1. Differentiate between the epidermis, dermis, and subcutaneous tissue as to structure and function

2. Describe how epithelial cells, melanocytes, and keratinocytes are related to the epidermis

3. Name and state the function of fibroblasts, macrophages, mast cells, and plasma cells as they relate to the dermis

4. Describe the structure and function of the hair and nails

5. Name and describe the function of the skin glands

6. Locate the structures of the skin and accessory organs on a diagram

7. Analyze, define, spell, and pronounce medical terms common to the skin

8. Define abbreviations common to the skin

INTRODUCTION

This is the first of the body system chapters in which you will learn medical terms in the context of the system studied.

The main title of this chapter is technically incorrect because the skin is actually only part of the system discussed. The proper name, the **integumentary** (in-**teg**-you-**MEN**-tah-ree) system, gets its name from the Latin word *integumentum*, meaning "covering." This system is the covering of the body. The skin is by far the major part, but also included are related structures such as hair, glands, and nails.

6.1   Anatomy and Physiology of the Skin

Most people do not think of the skin as an organ, but in fact, it is the largest organ of the body. It has two layers. The outer layer is the **epidermis** (ep-ih-**DER**-mis). The inner layer is the **dermis**. Underlying the dermis is the **subcutaneous** (sub-kyou-**TAY**-nee-us) layer, but it is not regarded as part of the skin. Figure 6-1 illustrates the skin.

Memory Key	The skin consists of the epidermis and the dermis.

EPIDERMIS

As described in Chapter 2, cells make up tissue and tissue makes up organs. The epidermis (an organ), consists primarily of **epithelial** (ep-ih-**THEE**-lee-al) cells. The tissue is known as epithelial tissue, or **epithelium** (ep-ih-**THEE**-lee-um). The epidermis not only covers the body but also lines body cavities and covers organs. Specialized cells called **melanocytes** (meh-**LAN**-oh-sights) are responsible for skin color. These cells produce **melanin** (**MEL**-ah-nin), a pigment. The more melanin produced, the darker the skin. **Keratinocytes** (keh-**RAT**-in-oh-sights), other specialized cells, are very important because they produce **keratin** (**KER**-ah-tin), a protein that infiltrates the outermost layer of epithelial cells and makes them tough, waterproof, and resistant to bacteria. The cells that have been filled with keratin are called **keratinized** cells.

There are four layers (strata) of epithelium in the epidermis covering most of the body, but there are five in the soles of the feet and palms of the hands because of the need for extra thickness. This extra layer causes the palms and soles to appear lighter than the rest of the skin, because the melanocytes are found in the deeper layers. At the deepest, or **basal cell**, layer of the epidermis, epithelial cells are constantly being produced, pushing the older cells toward the more superficial layers, where they die and become filled with keratin. This is a continuous process taking about 2 weeks. The most superficial layer is sometimes called the horny (hornlike) layer, and its medical name is the **stratum corneum** (**STRAY**-tum **KOR**-nee-um). The cells in this layer are continuously being shed.

There are no blood vessels or nerves in the epidermis.

Memory Key	The epidermis consists of epithelial cells, melanocytes, and keratinocytes. The tissue type is epithelium.

FIGURE 6-1
The skin

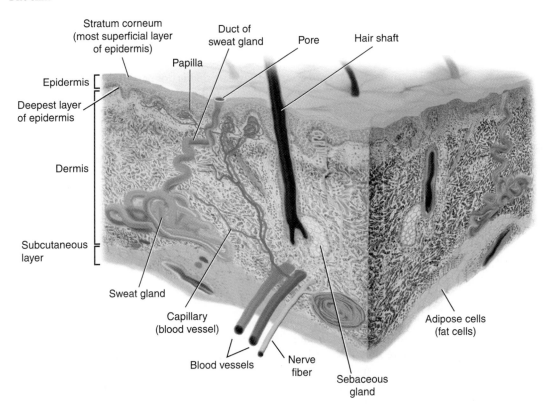

DERMIS

The dermis lies beneath the deepest layer of the epidermis. It is a thick area of **connective tissue** containing hair follicles, blood vessels, nerves, and glands. The dermis contains blood vessels and is therefore the nutrient supplier for the skin. These blood vessels also help control inner body temperature through a process called thermoregulation. When the body needs to lose heat, the vessels in the dermis dilate (expand), allowing a greater volume of blood to be cooled near the surface. When the body is cold, the same vessels constrict (contract), reducing heat loss. Sensory receptors in the dermis are responsible for our sense of touch. The glands secrete substances necessary for skin maintenance and function (see Glands in section 6.2).

The tissue of the dermis consists of four types of cells, which strengthen and protect the skin: **fibroblasts** (**FIGH**-broh-blasts), **macrophages** (**MACK**-roh-fay-jeez), **mast cells**, and **plasma cells**. These cells function to protect the body. Fibroblasts produce collagen, a protein that makes the skin tough and durable. Macrophages engulf bacteria and other potentially harmful foreign substances. Mast cells produce **histamine** (**HISS**-tah-meen), and plasma cells produce **antibodies**. Both histamine and antibodies act against foreign materials.

Memory Key	The dermis is connective tissue containing hair follicles, blood vessels, nerves, and glands. It consists of fibroblasts, macrophages, mast cells, and plasma cells.

SUBCUTANEOUS TISSUE

The subcutaneous tissue is a layer of connective tissue that is not part of the skin. It is important because it connects the dermis to the muscles and organs below. It also contains fatty tissue, which insulates inner structures from temperature extremes.

A summary of the anatomy and physiology of the skin is given in Table 6-1.

Memory Key	Subcutaneous tissue connects the dermis to inner structures and provides insulation.

6.2   Related Organs

The hair, nails, and glands are the other organs of the integumentary system.

HAIR

Hair consists of epidermal cells. They grow at the bottom of a tube called a **hair follicle**, which extends from the dermis through the epidermis. New epidermal cells push older ones up the follicle, where they die and become keratinized, forming the shaft of the hair. Hair color depends upon the amount of melanin present, as does the color of the skin. Because melanin production decreases with aging, the hair loses its color and turns gray. A hair follicle is illustrated in Figure 6-2.

TABLE 6-1

SUMMARY OF THE ANATOMY AND PHYSIOLOGY OF THE EPIDERMIS AND DERMIS

Epidermis		Dermis	
Cells:	epithelial melanocytes keratinocytes	**Cells:**	fibroblasts macrophages mast cells plasma cells
Tissue:	epithelial tissue	**Tissue:**	connective tissue
Function:	protection	**Function:**	temperature regulation sensation secretion nutrition protection

FIGURE 6-2
Hair and related structures

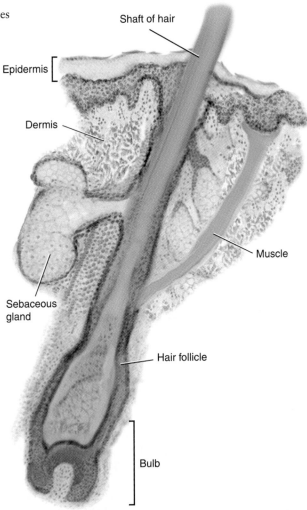

Shaft of hair

Epidermis

Dermis

Muscle

Sebaceous
gland

Hair follicle

Bulb

| Memory Key | Hair is formed in a hair follicle. The shaft of the hair consists of keratinized cells. |

NAILS

Nails are epithelial cells that have been keratinized. New cells form at the moon, or **lunula** (**LOO**-noo-lah), pushing the other cells toward the end of the finger or toe along the nailbed underlying the nail. A fingernail is illustrated in Figure 6-3. The cuticle, or **eponychium** (ep-oh-**NICK**-ee-um), overlaps onto the nail. It also consists of keratinized epithelial cells, but the keratin is much softer than on the rest of the nail.

| Memory Key | The nail and cuticle consist of keratinized epithelial cells. |

FIGURE 6-3
The nail: (A) posterior view, (B) fingernail and underlying structures

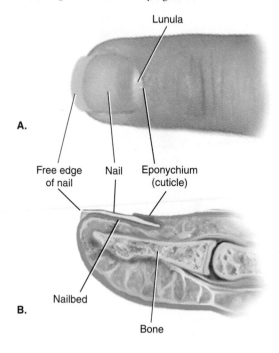

Lunula

A.

Free edge   Nail   Eponychium
of nail   (cuticle)

Nailbed
B.

Bone

GLANDS

The skin glands (see Figure 6-1) are very important to the maintenance of skin health and function. **Sebaceous** (seh-**BAY**-shus) **glands** secrete an oil called **sebum** (**SEE**-bum), which keeps the skin soft and waterproof. It also keeps the hair pliable; without sebum, the hair would become brittle and would break.

The **sudoriferous** (soo-dor-**IF**-er-us) **glands**, or sweat glands, play a role in thermoregulation by secreting sweat onto the surface of the skin. Evaporation of the sweat cools the skin.

The **ceruminous glands** (seh-**ROO**-min-us) produce **cerumen** (seh-**ROO**-men) in the ear, which is a waxy substance that helps prevent bacterial infection.

Memory Key	Sebaceous glands secrete sebum to lubricate the skin and hair. Sudoriferous glands secrete sweat to cool the skin. Ceruminous glands secrete cerumen in the ear to prevent infection.

6.3   Additional Word Elements

Use these additional word elements when studying the medical terms in this chapter.

Root	Meaning
cry/o	cold
leuk/o	white
papill/o	nipple-like
scler/o	hardening
xer/o	dry

Suffix	Meaning
-ism	process
-ium; -um	structure
-sis	state of; condition

6.4 Term Analysis and Definition

	albin/o	white
Term	**Term Analysis**	**Definition**
albinism (**AL**-bih-niz-um)	-ism = process	lack of pigment in the skin, hair, and eyes
	adip/o	**fat**
adipose (**AD**-ih-pohs)	-ose = pertaining to	pertaining to fat
	bi/o	**life**
skin biopsy (**BYE**-op-see)	-opsy = to view	removal of living tissue for microscopic examination

	cutane/o	skin
Term	**Term Analysis**	**Definition**
subcutaneous (**sub**-kyou-**TAY**-nee-us)	sub- = under -ous = pertaining to	pertaining to under the skin
	cyan/o	blue
cyanotic (**sigh**-ah-**NOT**-ick)	-tic = pertaining to	pertaining to a bluish discoloration of skin
	derm/o; dermat/o	skin
dermatitis (**der**-mah-**TYE**-tis)	-itis = inflammation	inflammation of the skin (see Figure 6-4)
dermatology (**der**-mah-**TOL**-oh-jee)	-logy = study	study of the skin and its diseases
dermatologist (**der**-mah-**TOL**-oh-jist)	-logist = one who specializes in the study of	one who specializes in the study of the skin and its diseases

FIGURE 6-4

Dermatitis caused by poison oak. *Courtesy of Timothy Berger, MD, Associate Clinical Professor, University of California, San Francisco*

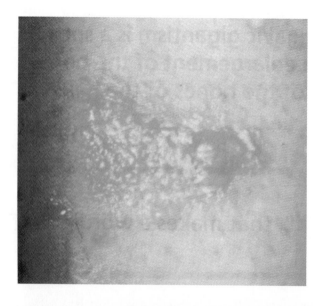

Term	Term Analysis	Definition
hypodermic (**high**-poh-**DER**-mick)	-ic = pertaining to hypo- = under; below	pertaining to below the skin; subcutaneous. *NOTE:* The prefixes hypo- and sub- cannot be interchanged. Hypo- is used with the root **derm/o**, and sub- is used with the root **cutane/o**.
dermatoplasty (der-**MA**-toh-**plast**-ee)	-plasty = surgical reconstruction	surgical reconstruction of the skin; surgical replacement of injured or diseased skin

	diaphor/e	**profuse sweating**
diaphoresis (**dye**-ah-foh-**REE**-sis)	-sis = state of; condition	state of profuse sweating

	electr/o	**electric**
electrolysis (**ee**-leck-**TROL**-ih-sis)	-lysis = breakdown; destruction	destruction of tissue by electricity. *NOTE:* Electrolysis is used to remove unwanted body hair.

	epitheli/o	**covering**
epithelium (**ep**-ih-**THEE**-lee-um)	-um = structure	structure made up of epithelial cells covering the internal and external surfaces of the body
epithelial (**ep**-ih-**THEE**-lee-al)	-al = pertaining to	pertaining to the epithelium

	erythemat/o	**red**
erythematous (**er**-ih-**THEM**-ah-tus)	-ous = pertaining to	pertaining to a redness of the skin. *NOTE:* erythematous is an adjective.

	erythr/o	**red**
erythema (**er**-ih-**THEE**-mah)		red discoloration to the skin. *NOTE:* erythema is a noun.

	hidr/o	sweat
Term	**Term Analysis**	**Definition**
anhidrosis (**an**-high-**DROH**-sis)	-osis = abnormal condition a(n)- = no; not; lack of	lack of sweat
hyperhidrosis (**high**-per-high-**DROH**-sis)	-osis = abnormal condition hyper- = excessive; above normal	excessive secretion of sweat
	kerat/o; keratin/o	**hard; hornlike**
hyperkeratosis (**high**-per-**ker**-ah-**TOH**-sis)	-osis = abnormal condition hyper- = excessive; above normal	excessive growth of the outer layer of skin (horny layer)
keratinocyte (ker-**RAT**-in-oh-sight)	-cyte = cell	cell that produces keratin
	lip/o	**fat**
lipoma (lih-**POH**-mah)	-oma = tumor; mass	tumor or mass containing fat
liposuction (**LIP**-oh-**suck**-shun)	suction = process of aspirating or withdrawing	withdrawal of fat from the subcutaneous tissue
	melan/o	**black**
melanocyte (mel-**LAN**-oh-sight)	-cyte = cell	cell that produces melanin
	myc/o	**fungus**
dermatomycosis (**der**-mah-toh-my-**KOH**-sis)	-osis = abnormal condition **dermat/o** = skin	fungal infection of the skin

	necr/o	death
Term	**Term Analysis**	**Definition**
necrotic tissue (neh-**KROT**-ick)	-tic = pertaining to	pertaining to death of tissues

NOTE: An example of necrotic tissue is a pressure sore, also known as a bedsore or decubitus ulcer. This is defined as dead skin, usually over a bony prominence, due to a lack of circulation and loss of oxygen to the skin. It may occur when a patient is kept in the same position, without being moved, for an extended length of time (see Figure 6-5).

	onych/o	nail
eponychium (**ep**-oh-**NICK**-ee-um)	-ium = structure epi- = upon; above	structure upon the nail; the cuticle
onychomycosis (**on**-ih-koh-my-**KOH**-sis)	-osis = abnormal condition myc/o = fungus	fungal infection of the nail
paronychia (**par**-oh-**NICK**-ee-ah)	-ia = condition para- = beside; near	inflammation of the tissue around the nail. *NOTE:* The suffix -itis, meaning "inflammation," is not used in this term (see Figure 6-6).

	pil/o	hair
pilosebaceous (**pye**-loh-seh-**BAY**-shus)	-ous = pertaining to seb/o = sebum	pertaining to hair follicles and sebaceous glands

FIGURE 6-5
Pressure sore. *Courtesy of Emory University Hospital, Atlanta, Ga.*

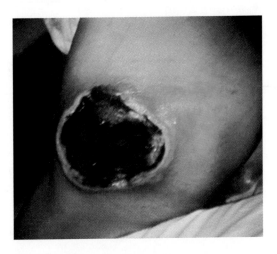

FIGURE 6-6
Paronychia

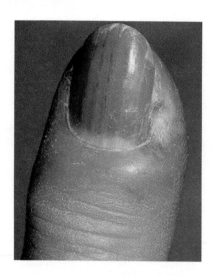

	py/o	pus
Term	**Term Analysis**	**Definition**
pyogenic (**pye**-oh-**JEN**-ick)	-genic = producing	pus producing
	ras/o	**scrape**
abrasion (ab-**RAY**-zhun)	-ion = process ab- = away from	scraping away of the superficial layers of injured skin; for example, injury from a floor burn
	rhytid/o	**wrinkle**
rhytidectomy (reye-tid-**EC**-tom-y)	-ectomy = surgical excision; removal	removal of wrinkles; facelift
	seb/o	**sebum**
seborrhea (**seb**-oh-**REE**-ah)	-rrhea = flow; discharge	increased discharge of sebum from the sebaceous glands
	steat/o	**fat**
steatoma (**stee**-ah-**TOH**-mah)	-oma = tumor; mass	fatty tumor of the sebaceous glands

	ungu/o	nail
Term	**Term Analysis**	**Definition**
periungual (**per**-ee-**UNG**-gwal)	-al = pertaining to peri- = around	pertaining to around the nail

PREFIXES

	derma-	skin
Term	**Term Analysis**	**Definition**
dermabrasion (**DERM**-ab-ray-zhun	-ion = process ab- = away from **ras/o** = scrape	scraping away of the top layers of skin using sandpaper or wire brushes to remove tattoos or disfigured skin. The skin then regenerates with little scarring.

SUFFIXES

	dermis; -derma	skin
Term	**Term Analysis**	**Definition**
epidermis (**ep**-ih-**DER**-mis)	epi- = upon; above	above the dermis
erythroderma (eh-**rith**-roh-**DER**-mah)	**erythr/o** = red	redness of the skin
leukoderma (**loo**-koh-**DER**-mah)	**leuk/o** = white	lack of pigmentation of the skin showing up as white patches; vitiligo
pyoderma (**pye**-oh-**DER**-mah)	**py/o** = pus	any pus-producing disease of the skin
scleroderma (**skleh**-roh-**DER**-mah)	**scler/o** = hardening	abnormal thickening of the dermis, usually starting in the hands and feet
xeroderma (**zer**-oh-**DER**-mah)	**xer/o** = dry	dry skin of a chronic (continuous) nature

	-oma	**tumor; mass**
adenoma (**ad**-eh-**NOH**-mah)	**aden/o** = gland	glandular tumor

Term	Term Analysis	Definition
carcinoma (**kar**-sih-**NOH**-mah)	**carcin/o** = cancerous	malignant tumor of epithelial cells. Examples include **basal cell carcinoma**, a malignant tumor that is the most common and least harmful type of skin cancer usually caused by overexposure to the sun (see Figure 6-7A), and **squamous cell carcinoma**, a malignant tumor that is more harmful and has a faster growing rate and tendency to metastasize to other body systems (see Figure 6-7B).
hemangioma (heh-**man**-jee-**OH**-mah)	**hem/o** = blood **angi/o** = vessel	a common, benign tumor of blood vessels most often seen in children or infants. Also known as birthmarks or nevi (singular = nevus) (see Figure 6-8)
melanoma (**mel**-ah-**NOH**-mah)	**melan/o** = black	tumor arising from the melanocytes; usually malignant (see Figure 6-9)
papilloma (**pap**-ih-**LOH**-mah)	**papill/o** = nipple-like	benign epithelial tumor
	-therapy	**treatment**
cryotherapy (**kri**-oh-**THER**-ah-pee)	**cry/o** = cold	destruction of tissue by freezing with liquid nitrogen

FIGURE 6-7

Carcinoma: (A) basal cell, (B) squamous cell. *Courtesy of Robert A. Silverman, MD, Clinical Associate Professor, Department of Pediatrics, Georgetown University.*

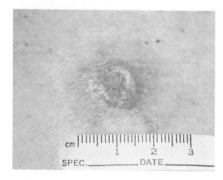

A.

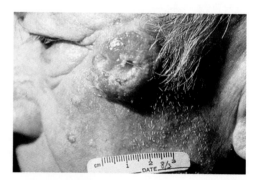

B.

FIGURE 6-8
Hemangioma

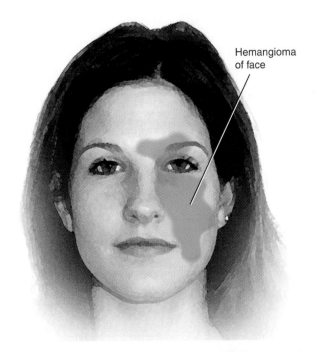

Hemangioma
of face

FIGURE 6-9
Melanoma. *Courtesy of the American Academy of Dermatology*

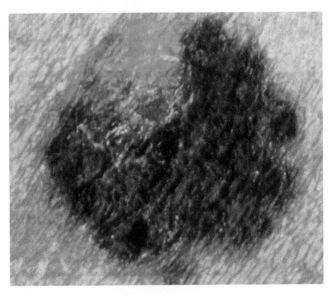

Term	Term Analysis	Definition
laser therapy (**LAY**-zer)	laser = intense beam of light	removal of skin lesions such as papillomas and hemangiomas, using an intense beam of light. *NOTE:* In this example, therapy is used as a word rather than a suffix.

6.5   Review of Terms

Define the terms in Tables 6-2 through 6-4 in the space provided.

TABLE 6-2

REVIEW OF ANATOMICAL TERMS

adipose	dermatologist	dermatology
epidermis	epithelial	epithelium
eponychium	hypodermic	keratinocyte
melanocyte	periungual	pilosebaceous
subcutaneous		

TABLE 6-3

REVIEW OF PATHOLOGICAL TERMS

adenoma	albinism	anhidrosis
carcinoma	cyanotic	dermatitis
dermatomycosis	diaphoresis	erythema
erythematous	erythroderma	hemangioma
hyperhidrosis	hyperkeratosis	leukoderma
lipoma	melanoma	necrotic
onychomycosis	papilloma	paronychia
pyoderma	pyogenic	scleroderma
seborrhea	steatoma	xeroderma

TABLE 6-4

REVIEW OF CLINICAL AND SURGICAL TERMS

cryotherapy	dermabrasion	electrolysis
laser therapy	liposuction	rhytidectomy
skin biopsy		

6.6   Abbreviations

Abbreviation	Meaning
bx	biopsy
SC; subq, subcut	subcutaneous
UV	ultraviolet
derm	dermatology

6.7   Putting It All Together

Exercise 6-1   FILL IN THE BLANK

1. The two layers of the skin are the _____ and _____ .

2. Another name for the skin is the _____ .

3. The epidermis is void of _____ and _____ .

4. The dermis consists of _____ tissue.

5. The main function of the epidermis is _____ .

6. Hair is formed at the _____ .

7. Name the glands found in the dermis and their secretions.

_____

_____

_____

Exercise 6-2   DEFINING ROOTS AND COMBINING FORMS

Underline the root or the combining form in the following words, then define each word.

1. subcutaneous _____
2. cyanotic _____
3. hypodermic _____
4. epithelial _____
5. erythematous _____
6. hyperhidrosis _____
7. leukoderma _____
8. necrotic _____
9. paronychia _____
10. seborrhea _____
11. steatoma _____
12. rhytidectomy _____
13. xeroderma _____
14. melanoma _____
15. albinism _____

Exercise 6-3   DEFINING SUFFIXES

Give the meaning of each of the following suffixes.

1. -oma _____
2. -ar _____
3. -derma _____
4. -rrhea _____
5. -genic _____
6. -ia _____
7. -ium _____
8. -osis _____
9. -cyte _____
10. -ion _____

11. -al   _____

12. -logy   _____

Exercise 6-4   BUILDING MEDICAL WORDS

Build the medical word for the following definitions.

1. excision of wrinkles   _____

2. pertaining to a bluish discoloration to the skin   _____

3. one who specializes in the study of the skin and its diseases   _____

4. lack of sweat   _____

5. cell that produces melanin   _____

6. fungal infection of the skin   _____

7. fungal infection of the nail   _____

8. hardening of the skin   _____

9. malignant tumor of epithelial cells   _____

10. malignant tumor arising from the melanocytes   _____

Exercise 6-5   MATCHING

Match the word element in Column A with its meaning in Column B.

Column A	**Column B**
_____ 1. albin/o	A. death
_____ 2. myc/o	B. sweat
_____ 3. hidr/o	C. hard; hornlike
_____ 4. kerat/o	D. white
_____ 5. melan/o	E. nipple-like
_____ 6. necr/o	F. fungus
_____ 7. onych/o	G. black
_____ 8. cry/o	H. cold
_____ 9. papill/o	I. dry
_____ 10. xer/o	J. nail

Exercise 6-6   MATCHING

Match the term in Column A with its definition in Column B.

Column A

_____ 1. subcutaneous

_____ 2. cyanotic

_____ 3. erythematous

_____ 4. hyperhidrosis

_____ 5. paronychia

_____ 6. seborrhea

_____ 7. periungual

_____ 8. steatoma

_____ 9. cryotherapy

_____ 10. papilloma

Column B

A. destruction of tissue by using liquid nitrogen, which freezes the tissue

B. benign epithelial tumor

C. inflammation of tissue around the nail

D. excessive secretion of sweat

E. pertaining to under the skin

F. pertaining to a bluish discoloration of the skin

G. red discoloration of the skin

H. fatty tumor of the sebaceous glands

I. increased discharge of sebum from sebaceous glands

J. pertaining to around the nail

Exercise 6-7   SPELLING PRACTICE

Circle any misspelled words in the list below. Correctly spell the misspelled words in the space provided.

1. cianotic   _____

2. dermatologist   _____

3. diaphoreses   _____

4. epithlial   _____

5. arythema   _____

6. dermatomycosis _____

7. necrotic   _____

8. hemangioma   _____

9. cryotherapy   _____

10. anhydrosis   _____

C H A P T E R

The Skeletal System

CHAPTER OBJECTIVES

On completion of this chapter, you will be able to do the following:

1. List the functions of the bones
2. Define terms relating to bone structure
3. Distinguish between the axial and appendicular skeletons
4. Name and locate the major bones of the body
5. Analyze, define, spell, and pronounce common terms of the skeletal system
6. Define common abbreviations of the skeletal system

INTRODUCTION

Many people think that bones are simply solid masses of nonliving tissue. Nothing could be further from the truth. Each of the 206 bones of the body is a complex, living organ. In this chapter, you will learn the anatomy and physiology of this fascinating body system, together with the terms associated with it.

7.1   Anatomy and Physiology of Bone

BONE FUNCTION

Height, width, and the basic shape of the body are determined by the length and thickness of the bones that make up the skeleton. But bones have other important functions. They make movement possible by acting as rigid and strong levers on which the muscles can exert force. They also provide protection and support for vital inner organs. Two examples are the skull bones (the cranium), which protect and support the brain, and the ribs, which do the same for the heart and lungs. Blood cells, which are essential to life, are produced by the red bone marrow, which lies in the inner portion of bone. Bones also play an important role in regulating the amount of essential minerals in the blood, particularly calcium and phosphorus. The bones store these minerals and release them into the bloodstream when required.

Memory Key	Bones provide protection and support, make movement possible, produce blood cells, and store and release calcium and phosphorus.

BONE STRUCTURE

As do all the other parts of the body, bones consist of cells. Mature bone cells are called **osteocytes** (**OS**-tee-oh-sights). They have a limited life span, because other cells, called **osteoclasts** (**OS**-tee-oh-klasts), are constantly breaking them down and reabsorbing the remaining material. New bone cells are created by a third type of cell called **osteoblasts** (**OS**-tee-oh-blasts). The process of bone formation is called **ossification** (os-ih-fih-**KAY**-shun) or **osteogenesis** (os-tee-oh-**JEN**-eh-sis). There is continual turnover of bone to ensure that bone tissue remains strong and that the bones mold themselves to match the stresses placed on them. This breakdown and renewal of bone is called **remodeling** and keeps the bones young and strong.

You may be surprised to learn that the process of remodeling changes the shape of bones, if the demands placed on the body require it. For example, if you start a weightlifting program, your bones will begin to thicken in certain areas to better cope with the new demands. Start jogging regularly, and a different change in bone shape will occur, to adjust to the unique requirements of running.

Memory Key	Osteoblasts create bone; osteoclasts reabsorb it. Mature bone cells are osteocytes. The process of bone formation is ossification. Breakdown and renewal of bone is called remodeling.

7.2   Description of the Skeleton

Figure 7-1 illustrates the anterior and posterior views of the skeleton. As you work your way through the material in this section, you will find it useful to regularly refer to this figure.

FIGURE 7-1
The human skeleton: (A) anterior view, (B) posterior view

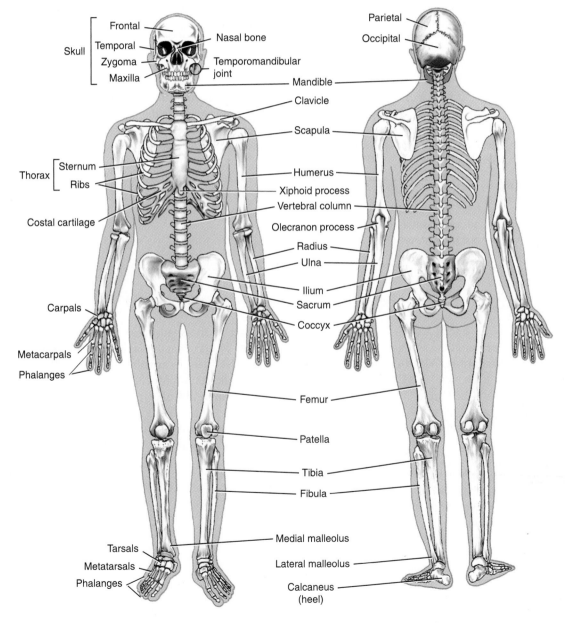

A. Anterior   B. Posterior

THE AXIAL AND APPENDICULAR SKELETONS

The group of bones that are related to the head and trunk is referred to as the **axial** (**ACKS**-ee-ul) **skeleton**. It consists of the **skull**, **vertebral** (**VER**-teh-bral) **column**, **thoracic** (thoh-**RAS**-ick) **cage**, and a special bone in the throat called the **hyoid** (**HIGH**-oid) **bone**. The **appendicular** (app-en-**DICK**-you-lar) **skeleton** consists of the **pectoral girdle** (which connects the arms to the thoracic cage), the **pelvic girdle** (which connects the legs to the axial skeleton), and the arms and legs.

Memory Key	The skull, vertebral column, thoracic cage, and hyoid bone make up the axial skeleton. The pectoral and pelvic girdles and the arms and legs make up the appendicular skeleton.

THE AXIAL SKELETON

The Cranial Bones   The cranial bones include the **frontal bone**, or **forehead**, the paired **parietal** (pah-**RYE**-eh-tal) **bones**, making up the crown of the skull, the two **temporal** (**TEM**-poh-ral) **bones** on either side of the cranium, the **occipital** (ock-**SIP**-ih-tal) **bone** at the back of the head, the **sphenoid** (**SFEE**-noid) **bone**, and the **ethmoid** (**ETH**-moid) **bone** (see Figure 7-2A).

Memory Key	The cranial bones are the:
	frontal bone
	parietal bones
	occipital bone
	temporal bones
	sphenoid bone
	ethmoid bone

The Facial Bones   The facial bones form part of the skull. They are the **nasal bone**, **zygomatic** (zye-goh-**MAT**-ick) **bone**, **vomer** (**VOH**-mer), **maxilla** (**MACK**-sih-lah), **mandible** (**MAN**-dih-bul), **nasal conchae** (**KONG**-kee) or **turbinates** (**TER**-bih-nayts), and **lacrimal** (**LACK**-rih-mal) **bones**. The mandible (commonly called the lower jaw) unites with the temporal bone of the skull at the **temporomandibular** (tem-poh-roh-man-**DIB**-you-lar) **joint** (**TMJ**) to form the only movable bone of the skull. The conchae extend from the lateral wall of the nasal cavity. In some people, these bones may become enlarged, blocking air passage through the nose and requiring surgical reduction (see Figure 7-2B).

Memory Key	The facial bones are the:
	nasal bones
	zygomatic bones
	vomer
	maxilla
	mandible
	nasal conchae (or turbinates)
	lacrimal bones

FIGURE 7-2
Bones of the skull

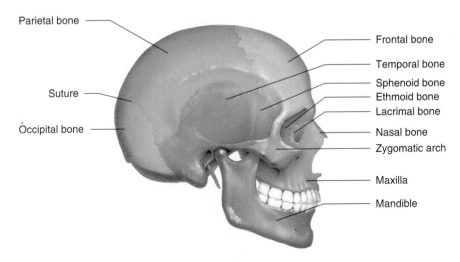

Parietal bone

Frontal bone

Temporal bone

Sphenoid bone

Ethmoid bone

Suture

Lacrimal bone

Occipital bone

Nasal bone

Zygomatic arch

Maxilla

Mandible

A. Lateral View

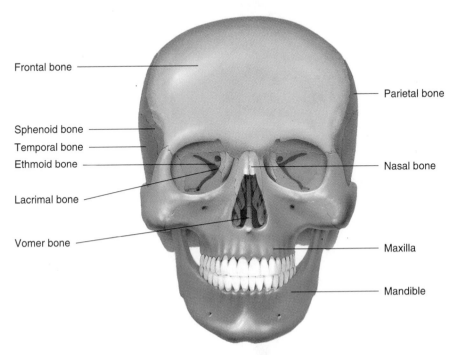

Frontal bone

Parietal bone

Sphenoid bone

Temporal bone

Ethmoid bone

Nasal bone

Lacrimal bone

Vomer bone

Maxilla

Mandible

B. Frontal View

The Vertebral Column Figure 7-3 illustrates the spine. The spine consists of 33 bones called **vertebrae** and thus is often referred to as the vertebral column. For ease of reference, the vertebrae are named by location. Just below the skull are the seven **cervical** (**SER**-vih-kal) vertebrae. Next in the chest area are 12 **thoracic** vertebrae (also called **dorsal** vertebrae), followed by five **lumbar** (**LUM**-bar) vertebrae in the lower back. Below that is the **sacrum** (**SAY**-krum), which consists of five fused bones, and the **coccyx** (**KOCK**-sicks), or tailbone, consisting of four fused bones. Except for the coccyx, the vertebrae are referred to by a letter followed by a number. The cervical vertebrae are C1–C7; the thoracic are T1–T12 (if dorsal is used, they are D1–D12); the lumbar are L1–L5; and the sacrum is S1–S5.

FIGURE 7-3
Vertebral column, lateral view

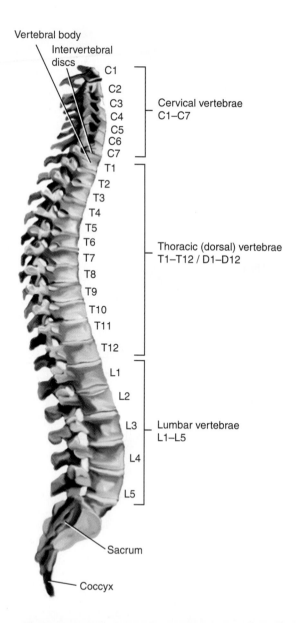

Vertebral body

Intervertebral discs

C1
C2
C3
C4
C5
C6
C7

Cervical vertebrae
C1–C7

T1
T2
T3
T4
T5
T6
T7
T8
T9
T10
T11
T12

Thoracic (dorsal) vertebrae
T1–T12 / D1–D12

L1
L2
L3
L4
L5

Lumbar vertebrae
L1–L5

Sacrum

Coccyx

Between the vertebrae are little round shock absorbers called **intervertebral discs**. Together, they absorb much of the shock of movement and jumping. The discs are made of cartilage. The tough outer layer is called the **annulus fibrosus** (**AN**-you-lus figh-**BROH**-sus). The soft, gel-like inner portion is called the **nucleus pulposus** (**NEW**-klee-us pul-**POH**-sus). The common and painful condition called a slipped or herniated (**HER**-nee-ay-ted) **disc** occurs when some of the gel material pushes the outer layer out of its normal position. When the layer is out of position, nerves are pinched, causing pain messages to be sent to the brain. Also, nerve impulses are sent to back muscles, causing them to painfully contract. This contraction is called a muscle spasm and contributes to the discomfort of a herniated disc (see Figure 7-4).

Memory Key	• There are 33 vertebrae. • The number of vertebrae in each segment of the vertebral column can be remembered by the following: eat breakfast at 7 A.M. (7 cervical), lunch at 12 noon (12 thoracic), and dinner at 5 P.M. (5 lumbar). • A slipped disc is a herniated disc.

The Thoracic Cage   Figure 7-1 illustrates the thoracic cage. Included are the breastbone, or **sternum** (**STER**-num), 12 pairs of ribs, **costal cartilage**, and thoracic vertebrae. Posteriorly, all of the ribs attach to the 12 thoracic vertebrae. Anteriorly, the top 10 pairs of ribs are connected by costal cartilage to the sternum. The other two pairs do not attach to the sternum and are therefore called **floating ribs**.

Memory Key	The thoracic cage consists of the sternum, 12 pairs of ribs, costal cartilage, and thoracic vertebrae.

THE APPENDICULAR SKELETON

Pectoral Girdle   The collarbones or **clavicles** (**KLAV**-ih-kulz), and shoulder blades or **scapulae** (**SKAP**-you-lee) make up the pectoral girdle. Refer to Figure 7-1 to view the clavicles and scapulae and their relationship to the thoracic cage.

FIGURE 7-4
Herniated disc

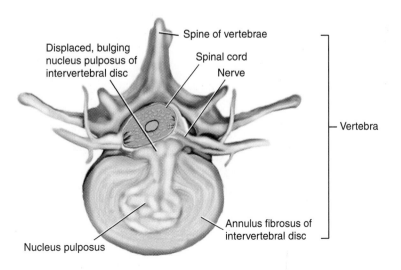

Displaced, bulging nucleus pulposus of intervertebral disc

Spine of vertebrae

Spinal cord

Nerve

Vertebra

Annulus fibrosus of intervertebral disc

Nucleus pulposus

Memory Key The pectoral girdle consists of the clavicles and scapulae.

Pelvic Girdle   The pelvic girdle protects the pelvic organs. It consists of the two hip, or **coxal** (**KOCKS**-al), bones. Each hip bone contains three segments that become fused: the **ilium** (**ILL**-ee-um), **ischium** (**ISS**-kee-um), and **pubis** (**PEW**-bis). Figure 7-5 illustrates the pelvis. The **acetabulum** (**ass**-eh-**TAB**-you-lum), or hip socket, allows the head of the femur to fit into it, forming the hip joint. The right and left hip bones form a circle by joining with each other anteriorly at the **symphysis** (**SIM**-fih-sis) **pubis** and posteriorly with the sacrum to form the **sacroiliac** (**say**-kroh-**ILL**-ee-ack) joint. In females, the symphysis pubis will stretch slightly to assist delivery of a baby.

Memory Key   The pelvic girdle consists of two coxal bones, joined anteriorly at the symphysis pubis and posteriorly at the sacrum.

Upper Extremity   The bones of the arm and hand make up the upper extremity. The arm bones include the upper arm or **humerus** (**HEW**-mer-us), and the two lower arm bones, the **ulna** (**ULL**-nah) and the **radius** (**RAY**-dee-us). The humerus, ulna, and radius can be seen in Figure 7-1. The bulge on the proximal end of the ulna is the elbow, also called the **olecranon** (oh-**LEK**-rah-non) **process**, and can be seen in Figure 7-1B.

Figure 7-6 illustrates the wrist and hand. The wrist is made up of eight **carpal** (**KAR**-pal) bones arranged in two rows. The hand bones are called **metacarpals** (met-a-**KAR**-palz) and are numbered I to V. The Roman numeral I indicates the metacarpal extending toward the thumb; V refers to the metacarpal extending toward the little finger. Small bones called **phalanges** (fah-**LAN**-jeez) make up the fingers. Each finger consists of three phalanges, except for the thumb, which has two. These bones are connected to each other at the **interphalangeal** (**in**-ter-fah-**LAN**-jee-al) **joints**, often referred to as **IP joints**.

FIGURE 7-5
Pelvis, anterior view

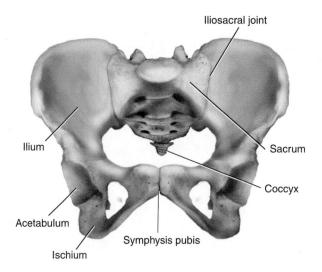

Iliosacral joint

Ilium

Sacrum

Coccyx

Acetabulum

Symphysis pubis

Ischium

FIGURE 7-6
Bone of the lower left arm, wrist, and hand

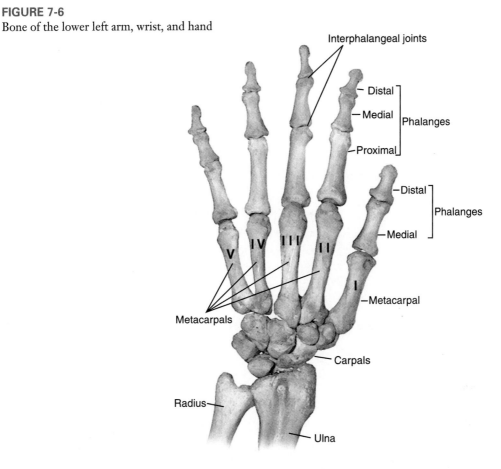

Lower Extremity   The bones of the leg and the foot make up the lower extremity. The bones of the leg include the thighbone, or **femur** (FEE-mur); the knee, or **patella** (pah-TEL-ah); the shin, or **tibia** (TIB-ee-ah); and the **fibula** (FIB-you-lah), which is the lateral bone of the lower leg. Refer to Figure 7-1 for an illustration.

The bones of the foot are illustrated in Figure 7-7. The ankle bones are called the **tarsals** (TAHR-salz). The foot bones are the **metatarsals** (met-ah-TAHR-salz). Like the metacarpals, the metatarsals are numbered I to V. The toes are called the **phalanges** (fah-LAN-jeez). The phalanges of the toes, like those of the fingers, are joined at the IP joints.

FIGURE 7-7
Dorsal view of foot

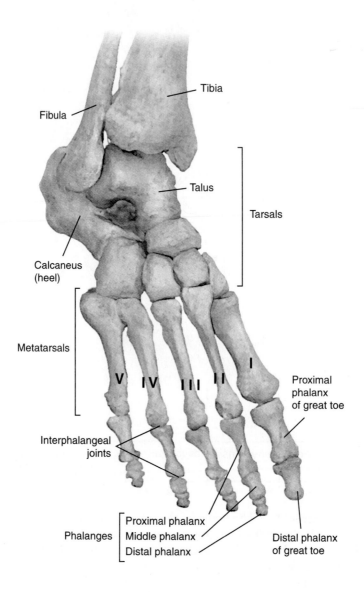

Tibia

Fibula

Talus

Tarsals

Calcaneus
(heel)

Metatarsals

V IV III II I

Proximal
phalanx
of great toe

Interphalangeal
joints

Phalanges · Proximal phalanx
Middle phalanx
Distal phalanx

Distal phalanx
of great toe

SUMMARY OF THE AXIAL AND APPENDICULAR SKELETONS

Table 7-1 summarizes the bones of the axial and appendicular skeletons.

TABLE 7-1

SUMMARY OF SKELETAL STRUCTURES

AXIAL SKELETON

Anatomical Name	Common Name
Cranial bones	**Skull**
• Frontal bone	Forehead
• Parietal bones	
• Temporal bones	Temples
• Occipital bone	
• Sphenoid bones (adj. sphenoidal)	
• Ethmoid bones (adj. ethmoidal)	
Facial bones	
• Zygoma (adj. zygomatic)	Cheek
• Vomer	
• Maxilla (adj. maxillary)	Upper jaw
• Mandible (adj. mandibular)	Lower jaw
• Conchae, or turbinates	
• Lacrimal bone	
Vertebral column	**Spine**
• Cervical vertabrae	
• Thoracic vertabrae	
• Lumbar vertabrae	
• Sacrum (adj. sacral)	
• coccyx (adj. coccygeal)	Tailbone
Thoracic cage (thorax)	**Chest, Torso**
• Sternum (adj. sternal)	Breastbone
• Ribs	
• Costal cartilage	

APPENDICULAR SKELETON

Anatomical Name	Common Name
Pectoral girdle	
• Clavicle (adj. clavicular)	Collarbone
• Scapula (adj. scapular)	Shoulder blade
Pelvic girdle	
• Ilium (adj. iliac)	Hip
• Ischium (adj. ischial)	
• Pubis (adj. pubic)	
Upper extremity	**Arm**
• Humerus (adj. humeral)	Upper arm
• Ulna (adj. ulnar)	Forearm
• Radius (adj. radial)	Forearm
• Olecranon (adj. olecranal)	Elbow
• Carpals	Wrist
• Metacarpals	
• Phalanges (adj. phalangeal)	Fingers
Lower extremity	**Leg**
• Femur (adj. femoral)	Thigh
• Tibia (adj. tibial)	Shin
• Fibula (adj. fibular)	
• Patella (adj. patellar)	Knee
• Tarsals	
• Malleolus (adj. malleolar)	
• Metatarsals	
• Phalanges (adj. phalangeal)	Toes
• Calcaneus (adj. calcaneal)	Heel

7.3   Joints

A joint is a place where bones unite. The most familiar joints are the movable joints, such as the shoulder and knee joints, but joints can also be stationary, as are those between the bones of the skull.

The movable joints are all similar in structure. **Articular cartilage** covers the ends of bones, preventing friction and allowing painless movement. Between the articular cartilages is the **joint cavity**. The joint cavity is lined with a **synovial membrane**, which secretes **synovial fluid** that acts as a joint lubricant. A **joint capsule**, strengthened by ligaments, encases the joint attaching bone to bone (see Figure 7-8). All of these structures work together to allow movement of body parts.

Joints are named for the bones that form the union. For example, the joint between the radius and the wrist is called the **radiocarpal** joint; the joint between the ilium and the femur is called the **iliofemoral** joint.

Memory Key	
• A joint is the union between two bones.	
• Joint structures consist of: articular cartilage	synovial fluid
joint cavity	joint capsule
synovial membrane	
• Joints are named after the bones that form the union.	

FIGURE 7-8
A synovial joint

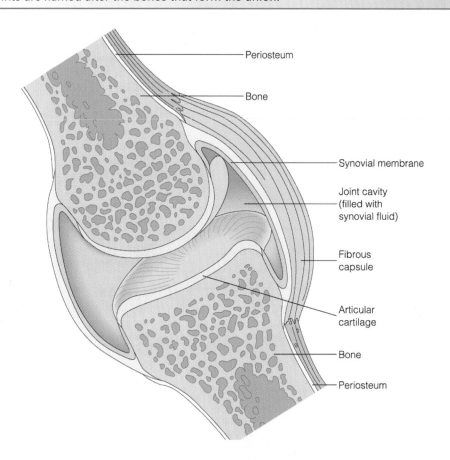

Periosteum

Bone

Synovial membrane

Joint cavity (filled with synovial fluid)

Fibrous capsule

Articular cartilage

Bone

Periosteum

7.4   Additional Word Elements

Use these additional word elements when studying the medical terms in this chapter.

Root	Meaning
kyph/o	humpback
lord/o	swayback
ped/o	child
scoli/o	curved
tempor/o	temporal bone

Suffix	Meaning
-porosis	porous

7.5   Term Analysis and Definition

A lengthy list of terms follows. Whenever possible, the adjectival form is given because it is the most common. The format will help you visualize the root with different suffixes and prefixes, observe how the word is formed, and learn the definition. Notice the variety of adjectival endings. Remember from Chapter 3 that adjectival suffixes usually cannot be interchanged: for example, cranial cannot be changed to cranious.

GENERAL BONE TERMINOLOGY

	myel/o	bone marrow; spinal cord
Term	**Term Analysis**	**Definition**
myeloma (my-el-**LOH**-mah)	-oma = tumor; mass	benign tumor of the bone marrow
osteomyelitis (**oss**-tee-oh-**my**-eh-**LYE**-tis)	-itis = inflammation **oste/o** = bone	inflammation of bone and bone marrow

Memory Key   Do not confuse **my/o**, meaning "muscle," with **myel/o**, meaning "bone marrow" or "spinal cord."

	osse/o; oste/o	bone
Term	**Term Analysis**	**Definition**
osteitis (os-tee-**EYE**-tis)	-itis = inflammation	inflammation of the bone
osteochondritis (**os**-tee-oh-kon-**DRYE**-tis)	-itis = inflammation **chondr/o** = cartilage	inflammation of bone and cartilage
osteocyte (**OS**-tee-oh-sight)	-cyte = cell	mature bone cell
osteoma (os-tee-**OH**-mah)	-oma = tumor; mass	benign tumor of bone
osteotome (**OS**-tee-oh-tohm)	-tome = instrument used to cut	instrument used to cut bone
osteotomy (**oss**-tee-**OT**-oh-mee)	-tomy = process of cutting; incision	process of cutting bone
endosteum (en- **DOS**-tee-um)	-um = structure endo- = within	inner lining of the shaft (long slender portion) of a long bone such as the tibia or ulna
periosteum (**per**-ee-**OS**-tee-um)	-um = structure peri- = around	the structure around the shaft of a long bone

AXIAL SKELETON

The axial skeleton includes bones of the skull, face, and thorax; the vertebrae; and the hyoid bone (see Figures 7-1, 7-2, and 7-3).

Skull and Facial Bones

	crani/o	skull
Term	**Term Analysis**	**Definition**
craniofacial (**kray**-nih-oh-**FAY**-shahl)	-al = pertaining to **faci/o** = face	pertaining to the skull and face
cranioplasty (**KRAY**-nee-oh-**plas**-tee)	-plasty = surgical repair or reconstruction	surgical repair of the skull
craniotomy (kray-nee-**OT**-oh-mee)	-tomy = incision	incision into the skull

	mandibul/o	mandible; lower jaw

Term	Term Analysis	Definition
mandibular (man-**DIB**-you-lar)	-ar = pertaining to	pertaining to the lower jaw
temporomandibular joint (TMJ) (**tem**-poh-roh-man--**DIB**-you-lar)	-ar = pertaining to **tempor/o** = temporal bone	pertaining to the joint between the temporal bone and the lower jaw

	maxill/o	maxilla; upper jaw

maxillary (**MACK**-sih-**ler**-ee)	-ary = pertaining to	pertaining to the upper jaw

Memory Key   To remember that *maxilla* means upper jaw, think of maximum, meaning the greatest, highest, or uppermost.

Thoracic Cage

The sternum, ribs, costal cartilage, and thoracic vertebrae make up the thoracic cage (see Figure 7-1).

	chondr/o	cartilage

Term	Term Analysis	Definition
achondroplasia (ah-**kon**-droh-**PLAY**-zee-ah)	-plasia = development; formation a- = no; not; inadequate	inadequate cartilage formation, resulting in a type of dwarfism
chondrocyte (**KON**-droh-sight)	-cyte = cell	cartilage cell
chondroma (kon-**DROH**-mah)	-oma = tumor; mass	benign tumor of cartilage

	cost/o	rib

costochondral (**kos**-toh-**KON**-drahl)	-al = pertaining to **chondr/o** = cartilage	pertaining to the ribs and cartilage
subcostal (sub-**KOS**-tal)	-al = pertaining to sub- = under	pertaining to under the ribs

	stern/o	sternum; breastbone
Term	**Term Analysis**	**Definition**
costosternal (**kos**-toh-**STER**-nal)	-al = pertaining to **cost/o** = ribs	pertaining to the ribs and sternum

	xiph/o	sword
xiphoid (**ZIGH**-foid)	-oid = resembling	resembling a sword; refers to the xiphoid process of sternum

Vertebrae

The vertebrae include the cervical, thoracic, lumbar, sacral, and coccygeal bones (see Figure 7-3).

	cervic/o	neck
Term	**Term Analysis**	**Definition**
cervical (**SER**-vih-kal)	-al = pertaining to	pertaining to the neck

	coccyg/o	coccyx; tailbone
coccygeal (kock-**SIJ**-ee-al)	-eal = pertaining to	pertaining to the tailbone

	lumb/o	lower back; loins
lumbodynia (**lum**-boh-**DIN**-ee-ah)	-dynia = pain	pain in the lower back; also known as lumbago
lumbosacral joint (**lum**-boh-**SAY**-kral)	-al = pertaining to **sacr/o** = sacrum	pertaining to the joint between the last lumbar vertebra and the sacrum

	sacr/o	sacrum
sacrococcygeal joint (**say**-kro-kock-**SIJ**-ee-al)	-eal = pertaining to **coccyg/o** = tailbone	pertaining to the joint between the sacrum and the coccyx

	spondyl/o	vertebra
Term	**Term Analysis**	**Definition**
spondylitis (**spon**-dih-**LYE**-tis)	-itis = inflammation	inflammation of the vertebrae
spondylopathy (**spon**-dil-**OP**-ah-thee)	-pathy = disease	any disease of the vertebrae

Memory Key | **Spondyl/o** is most often used in words referring to conditions of the vertebrae. Compare with **vertebr/o**, which is most often used in words to describe structure.

	thorac/o	chest
thoracolumbar (thoh-**rack**-oh-**LUM**-bar)	-ar = pertaining to **lumb/o** = lower back; loins	pertaining to the chest and lower back

	vertebr/o	vertebra
costovertebral joint (**kos**-toh-**VER**-teh-brahl)	-al = pertaining to **cost/o** = rib	pertaining to the joint between a rib and a vertebra
intervertebral (**in**-ter-**VER**-te-bral)	-al = pertaining to inter- = between	pertaining to between the vertebrae

APPENDICULAR SKELETON

The appendicular skeleton includes the pectoral and pelvic girdles and the upper and lower extremities (see Figure 7-1).

Pectoral Girdle

	clavicul/o	clavicle; collarbone
Term	**Term Analysis**	**Definition**
sternoclavicular joint (**ster**-noh-klah-**VICK**-you-lar)	-ar = pertaining to **stern/o** = sternum; breastbone	pertaining to the joint between the sternum and clavicle

	scapul/o	scapula
Term	**Term Analysis**	**Definition**
subscapular (sub-**SKAP**-you-lar)	-ar = pertaining to sub- = under; below	below the scapula

Upper Extremities

	brachi/o	arm
Term	**Term Analysis**	**Definition**
brachial (**BRAY**-kee-al)	-al = pertaining to	pertaining to the arm
brachiocephalic (**bray**-kee-oh-seh-**FAL**-ick)	-ic = pertaining to **cephal/o** = head	pertaining to the arm and head

	carp/o	wrist
carpectomy (kar-**PECK**-toh-mee)	-ectomy = excision; surgical removal	excision of a carpal (wrist) bone

	olecran/o	olecranon (elbow)
olecranal (oh-**LEK**-ran-al)	-al = pertaining to	pertaining to the olecranon, a bony projection on the ulna

	phalang/o	**phalanx; one of the bones making up the fingers or toes**
interphalangeal joint (IP) (**in**-ter-fah-**LAN**-jee-al)	-eal = pertaining to inter- = between	pertaining to the joint between the phalanges

	radi/o	radius (one of the bones of the lower arm)
Term	**Term Analysis**	**Definition**
radiocarpal joint (**ray**-dee-oh-**KAR**-pal)	-al = pertaining to **carp/o** = wrist	pertaining to the joint between the radius and wrist
	uln/o	ulnar (one of the bones of the lower arm)
ulnar (**UL**-nar)	-ar = pertaining to	pertaining to the ulna

Pelvic Girdle

	acetabul/o	acetabulum; hip socket
Term	**Term Analysis**	**Definition**
acetabular (**ass**-eh-**TAB**-you-lar)	-ar = pertaining to	pertaining to the hip socket
acetabuloplasty (**ass**-eh-**TAB**-you-loh-**plas**-tee)	-plasty = surgical repair or reconstruction	surgical repair of the hip socket

Memory Key	The hip socket resembles a cup that the Romans used to hold vinegar. *Acetum* is Latin for vinegar.

	ili/o	hip
iliosacral joint (**ill**-ee-oh-**SAY**-kral)	-al = pertaining to **sacr/o** = sacrum	pertaining to the joint between the hip and sacrum; also known as the sacroiliac (**say**-kroh-**ILL**-ee-ack) joint
	pelv/i; pelv/o	pelvis
pelvic (**PEL**-vick)	-ic = pertaining to	pertaining to the pelvis

Lower Extremities

	calcane/o	heel
Term	**Term Analysis**	**Definition**
calcaneal (kal-**KAY**-nee-al)	-eal = pertaining to	pertaining to the heel

	femor/o	femur; thigh bone
iliofemoral joint (**ill**-ee-oh-**FEM**-or-al)	-al = pertaining to ili/o = hip	pertaining to the joint between the hip and femur

	fibul/o	fibula
fibulocalcaneal (**fib**-you-loh-kal-**KAY**-nee-al)	-eal = pertaining to calcane/o = heel	pertaining to the fibula and heel

Memory Key | *Fibula* is Latin for clasp or pin. The fibula is pinned to the tibia like a brooch.

	patell/a; patell/o	patella; kneecap
patellapexy (pa-**TEL**-ah-**peck**-see)	-pexy = surgical fixation	surgical fixation of the kneecap
infrapatellar (**in**-frah-pah-**TEL**-ar)	-ar = pertaining to infra- = below	pertaining to below the kneecap
suprapatellar (**sue**-prah-pah-**TEL**-ar)	-ar = pertaining to supra- = above	pertaining to above the kneecap

	tibi/o	tibia; shin
tibiofibular joint (**tib**-ee-oh-**FIB**-you-lar)	-ar = pertaining to fibul/o = fibula	pertaining to the joint between the tibia and fibula

Joints

	arthr/o; articul/o	joint
Term	**Term Analysis**	**Definition**
arthralgia (ar-**THRAL**-jee-ah)	-algia = pain	joint pain; also known as arthrodynia (ar-throh-**DIN**-ee-ah)
arthritis (ar-**THRIGH**-tis)	-itis = inflammation	inflammation of a joint *NOTE:* Types include: **osteoarthritis (OA)**, which is degeneration of the articular cartilage due to overuse and resulting in painful movement of the joint (see Figure 7-9), **rheumatoid arthritis (RA)**, an autoimmune (protection or immunity against one's self) disease in which the body's immune system fails to recognize its own cells as normal and the body's tissues are attacked as if they were foreign invaders, resulting in the degeneration of the joint (see Figure 7-10).

FIGURE 7-9

Osteoarthritis: (A) normal joint; (B) early signs of osteoarthritis with degeneration of the articular cartilage; (C) late stages of osteoarthritis with complete breakdown of the joint, thickened bone, and exposed bone

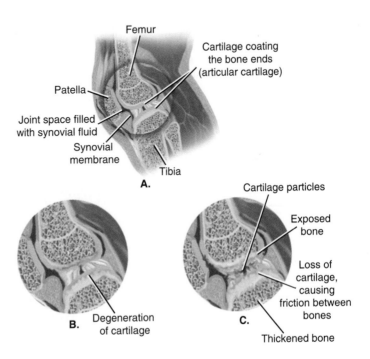

FIGURE 7-10
Rheumatoid hand deformity

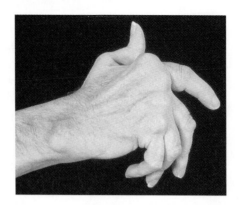

Term	Term Analysis	Definition
arthropathy (ar-**THROP**-ah-thee)	-pathy = disease	any disease of a joint
arthroplasty (**ar**-throh-**plas**-tee)	-plasty = surgical repair or reconstruction	surgical repair of a joint; usually refers to the total or partial replacement of the knee or hip joints with a **prosthetic** (artificial) device (see Figure 7-11).

FIGURE 7-11
Arthroplasty: (A) total hip replacement; (B) total knee replacement. A strong plastic called poly-ethylene takes the place of articular cartilage, preventing friction between bones.

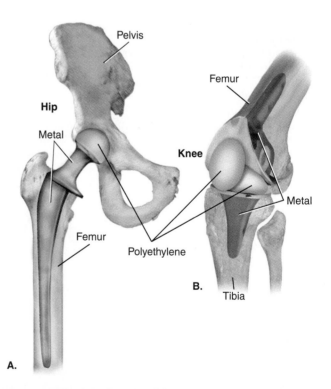

Term	Term Analysis	Definition
arthroscopy (ar-**THROS**-koh-pee)	-scopy = process of visual examination	process of visually examining the joint cavity by using an arthroscope (see Figure 7-12). *NOTE:* In arthroscopic surgery, a video camera takes images of a joint cavity and displays these images onto a TV monitor. With this technique, the joint can be worked upon under local anesthetic with good visualization of the entire joint. Recovery time is minimal and hospital stay is reduced.

FIGURE 7-12
(A) Arthroscopic surgery; (B) a picture of the inside of the knee joint as seen through an arthroscope

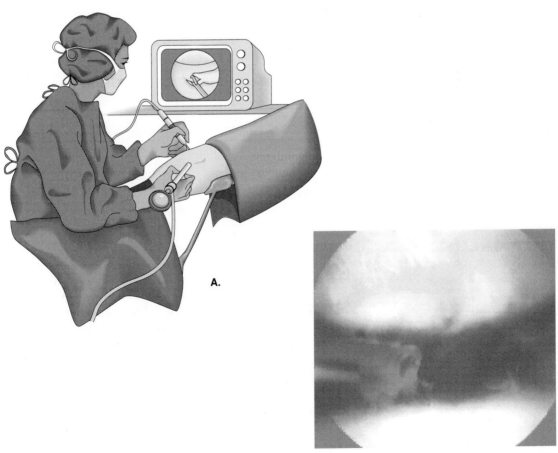

A.

B.

Term	Term Analysis	Definition
interarticular (**in**-ter-ar-**TICK**-you-lar)	-ar = pertaining to inter- = between	pertaining to between the joints
	burs/o	**bursa (sac filled with synovial fluid located around joints)**
bursitis (ber-**SIGH**-tis)	-itis = inflammation	inflamed bursa
bursectomy (ber-**SECK**-toh-mee)	-ectomy = excision	excision of the bursa

SUFFIXES

	-blast	**immature**
Term	**Term Analysis**	**Definition**
osteoblast (**OS**-tee-oh-blast)	**oste/o** = bone	immature bone cell
	-centesis	**surgical puncture to remove fluid; aspiration**
arthrocentesis (**ar**-throh-sen-**TEE**-sis)	**arthr/o** = joint	surgical puncture of a joint to remove fluid; aspiration of a joint cavity
	-clasis	**surgical fracture or refracture**
osteoclasis (os-tee-**OCK**-lah-sis)	**oste/o** = bone	surgical fracture or refracture of bone
	-clast	**breakdown**
osteoclast (**OS**-tee-oh-clast)	**oste/o** = bone	bone cell that breaks down bone

	-desis	**surgical fusion; surgical binding**
Term	**Term Analysis**	**Definition**
arthrodesis (ar-throh-**DEE**-sis)	**arthr/o** = joint	surgical fusion of a joint
	-genesis	**formation**
osteogenesis (**os**-tee-oh-**JEN**-eh-sis)	**oste/o** = bone	bone formation; also known as ossification
	-malacia	**softening**
chondromalacia (**kon**-droh-mah-**LAY**-shee-ah)	**chondr/o** = cartilage	softening of cartilage
osteomalacia (**os**-tee-oh-mah-**LAY**-shee-ah)	**oste/o** = bone	softening of bone
	-osis	**abnormal condition**
kyphosis (kye-**FOH**-sis)	**kyph/o** = humpback	exaggerated posterior curvature of the thoracic spine; humpback (see Figure 17-13A)
lordosis (lor-**DOH**-sis)	**lord/o** = swayback	exaggerated anterior curvature of the lumbar spine; swayback (see Figure 17-13B)
osteoporosis (**os**-tee-oh-poh-**ROH**-sis)	**oste/o** = bone -porosis = porous	loss of bone density resulting in open spaces within bony substance
scoliosis (**skoh**-lee-**OH**-sis)	**scoli/o** = curved	abnormal lateral curvature of the spine (see Figure 17-13C)
	-sarcoma	**malignant tumor of connective tissue**
chondrosarcoma (**kon**-droh-sar-**KOH**-mah)	**chondr/o** = cartilage	malignant tumor of cartilage

FIGURE 7-13
(A) Kyphosis; (B) lordosis; (C) scoliosis

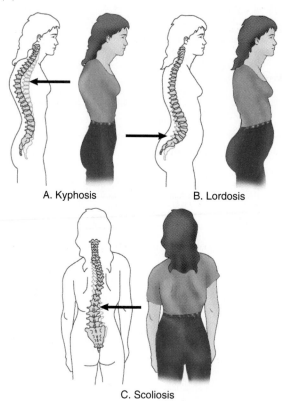

A. Kyphosis   B. Lordosis

C. Scoliosis

Term	Term Analysis	Definition
osteosarcoma (**os**-tee-oh-sar-**KOH**-mah)	**oste/o** = bone	malignant tumor of bone; also known as osteogenic sarcoma

PREFIXES

	ortho-	straight
Term	**Term Analysis**	**Definition**
orthopedics (**or**-thoh-**PEE**-dicks)	-ic = pertaining to **ped/o** = child	surgical specialty dealing with the correction of deformities and dysfunctions of the skeletal system

7.6   Review of Terms

Define the terms in Tables 7-2 through 7-6 in the space provided.

TABLE 7-2

REVIEW OF ANATOMICAL TERMS

acetabular	brachial	brachiocephalic
calcaneal	cervical	chondrocyte
costochondral	costosternal	craniofacial
infrapatellar	interarticular	interphalangeal
intervertebral	lumbosacral	mandibular
maxillary	olecranal	orthopedics
osteoblast	osteoclast	osteocyte
osteogenesis	pelvic	subcostal
subscapular	suprapatellar	thoracolumbar
ulnar	vertebral	vertebrofemoral
xiphoid		

TABLE 7-3

REVIEW OF PATHOLOGIC TERMS

achondroplasia	arthralgia	arthritis
arthropathy	chondroma	chondromalacia

continued on page 132

Table 7-3 *continued from page 131*

chondrosarcoma	kyphosis	lordosis
lumbodynia	myeloma	osteoarthritis
osteitis	osteochondritis	osteoma
osteomalacia	osteomyelitis	osteoporosis
osteosarcoma	scoliosis	spondylitis
spondylopathy		

TABLE 7-4

REVIEW OF DIAGNOSTIC TERMS

arthrocentesis	arthroscopy

TABLE 7-5

REVIEW OF SURGICAL TERMS

acetabuloplasty	arthrodesis	arthroplasty
carpectomy	cranioplasty	craniotomy
osteoclasis	osteotome	osteotomy
patellapexy		

TABLE 7-6

REVIEW OF JOINTS

bursectomy	bursitis	costovertebral
fibulocalcaneal	iliofemoral	iliosacral; sacroiliac
interphalangeal	lumbosacral	radiocarpal
sacrococcygeal	sternoclavicular	temporomandibular
tibiofibular		

7.7   Abbreviations

Abbreviation	Meaning
C	cervical
C1, C2 . . . C7	first cervical vertebra, second cervical vertebra . . . seventh cervical vertebra
DDD	degenerative disc disease
IP	interphalangeal
L	lumbar
L1, L2 . . . L5	first lumbar vertebra, second lumbar vertebra . . . fifth lumbar vertebra
LDD	lumbar disc disease
MCP	metacarpophalangeal
MSS	musculoskeletal system

continued on page 134

continued from page 133

Abbreviation	Meaning
OA	osteoarthritis
ortho	orthopedics
RA	rheumatoid arthritis
S1, S2 . . . S5	first sacral vertebra, second sacral vertebra . . . fifth sacral vertebra
T	thoracic
T1, T2 . . . T12 (also D1, D2 . . . D12 if *dorsal* is used)	first thoracic vertebra, second thoracic vertebra . . . twelfth thoracic vertebra
TKR	total knee replacement
TMJ	temporomandibular joint

7.8   Putting It All Together

Exercise 7-1   SHORT ANSWER

1. The bony structure protecting the brain is the _____ .

2. Name five functions of the skeletal system _____

_____ .

3. Two minerals found in bone are _____ and _____ .

4. Distinguish between osteoclasts, osteocytes, and osteoblasts.

_____

_____

Exercise 7-2   CLASSIFICATION

Classify the following bones as part of the axial or appendicular skeleton.

1. skull   _____

2. arms   _____

3. rib cage _____

4. femur _____

5. hyoid bone _____

6. clavicle _____

7. ilium _____

Exercise 7-3   IDENTIFICATION

Identify the location of individual bones using the following list.

a. skull

b. thoracic cage

c. pelvic girdle

d. face

e. upper extremity

f. pectoral girdle

g. vertebral column

h. lower extremity

1. maxilla _____

2. carpals _____

3. femur _____

4. phalanges _____

5. parietal bone _____

6. costal cartilage _____

7. humerus _____

8. lumbar _____

9. occipital bone _____

10. patella _____

11. xiphoid process _____

12. radius _____

13. fibula _____

14. zygoma _____

15. cervical _____

16. ilium _____

17. calcaneus _____

18. mandible _____

19. coccyx _____

20. ischium _____

21. metatarsals _____

22. olecranon _____

23. sternum _____

24. tarsals _____

25. ulna _____

26. clavicle _____

Exercise 7-4   BUILDING MEDICAL WORDS

I. Use **myel/o** to build medical terms for the following definitions.

1. benign tumor of the bone marrow _____

2. inflammation of the bone and
   bone marrow _____

II. Use **oste/o** to build medical terms for the following definitions.

3. inflammation of bone and joints _____

4. immature bone cell   _____

5. inflammation of bone and cartilage   _____

6. mature bone cell   _____

7. bone formation   _____

8. benign tumor of bone   _____

9. malignant tumor of bone   _____

III. Use **crani/o** to build medical terms for the following definitions.

10. incision into the skull   _____

11. surgical repair of the skull   _____

12. pertaining to the skull and face   _____

IV. Use **chondr/o** to build medical terms for the following definitions.

13. cartilage cell   _____

14. benign tumor of cartilage   _____

15. malignant tumor of cartilage   _____

V. Use **cost/o** to build medical terms for the following definitions.

16. pertaining to the ribs and cartilage   _____

17. pertaining to the rib and vertebra   _____

18. pertaining to under the ribs   _____

VI. Use **arthr/o** to build medical terms for the following definitions.

19. joint pain   _____

20. inflammation of a joint   _____

21. any disease of a joint   _____

22. surgical repair of a joint   _____

23. process of visually examining a joint   _____

Exercise 7-5   TERMS FOR BONES

Give the common name for the following bones.

1. thorax   _____

2. clavicle   _____

3. carpals   _____

4. humerus   _____

5. olecranon _____

6. ilium _____

7. calcaneus _____

8. femur _____

9. tibia _____

Exercise 7-6   IDENTIFY SURGICAL PROCEDURES

Mark with an **X** the terms indicating surgical procedures.

1. myeloma _____

2. osteoclasis _____

3. lordosis _____

4. arthrodesis _____

5. osteoporosis _____

6. acetabular _____

7. brachial _____

8. lumbodynia _____

9. orthopedics _____

10. cranioplasty _____

Exercise 7-7   SPELLING

Circle any misspelled words in the list below and correctly spell them in the space provided.

1. calcaneous _____

2. tibula _____

3. hyoid _____

4. myloma _____

5. temperomandibular _____

6. ileosacral _____

7. osteogeneses _____

8. craniofacial _____

9. maleolus _____

10. coccx   _____

11. humerous   _____

12. olecranal   _____

13. parietal   _____

14. arthrodeses   _____

15. patella   _____

Exercise 7-8   ADJECTIVES

Give the adjective for each of the following.

1. cranium   _____

2. face   _____

3. ethmoid   _____

4. mandible   _____

5. maxilla   _____

6. zygoma   _____

7. sternum   _____

8. coccyx   _____

9. malleolus   _____

10. sacrum   _____

11. vertebra   _____

12. thorax   _____

13. clavicle   _____

14. scapula   _____

15. olecranon   _____

16. radius   _____

17. acetabulum   _____

18. ischium   _____

19. calcaneus   _____

20. fibula   _____

Exercise 7-9   **REVIEW OF PATHOLOGY**

Below is a list of pathology from this chapter. Define each word in the space provided.

1. achondroplasia _____

2. chondroma _____

3. chondrosarcoma _____

4. lumbodynia _____

5. spondylitis _____

6. osteitis _____

7. osteoarthritis _____

8. osteomalacia _____

9. kyphosis _____

10. lordosis _____

11. scoliosis _____

12. osteoporosis _____

13. lumbodynia _____

14. chondromalacia _____

15. myeloma _____

16. osteomyelitis _____

17. osteochondritis _____

18. osteoma _____

19. osteosarcoma _____

Exercise 7-10   **REVIEW OF DIAGNOSTIC PROCEDURES**

Below is a list of diagnostic procedures from this chapter. Define each term in the space provided.

1. arthroscopy _____

2. arthrocentesis _____

Exercise 7-11   REVIEW OF SURGICAL PROCEDURES

Below is a list of surgical procedures from this chapter. Define each term in the space provided.

1. craniotomy _____

2. cranioplasty _____

3. carpectomy _____

4. acetabuloplasty _____

5. patellapexy _____

6. arthroplasty _____

7. osteotome _____

8. osteotomy _____

9. osteoclasis _____

10. arthrodesis _____

Exercise 7-12   REVIEW OF BONE STRUCTURE

Below is a list of terms relating to structure. Define each term in the space provided.

1. brachiocephalic _____

2. articular cartilage _____

3. cervical _____

4. craniofacial _____

5. costochondral _____

6. sphenoid _____

7. costovertebral _____

8. orthopedics _____

9. calcaneal _____

10. maxillary _____

C H A P T E R

The Muscular System

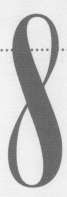

CHAPTER ORGANIZATION

This chapter will help you understand the muscular system. It is divided into the following sections:

CHAPTER OBJECTIVES

On completion of this chapter, you will be able to do the following:

1. Differentiate between voluntary, involuntary, skeletal, cardiac, and visceral muscles

2. Define terms relating to skeletal attachments

3. Name and locate common skeletal muscles

4. Pronounce, analyze, define, and spell terms relating to the muscular system

5. Define abbreviations relating to the muscular system

INTRODUCTION

Grip your right forearm with your left hand. Move the right hand up and down, then rotate it. What you are feeling are the various contractions of your forearm muscles as they respond to your mental command to move. While you were doing this simple exercise, your heart continued to beat. This action, too, involves muscular contraction, but were you mentally willing it to happen? Of course not. The difference is that the muscles of your forearm are known as **voluntary** muscles, because they perform movement on command. The heart is an **involuntary** muscle. It performs without conscious command.

All bodily movement—whether it involves the lifting of a skeletal part such as an arm, the beating of the heart, or the action of the diaphragm during breathing—involves the contraction and expansion of voluntary or involuntary muscle. Skeletal movement is performed by **skeletal** muscles. Heartbeats are performed by **cardiac** muscle. Breathing, digestion, and other movements involving internal organs are performed by muscles within the organ itself called **visceral** muscles.

In this chapter, you will learn the terms associated with the skeletal muscles. Cardiac and visceral muscles will be addressed in other chapters.

Memory Key | Skeletal muscle is voluntary. Cardiac and visceral muscles are involuntary.

8.1   Skeletal Attachments

Bones are connected to other bones by tough connective tissue called **ligaments**. Muscles are connected to bones by equally tough connective tissue called **tendons**. There are tendons on each end of skeletal muscles because they need to be attached to two bones to make movement possible. To illustrate this concept to yourself, lift you forearm, starting from a 90 degree angle with your upper arm (Figure 8-1). Do you see the similarity to a drawbridge? Just as the deck of a bridge cannot be lifted without being pulled up by something that is attached to a structure that does not move, neither can your forearm. The muscle that moves the forearm is the **biceps brachii** (**BRAY**-kee-eye). It lies over the humerus and is attached at one end to the scapula, which does not move when the biceps contracts. The other end of the biceps is attached to the radius and moves when the biceps contracts. The point of attachment of the biceps to the scapula is called the **origin**. This is the term used for muscle attachment to the bone that does not move when the muscle contracts. The point of attachment to the bone that does move, in this example the radius, is called the **insertion**. This is the term used for muscle attachment to the bone that moves when the muscle contracts.

Memory Key | Muscles attach to the stable bone at the origin and to the moving bone at the insertion.

8.2   Major Skeletal Muscles

Figure 8-2 illustrates the major superficial muscles of the body.

FIGURE 8-1
Movement of the forearm by the biceps brachii

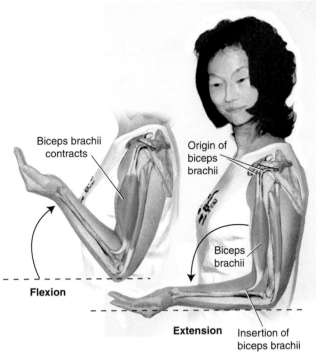

Biceps brachii contracts

Origin of biceps brachii

Biceps brachii

Flexion

Extension   Insertion of biceps brachii

8.3   Additional Word Elements

Use these additional word elements when studying the medical terms in this chapter.

Root	Meaning
flex/o	bend
pronati/o	facing backward
supinati/o	facing forward
tens/o	stretch

Prefix	Meaning
dorsi-	back

FIGURE 8-2
Major superficial muscles of the body: (A) anterior view, (B) posterior view

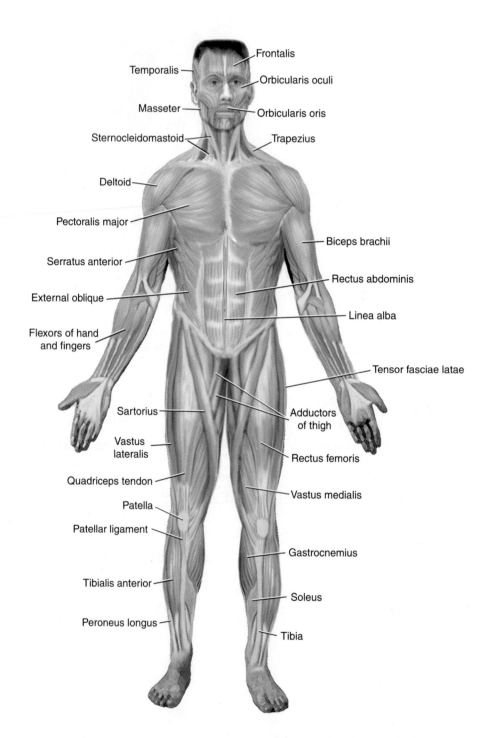

A.

FIGURE 8-2
continued

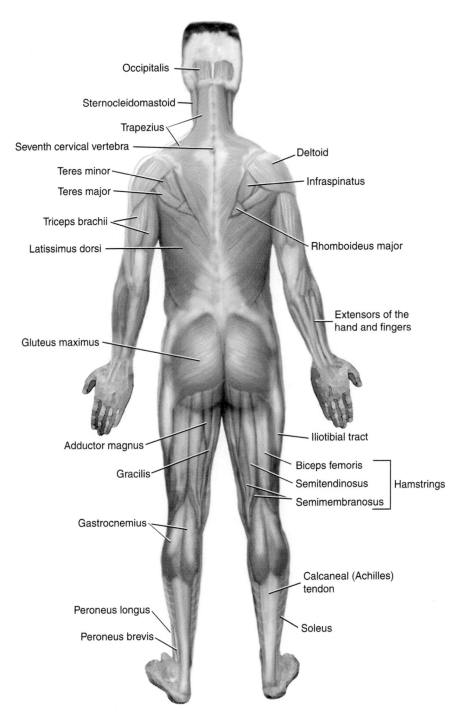

Occipitalis

Sternocleidomastoid

Trapezius

Seventh cervical vertebra

Deltoid

Teres minor

Infraspinatus

Teres major

Triceps brachii

Latissimus dorsi

Rhomboideus major

Extensors of the
hand and fingers

Gluteus maximus

Adductor magnus

Iliotibial tract

Gracilis

Biceps femoris

Semitendinosus

Semimembranosus

Hamstrings

Gastrocnemius

Calcaneal (Achilles)
tendon

Peroneus longus

Soleus

Peroneus brevis

B.

8.4 Term Analysis and Definition

	duct/o	to draw
Term	**Term Analysis**	**Definition**
abductor (ab-**DUCK**-tor)	-or = person or thing that does something ab- = away from	muscles that move a part away from the midline
adductor (ah-**DUCK**-tor)	-or = person or thing that does something ad- = toward	muscles that move a part toward the midline

	electr/o	electric
electromyography (EMG) (ee-**leck**-troh-my-**OG**-rah-fee)	-graphy = process of recording **my/o** = muscle	recording of the electrical characteristics of muscle. *NOTE:* Electrical activity is produced in a muscle when it is stimulated by a nerve.

	ton/o	tone; tension
atonic (a-**TON**-ick)	-ic = pertaining to a- = no; not; lack of	a muscle that has no tone or tension; atony
dystonia (dis-**TOH**-nee-ah)	-ia = condition dys- = bad; difficult; painful	abnormal muscle tone or tension
myotonia (**my**-oh-**TOH**-nee-ah)	-ia = condition **my/o** = muscle	inability of the muscle to relax after increased muscular contraction
tonic (**TON**-ick)	-ic = pertaining to	pertaining to tone; tension

	fasci/o	**fascia (band of tissue surrounding the muscle)**
fascial (**FASH**-ee-al)	-al = pertaining to	pertaining to the fascia
fasciectomy (fash-ee-**ECK**-toh-mee)	-ectomy = excision; surgical removal	excision of fascia

Term	Term Analysis	Definition
fasciitis; fascitis (**fas**-ee-**EYE**-tis); (fah-**SIGH**-tis)	-itis = inflammation	inflammation of fascia
fasciorrhaphy (**fash**-ee-**OR**-ah-fee)	-rrhaphy = suture	suturing the fascia
	kinesi/o	**movement**
kinesiology (kih-**nee**-see-**OL**-oh-jee)	-logy = study of	study of movement
kinesimeter (**kin**-eh-**SIM**-eh-ter)	-meter = instrument used to measure	instrument used to measure movement
	lei/o	**smooth**
leiomyoma (**lye**-oh-my-**OH**-mah)	-oma = tumor; mass **my/o** = muscle	benign tumor of smooth muscle. *NOTE:* The visceral muscles are smooth, whereas the skeletal and cardiac muscles are striated because they appear striped under the microscope.
leiomyosarcoma (**lye**-oh-**my**-oh-sar-**KOH**-mah)	-sarcoma = malignant tumor of connective tissue **my/o** = muscle	malignant tumor of smooth muscle. *NOTE:* Muscle is composed of connective tissue
	muscul/o	**muscle**
muscular (**MUS**-kyou-lar)	-ar = pertaining to	pertaining to muscle
musculoskeletal (**mus**-kyou-loh-**SKEL**-eh-tal)	-al = pertaining to **skelet/o** = skeleton	pertaining to the muscle and skeleton
	my/o	**muscle**
electromyogram (ee-**leck**-troh-**MY**-oh-gram)	-gram = record **electr/o** = electric	record of the electrical currents in a muscle
fibromyalgia (**figh**-broh-my-**AL**-jee-ah)	-algia = pain **fibr/o** = fiber	pain in fibrous tissues muscles, tendons, and ligaments

Term	Term Analysis	Definition
myalgia (my-**AL**-jee-ah)	-algia = pain	muscle pain
myopathy (my-**OP**-pah-thee)	-pathy = disease	any muscular disease
	myos/o	**muscle**
myositis (**my**-oh-**SIGH**-tis)	-itis = inflammation	inflammation of muscle
polymyositis (**pol**-ee-**my**-oh-**SIGH**-tis)	-itis = inflammation poly- = many	inflammation of many muscles
	rhabd/o	**rod-shaped; striped; striated**
rhabdomyoma (**rab**-doh-my-**OH**-mah)	-oma = tumor; mass **my/o** = muscle	benign tumor of striated muscle
rhabdomyosarcoma (**rab**-doh-**my**-oh-sar-**KOH**-mah)	-sarcoma = malignant tumor of connective tissue **my/o** = muscle	malignant tumor of striated muscle tissue
	tendin/o; ten/o	**tendon**
tendinitis (**ten**-dih-**NIGH**-tis)	-itis = inflammation	inflammation of a tendon
tendinous (**TEN**-dih-nus)	-ous = pertaining to	pertaining to a tendon
tenodesis (ten-**ODD**-eh-sis)	-desis = surgical fixation	surgical fixation of a tendon
tenotomy (teh-**NOT**-oh-me)	-tomy = to cut	cutting of a tendon
	tenosynovi/o	**tendon sheath (covering of a tendon)**
tenosynovitis (**teh**-noh-**sin**-oh-**VIGH**-tis)	-itis = inflammation	inflammation of a tendon sheath

SUFFIXES

	-asthenia	no strength
Term	**Term Analysis**	**Definition**
myasthenia (**my**-as-**THEE**-nee-ah)	**my/o** = muscle	no muscle strength
	-clonus	turmoil
myoclonus (**my**-oh-**KLOH**-nus) (my-**OCK**-loh-nus)	**my/o** = muscle	alternate muscular relaxation and contraction in rapid succession
	-ion	process of

The following terms are used when describing muscle action (see Figure 8-3).

abduction (ab-**DUCK**-shun)	ab- = away from **duct/o** = to draw	process of drawing away from; opposite of adduction
adduction (ah-**DUCK**-shun)	ad- = toward **duct/o** = to draw	process of drawing toward; opposite of abduction
circumduction (**ser**-kum-**DUCK**-shun)	circum- = around **duct/o** = to draw	process of drawing a part in a circular motion
dorsiflexion (**door**-see-**FLECK**-shun)	dorsi- = back **flex/o** = bend	bending the ankle joint so that the foot bends backward (upward); opposite of plantar flexion
plantar flexion (**PLAN**-tar **FLECK**-shun)	**flex/o** = bend plantar = the sole of the foot	bending the ankle joint so that the foot bends toward the sole of the foot
extension (eck-**STEN**-shun)	ex- = out **tens/o** = stretch	to stretch out; stretching out of a limb; increasing the angle between two bones; opposite of flexion
flexion (**FLECK**-shun)	**flex/o** = bend	bending a limb; decreasing the angle between two bones; opposite of extension
pronation (pro-**NAY**-shun)	**pronati/o** = facing backward	as applied to the hand, process of turning the palm backward; opposite of supination
supination (**sue**-pih-**NAY**-shun)	**supinati/o** = facing forward	as applied to the hand, the process of turning the palm forward; opposite of pronation

FIGURE 8-3

Types of muscle action

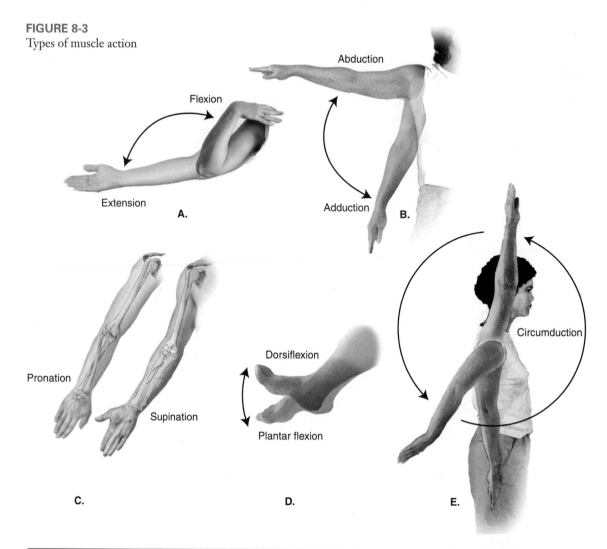

	-kinesia	**movement; motion**
Term	**Term Analysis**	**Definition**
bradykinesia (**brad**-ee-kih-**NEE**-zee-ah) (**brad**-ee-kih-**NEE**-shuh)	brady- = slow	slow movement
dyskinesia (**dis**-kih-**NEE**-zee-ah)	dys- = bad; difficult; painful; poor	impairment of muscle movement
hyperkinesia (**high**-per-kye-**NEE**-zee-ah)	hyper- = excessive; above normal	excessive movement

	-trophy	nourishment
Term	**Term Analysis**	**Definition**
atrophy (**AH**-troh-fee)	a- = no; not	wasting away of the muscle
dystrophy (**DIS**-troh-fee)	dys- = poor; bad; difficult; painful	abnormal development, especially muscular dystrophy
hypertrophy (high-**PER**-troh-fee)	hyper- = excessive; above normal	enlargement of an organ due to an increase in the size of cells
	-thermy	heat
diathermy (**DYE**-ah-**ther**-mee)	dia- = complete; through	heat applied to deep tissues

8.5   Review of Terms

Define the terms in Tables 8-1 through 8-5 in the space provided.

TABLE 8-1

REVIEW OF ANATOMICAL TERMS

abductor	adductor	fascial
kinesiology	muscular	musculoskeletal
tendinous	tonic	

TABLE 8-2

REVIEW OF PATHOLOGIC TERMS

atonic	atrophy	bradykinesia
dyskinesia	dystonia	dystrophy

continued on page 152

Table 8-2 *continued from page 151*

fasciitis	fascitis	fibromyalgia
hyperkinesia	hypertrophy	leiomyoma
leiomyosarcoma	myalgia	myasthenia
myoclonus	myopathy	myositis
myotonia	polymyositis	rhabdomyoma
rhabdomyosarcoma	tendinitis	tenosynovitis

TABLE 8-3

REVIEW OF DIAGNOSTIC TERMS

electromyogram	electromyography	kinesimeter

TABLE 8-4

REVIEW OF CLINICAL AND SURGICAL TERMS

bursectomy	diathermy	fasciectomy
fasciorrhaphy	tenodesis	tenotomy

TABLE 8-5

REVIEW OF MUSCLE MOVEMENTS

abduction	adduction	circumduction

continued on page 153

Table 8-5 *continued from page 152*

dorsiflexion	extension	flexion
plantar flexion	pronation	supination

8.6   Abbreviations

Abbreviation	Meaning
EMG	electromyography
IM	intramuscular
ROM	range of motion (degree to which a joint can be moved. Range is measured in degrees. Full range is 360 degrees. Limited movement may be 60 degrees.)
RICE	rest, ice, compression, elevation
SLR	straight leg raising

8.7   Putting It All Together

Exercise 8-1   **SHORT ANSWER**

1. Differentiate between the following terms in each group.

   (a) voluntary and involuntary muscles

   _____

   (b) cardiac, skeletal, and visceral muscles

   _____

   (c) origin and insertion

   _____

   (d) ligaments and tendons

   _____

Exercise 8-2   BUILDING TERMS

I. Use **my/o** or **myos/o** to build terms for the following definitions.

1. record of the electric currents in a muscle

    _____

2. muscle pain

    _____

3. inflammation of a muscle

    _____

4. any muscle disease

    _____

5. inflammation of many muscles

    _____

II. Use the suffix -kinesia to build terms for the following definitions.

6. slow movement

    _____

7. impaired movement

    _____

8. excessive movement

    _____

III. Use the suffix -trophy to build terms for the following definitions.

9. wasting away of the muscle

    _____

10. abnormal development

    _____

11. enlargement of an organ (due to an increase in the size of cells)

    _____

Exercise 8-3   DEFINITIONS

Define the following:

A. Anatomical Terms

1. adductor   _____

2. abductor   _____

3. fascial   _____

4. tendinous   _____

B. Pathologic Terms

5. dystonia   _____

6. leiomyoma   _____

7. rhabdomyosarcoma _____

8. tendinitis _____

9. myasthenia _____

C. Diagnostic Terms

    10. electromyogram   _____

    11. kinesimeter   _____

D. Surgical and Clinical Procedures

    12. diathermy   _____

    13. fasciorrhaphy   _____

    14. tenodesis   _____

Exercise 8-4   SPELLING PRACTICE

Circle any misspelled words in the list below and correctly spell them in the space provided.

  1. maseter   _____

  2. sternocliedomastoid   _____

  3. serratus   _____

  4. rectus abdominis   _____

  5. transversus   _____

  6. trapezious   _____

  7. latisimus dorsi   _____

  8. terres major   _____

  9. rhomdoideus   _____

10. semitendinosus   _____

11. gastrocnemius   _____

12. Achiles   _____

Exercise 8-5   OPPOSITES

State the opposite muscle action in the space provided.

  1. abduction   _____

  2. extension   _____

  3. plantar flexion   _____

  4. supination   _____

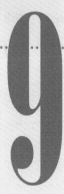

CHAPTER

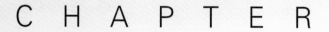

The Nervous System

CHAPTER ORGANIZATION

This chapter will help you understand the nervous system. It is divided into the following sections:

CHAPTER OBJECTIVES

On completion of this chapter, you will be able to do the following:

1. Name and describe the divisions of the nervous system
2. State the major functions of the nervous system
3. Name and state the function of nerve cells
4. Differentiate between the cell body, the axon, and dendrites
5. Define *synapse*
6. List and describe the major portions of the brain
7. Describe the spinal cord
8. Name the protective covering of the brain and spinal cord
9. Differentiate between the somatic and autonomic nervous systems
10. Pronounce, analyze, define, and spell common terms of the nervous system
11. Define common abbreviations of the nervous system

INTRODUCTION

The nervous system allows the body to adjust to the requirements of internal and external environments. As soon as a change in the environment is sensed, the brain is notified. It then formulates an appropriate response and sends signals to the body to bring about the needed change. This is not a simple task. A vastly complex system is required to maintain bodily equilibrium. In fact, the human nervous system is far more complex than the most complicated computer. In this chapter, you will learn the terms associated with this amazing system.

9.1   Divisions of the Nervous System

As you study this section, you will find it helpful to refer to Figure 9-1, which diagrammatically represents the divisions of the nervous system.

There are two parts to the nervous system: the **central nervous system** (CNS) and the **peripheral nervous system** (PNS). The CNS consists of the spinal cord, which is the body's information superhighway, and the brain, which is the information-processing center. The PNS is mostly made up of nerve tissue, commonly referred to as **nerves**. As are all body tissues, nerves are made up of cells. The cells of the nerves are called **neurons** (**NEW**-ronz).

The PNS is made up of both **sensory** and **motor neurons**. Sensory neurons detect external and internal environmental influences and carry **sensory impulses** about those influences to the brain. Motor neurons carry messages called **motor impulses** from the brain to various parts of the body.

Memory Key	• The CNS consists of the spinal cord and brain.
	• The PNS consists of the sensory and motor nerves.
	• Neurons are the cells that make up nerves.

9.2   Functions of the Nervous System

The work of the sensory neurons is called the **sensory function** of the nervous system. When the brain receives a sensory impulse, it determines what sort of reaction is needed, if any. This analytical process is very complex and is called the **integrative function** of the nervous system. The **motor function** takes over when the brain has decided that a response is needed. A motor impulse is sent through the motor neurons to the skeletal muscles, or to an organ such as the heart, or to a gland such as the adrenal gland. These motor impulses stimulate the muscle, organ, or gland to initiate some needed change. The muscle, organ, or gland involved is called an **effector**, because it effects the required change.

Memory Key	The nervous system has sensory, integrative, and motor functions.

FIGURE 9-1

Divisions of the central nervous system and peripheral nervous system

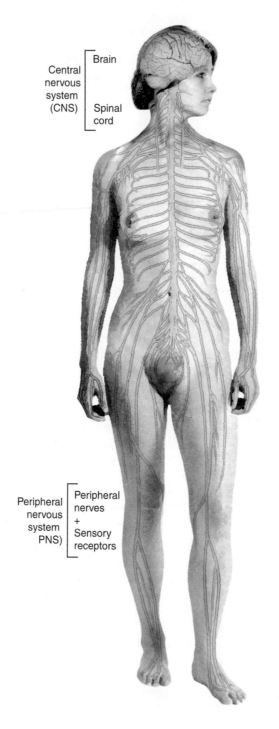

Central
nervous
system
(CNS)

Brain

Spinal
cord

Peripheral
nervous
system
PNS)

Peripheral
nerves
+
Sensory
receptors

9.3   Nerve Cells

Neurons, which carry impulses, are one of two types of cell that make up nervous tissue. The other type is the **neuroglia** (new-**ROG**-lee-ah). These cells are found between the neurons. They do not carry electrical impulses but protect the neurons by engulfing unwanted substances. This process is called **phagocytosis** (**fag**-oh-sigh-**TOH**-sis). Neuroglia also provide nutrients by attaching blood vessels to the neurons.

Figure 9-2 illustrates a neuron. Although neurons vary greatly in size (some are as long as 3 feet, or 90 centimeters), every neuron has a **cell body**, an **axon** (**ACK**-son), and many **dendrites** (**DEN**-drytes). The cell body performs the work of maintaining the neuron. The axon is the part that transmits electrical impulses. The dendrites look like the branches of a tree. They are responsible for receiving information from the internal and external environments and transmitting it to the cell body. Some axons, but not all, are covered by a white fatty **myelin sheath**. These axons are said to be **myelinated** (see Figure 9-2). These

FIGURE 9-2
Structures of a neuron

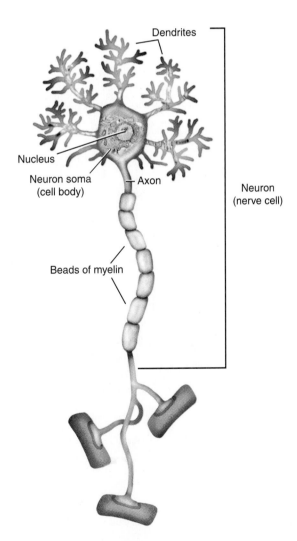

Dendrites

Nucleus

Neuron soma
(cell body)

Axon

Beads of myelin

Neuron
(nerve cell)

myelinated axons are referred to as white matter. Some axons look gray because they do not have the myelin sheath. Those axons are referred to as gray matter.

Memory Key	• Nervous tissue consists of neurons and neuroglia. • Neuroglia protect neurons through phagocytosis and attach blood vessels to neurons. • Every neuron has a cell body, an axon, and many dendrites.

9.4   Synapses

Neurons need a way to transmit electrical impulses to another neuron or to a muscle. This transmission is done at a junction called a **synapse** (**SIN**-apps). When an electrical impulse travels down the neuron and reaches the synapse, a chemical referred to as a **neurotransmitter** (**new**-roh-trans-**MIT**-er) is released from a little sac at the end of the nerve. The

FIGURE 9-3
Synapse between a nerve and a muscle

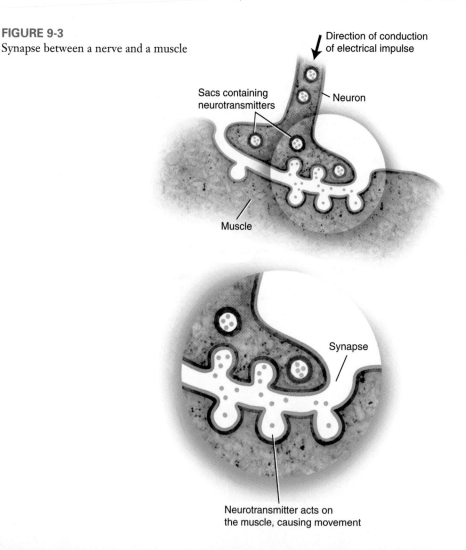

neurotransmitter travels across the synapse and acts on the muscle, causing it to generate its own electrical impulse that produces muscle movement. Figure 9-3 illustrates a synapse.

| Memory Key | Synapses transmit impulses from neuron to neuron or from neuron to muscle. |

9.5   The Central Nervous System

THE BRAIN

The central nervous system (CNS) consists of the brain and the spinal cord. The structures of the brain are illustrated in Figure 9-4.

The **cerebrum** (seh-**REE**-brum) is the largest part of the brain. It receives sensory impulses from the peripheral nerves and initiates motor impulses to the viscera, especially muscles. It is the site of higher intellectual functioning. The cerebrum is divided into right and left **hemispheres** by a deep gap known as the **longitudinal fissure**. Bundles of nerve fibers called the **corpus callosum** (**KOR**-pus kah-**LOH**-sum) connect the two hemispheres, allowing them to share information (see Figure 9-5). If the corpus callosum is severed, each hemisphere functions independently and functions are not properly integrated because the only communication link is gone.

The outer layer of the cerebrum is covered by gray matter called the **cerebral cortex** (seh-**REE**-bral **KOR**-tecks), which is involved in sensory and motor functions as well as thought, judgment, and perception (see Figure 9-5). The surface of the cerebrum has the appearance of little gray bulges that look like sausages, which are called **gyri** (**JIGH**-rye) or **convolutions**. Each gyrus (**JIGH**-rus) is separated by shallow grooves called **sulci** (**SUL**-sigh) or by deeper grooves called **fissures**. The fissures divide the cerebrum into lobes named after the bones of the skull above them: **frontal lobe**, **parietal** (pah-**RYE**-eh-tal) **lobe**, **temporal lobe**, and **occipital** (ock-**SIP**-ih-tal) **lobe**.

The **thalamus** (**THAL**-ah-mus) (see Figure 9-4) acts as a relay station for incoming sensory stimuli. Once it recognizes stimuli as pain, temperature, touch, and so on, it transmits them to specific areas of the cerebral cortex for interpretation and then transmits motor impulses from the different cortex areas to the spinal cord for distribution to the appropriate motor neurons.

The **hypothalamus** (high-poh-**THAL**-ah-mus) (see Figure 9-4) is located below the thalamus. It helps regulate appetite, thirst, and temperature. It is also associated with the endocrine system and is involved with emotional and basic behavior patterns.

The **brain stem** is sometimes referred to as the ancient brain or the animal brain. It is the site of basic life functions such as arousal, respiration, heart rate, blood pressure, and visual and auditory reflexes (moving the eyes and head to view objects or to hear sounds). It is also the center for nonvital reflexes such as coughing, sneezing, and swallowing. The brain stem also serves as a pathway for impulses traveling to and from the brain and spinal cord. The nerve fibers extend through the **midbrain**, **pons** (**PONZ**), and **medulla oblongata** (meh-**DULL**-ah ob-long-**GAH**-tah). The nerves cross over at the pons. Therefore, the right side of the brain controls the left side of the body, and the left side of the brain controls the right side of the body.

The **cerebellum** (ser-eh-**BELL**-um) lies under the occipital lobe of the cerebrum and protrudes dorsally. It is important in maintaining balance, muscle coordination, and equilibrium.

FIGURE 9-4
Lateral view of the brain: (A) internal brain structure, (B) external brain structure

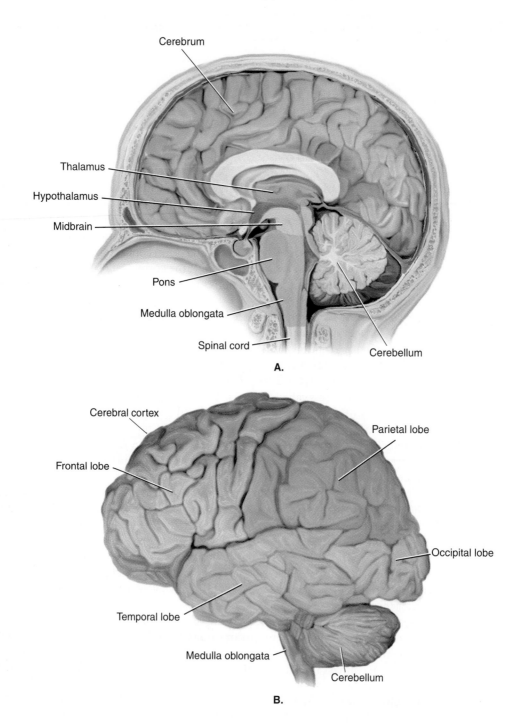

FIGURE 9-5
Anatomical structures of the cerebrum

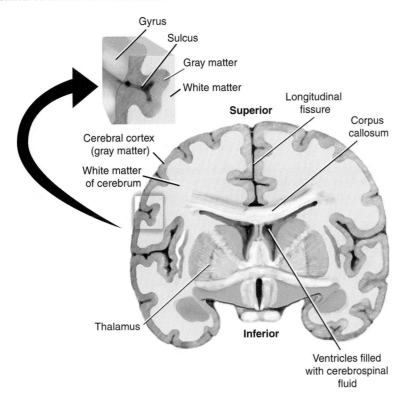

• The brain consists of the
  cerebrum
  thalamus (a relay station for sensory and motor impulses)
  hypothalamus (helps regulate appetite, thirst, emotions, and basic behavior patterns)
  brain stem (midbrain, pons, medulla oblongata; involved with visual and auditory
    reflexes, respiration, heart rate, blood pressure, and arousal)
  cerebellum (involved with maintaining balance, muscle coordination, and
    equilibrium)

• The lobes of the cerebrum are:
  frontal
  parietal
  temporal
  occipital

• The cerebrum is covered by the cerebral cortex, which is divided into right and left
  hemispheres by the longitudinal fissures but is joined by the corpus callosum.

THE SPINAL CORD

The **spinal cord** consists of nerves. It is encased within the vertebrae for protection, extending from the medulla oblongata to the second lumbar vertebra and ending in a cone-shaped structure called the **conus medullaris** (**KO**-nus med-you-**LAR**-is). The nerves extend downward from the conus medullaris, looking somewhat like a horse's tail. This is referred to as the **cauda equina** (**KAW**-dah ee-**KWI**-nah).

The spinal cord branches into 31 pairs of spinal nerves. Each pair extends from the spinal cord bilaterally throughout its entire length. Eight pairs are cervical, 12 pairs are thoracic, 5 pairs are lumbar, 5 pairs are sacral, and 1 pair is coccygeal (see Figure 9-6).

Memory Key	The spinal cord starts at the medulla oblongata, extends through the vertebrae, and ends at the conus medullaris, from which the nerves extend (cauda equina). Thirty-one pairs extend from the spinal cord (8 cervical, 12 thoracic, 5 lumbar, 5 sacral, and 1 coccygeal).

PROTECTIVE COVERINGS

The most obvious protection for the brain and spinal cord are the skull bones and the vertebrae. However, three membranes called **meninges** (meh-**NIN**-jeez) also serve as protective coverings. The outermost covering is the tough and thick **dura mater** (**DOO**-rah **MAY**-ter). The middle layer is the **arachnoid membrane** (ah-**RACK**-noid **MEM**-brain), and the inner one the **pia mater** (**PEE**-yah **MAY**-ter). Figure 9-7 shows the meninges. Note also the **subdural space** below the dura mater and the **subarachnoid space** below the arachnoid membrane.

Another form of protection is the **cerebrospinal fluid (CSF)**, a colorless liquid that continually circulates within the subarachnoid space around the brain and spinal cord, in the central canal inside the spinal cord, and in hollow cavities inside the brain called **ventricles** (see Figure 9-5). Because the brain and spinal cord float in the CSF, the central nervous system is cushioned, absorbing shocks.

The brain has a third type of protection, the **blood-brain barrier** (BBB), which is a protective mechanism that prevents toxic substances from entering the brain while allowing necessary substances such as oxygen and glucose to enter.

Memory Key	The CNS is protected by bone, meninges, CSF, and the BBB.

FIGURE 9-6
Spinal cord, posterior view

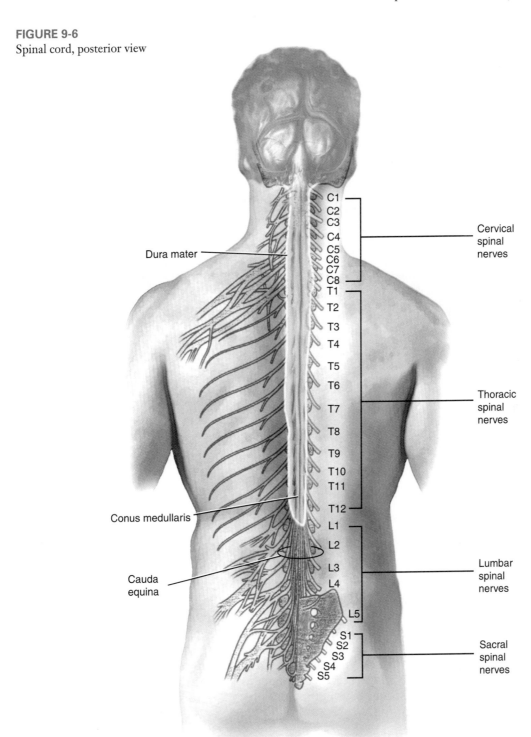

FIGURE 9-7
Meninges

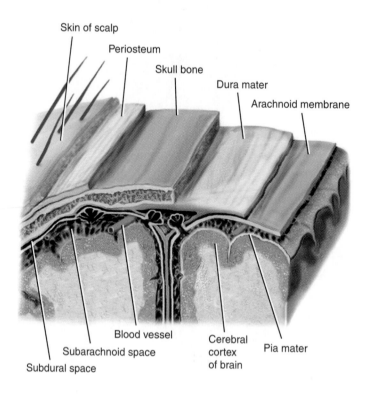

9.6   The Peripheral Nervous System

Twelve pairs of **cranial nerves** emerge bilaterally from the base of the skull, carrying nerve impulses to the muscles of the upper regions of the body, such as the tongue, larynx, thorax, abdominal viscera, eyes, face, pharynx, and mouth. Thirty-one pairs of **spinal nerves** emerge from the spinal cord bilaterally, carrying nerve impulses to a variety of organs. Figure 9-8 illustrates some spinal nerves as they extend from the spinal cord to peripheral sites. The names given to these nerves as they extend through the body reflect the artery closest to them or the organ or structure the nerve serves. For example, the radial nerve stimulates the muscles attaching to the radius bone of the arm.

| Memory Key | There are 12 pairs of cranial nerves and 31 pairs of spinal nerves in the PNS. |

FIGURE 9-8
Peripheral nerves

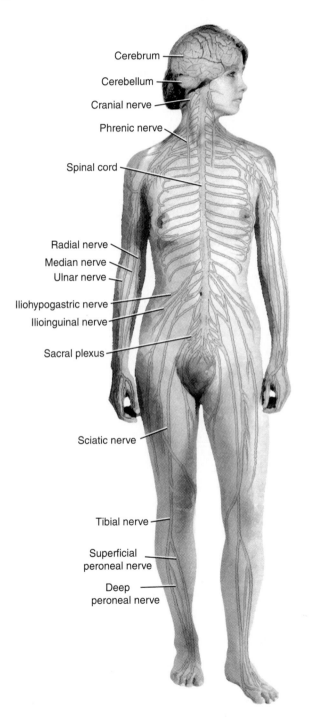

Cerebrum

Cerebellum

Cranial nerve

Phrenic nerve

Spinal cord

Radial nerve

Median nerve

Ulnar nerve

Iliohypogastric nerve

Ilioinguinal nerve

Sacral plexus

Sciatic nerve

Tibial nerve

Superficial
peroneal nerve

Deep
peroneal nerve

9.7   Additional Word Elements

Use these additional word elements when studying the medical terms in this chapter.

Root	Meaning
ech/o	sound
gli/o	glue
myelin/o	myelin sheath
tom/o	to cut

Suffix	Meaning
-schisis	cleft; splitting
-us	condition; thing

Prefix	Meaning
para-	abnormal
polio-	gray

9.8   Term Analysis and Definition

	cerebell/o	cerebellum
Term	**Term Analysis**	**Definition**
cerebellar (**ser**-eh-**BEL**-ar)	-ar = pertaining to	pertaining to the cerebellum
cerebellitis (**ser**-eh-bel-**EYE**-tis)	-itis = inflammation	inflammation of the cerebellum

	cerebr/o	brain
Term	**Term Analysis**	**Definition**
cerebral (seh-**REE**-bral)	-al = pertaining to	pertaining to the brain
cerebrospinal (**ser**-eh-broh-**SPYE**-nal)	-al = pertaining to **spin/o** = spine	pertaining to the brain and spine
cerebrovascular (**ser**-eh-broh-**VAS**-kyou-lar)	-ar = pertaining to **vascul/o** = vessel	pertaining to the brain and blood vessels

	cortic/o	cortex; outer covering
cortical (**KOR**-tih-kal)	-al = pertaining to	pertaining to the cortex
corticospinal (kor-ti-koh-**SPYE**-nal)	-al = pertaining to **spin/o** = spine	pertaining to the cerebral cortex and spine

	dur/o	dura mater (one of the membranes surrounding the brain)
epidural (**ep**-ih-**DOO**-ral)	-al = pertaining to epi- = on; upon; above	upon the dura mater
subdural (sub-**DOO**-ral)	-al = pertaining to sub- = below; under	under the dura mater

	encephal/o	brain
electroencephalogram (ee-**leck**-troh-en-**SEF**-ah-loh-gram)	-gram = record **electr/o** = electric	record of the electrical activity of the brain. *NOTE:* Brain waves can be **alpha waves** (typical of the awake person at rest), **beta waves** (typical of increased activity), **delta waves** (typical of deep sleep). In conditions such as **seizure disorders** (**epilepsy**), the brain waves are abnormal in that they are uncoordinated and unorganized (see Figure 9-9)
electroencephalograph (ee-**leck**-troh-en-**SEF**-ah-loh-graf)	-graph = instrument used to record **electr/o** = electric	instrument used to record the electrical activity of the brain

FIGURE 9-9

Brain waves: (A) normal brain waves are usually consistent in height and width, (B) abnormal brain waves. Note the inconsistent height and width of the brain waves as seen in patients with seizure disorders (epilepsy).

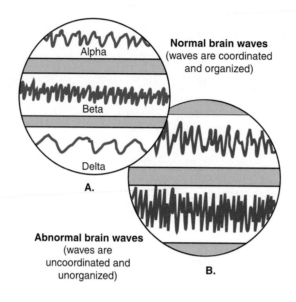

Term	Term Analysis	Definition
encephalitis (en-**sef**-ah-**LYE**-tis)	-itis = inflammation	inflammation of the brain
encephalomalacia (en-**sef**-ah-loh-mah-**LAY**-see-ah)	-malacia = softening	softening of the brain
encephalopathy (en-**sef**-ah-**LOP**-ah-thee)	-pathy = disease	any disease of the brain
	hydr/o	**water**
hydrocephalus (**high**-droh-**SEF**-ah-lus)	-us = condition; thing **cephal/o** = head	accumulation of fluid in the brain (see Figure 9-10)
	magnet/o	**magnet**
magnetic resonance imaging (MRI) (mag-**NET**-ik **RES**-oh-nance)	-tic = pertaining to resonance = magnification imaging = a picture	a picture of the brain produced by using magnetic waves (see Figure 9-11). *NOTE:* Radiation is not used to produce an image.

FIGURE 9-10
Hydrocephalus. *Courtesy of Armed Forces Institute of Pathology*

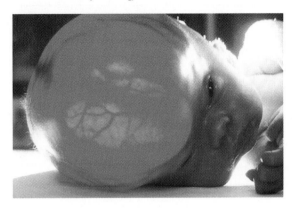

FIGURE 9-11
Schematic of magnetic resonance imaging

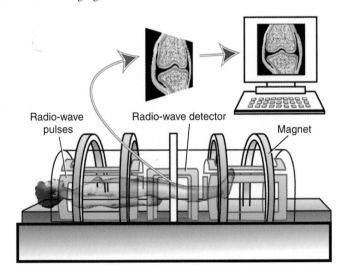

	mening/o	**meninges; membrane**
Term	**Term Analysis**	**Definition**
meningitis (**meh**-nin-**JIGH**-tis)	-itis = inflammation	inflammation of the meninges
meningoencephalitis (meh-**NING**-goh-en-**sef**-ah-**LYE**-tis)	-itis = inflammation **encephal/o** = brain	inflammation of the meninges and brain

	myel/o	spinal cord, bone marrow
Term	**Term Analysis**	**Definition**
myelogram (**MY**-eh-loh-gram)	-gram = record	record of the spinal cord
myeloschisis (my-eh-**LOS**-kih-sis)	-schisis = cleft; splitting	splitting of the spinal cord
poliomyelitis (**poh**-lee-oh-my-eh-**LYE**-tis)	-itis = inflammation polio- = gray	inflammation of the gray matter of the spinal cord

	neur/o	nerve
myoneural (**my**-oh-**NEW**-ral)	-al = pertaining to **my/o** = muscle	pertaining to the muscle and nerve; also known as neuromuscular
neuralgia (new-**RAL**-jee-ah)	-algia = pain	nerve pain
neurology (new-**ROL**-oh-jee)	-logy = study of	the study of the nervous system including diseases and treatment
neurologist (new-**ROL**-oh-jist)	-logist = a specialist in the study of	a specialist in the study of the diagnosis and treatment of nervous system disorders
neurolysis (new-**ROL**-is-is)	-lysis = destruction, breakdown; separation	nerve destruction
polyneuritis (**pol**-ee-new-**RYE**-tis)	-itis = inflammation poly- = many	inflammation of many nerves

	radicul/o	nerve roots
myeloradiculitis (**my**-eh-loh-rah-**dick**-you-**LYE**-tis)	-itis = inflammation **myel/o** = spinal cord	inflammation of the spinal cord and nerve roots

	spin/o	spine
spinal tap (**SPYE**-nal)	-al = pertaining to tap = draining of fluid	insertion of a needle into the subarachnoid space below the third lumbar vertebra to withdraw cerebrospinal fluid for diagnostic purposes; also known as lumbar puncture (see Figure 9-12)

FIGURE 9-12
Lumbar puncture

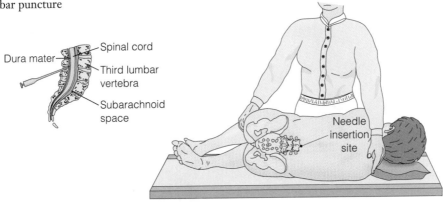

Dura mater
Spinal cord
Third lumbar vertebra
Subarachnoid space
Needle insertion site

	thalam/o	**thalamus**
Term	**Term Analysis**	**Definition**
thalamocortical (**thal**-ah-moh-**KOR**-tih-kal)	-al = pertaining to **cortic/o** = cortex	pertaining to the thalamus and cerebral cortex

	ventricul/o	**ventricles**
ventriculostomy (ven-**trick**-you-**LOS**-toh-me)	-stomy = new opening	new opening in the ventricles

SUFFIXES

	-cele	**hernia (protrusion)**
Term	**Term Analysis**	**Definition**
meningocele (meh-**NING**-goh-**seel**)	**mening/o** = meninges; membrane	hernia of the meninges; displacement of the meninges from its normal position (see Figure 9-13A)
myelomeningocele (**my**-eh-loh-meh-**NING**-goh-**seel**)	**myel/o** = spinal cord **mening/o** = meninges; membrane	hernia of the spinal cord and meninges; displacement of the spinal cord and meninges from their normal position (see Figure 9-13B)

FIGURE 9-13
Meningocele and myelomeningocele

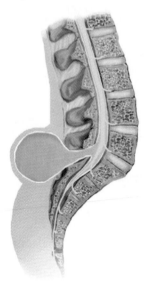 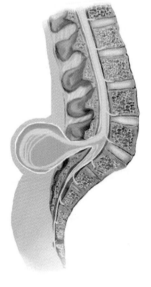

A. Meningocele   B. Myelomeningocele

	-esthesia	sensation
Term	**Term Analysis**	**Definition**
anesthesia (**an**-es-**THEE**-zee-ah)	an- = no; not	loss of sensation
hypoesthesia (**high**-poh-es-**THEE**-zee-ah)	hypo- = below; under; decrease	decreased sensation
hyperesthesia (**high**-per-es-**THEE**-zee-ah)	hyper- = excessive; above	increased sensation
dysesthesia (**dis**-es-**THEE**-zee-ah)	dys- = bad; painful difficult	irritating sensation in response to normal stimuli
paresthesia (**par**-es-**THEE**-zee-ah)	para- = abnormal	abnormal sensation such as numbness and tingling

	-graphy	process of recording; process of producing images
Term	**Term Analysis**	**Definition**
cerebral angiography (**SER**-eh-bral **an**-jee-**OG**-rah-fee)	**angi/o** = vessel -al = pertaining to **cerebr/o** = brain	the cerebral arteries are visualized after injection of a contrast medium (a dye used to highlight structures being studied) (to see an angiogram, refer to Figure 12-10)
computed tomography (CT scan) (toh-**MOG**-rah-fee)	**tom/o** = to cut	x-ray beam rotates around the patient, detailing the structure at various depths. The information is computer analyzed and converted to a picture of the body part. Common body parts studied in this fashion include the abdomen, kidneys, brain, and chest (see Figure 9-14)
echoencephalography (**eck**-oh-en-**sef**-ah-**LOG**-rah-fee)	**ech/o** = sound **encephal/o** = brain	process of producing an image of the brain using ultrasound
electroencephalography (EEG) (ee-**leck**-troh-en-**sef**-ah-**LOG**-rah-fee)	**electr/o** = electric **encephal/o** = brain	process of recording the electrical impulses of the brain
myelography (**my**-eh-**LOG**-rah-fee)	**myel/o** = spinal cord	image of the spinal cord is produced using x-rays after injection of a contrast medium

FIGURE 9-14
Computed tomography and conventional x-ray procedure

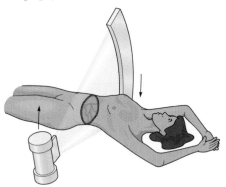

A. Computed tomography

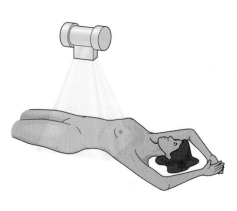

B. Conventional x-ray

	-kinesia;-kinesis	movement; motion
Term	**Term Analysis**	**Definition**
hyperkinesis (**high**-per-kih-**NEE**-sis)	hyper- = excessive; above	excessive motion; hyperactivity
dyskinesia (**dis**-kih-**NEE**-zee-ah)	dys- = bad; difficult	impaired movement
bradykinesia (**brad**-ee-kih-**NEE**-zee-ah) (**brad**-ee-kih-**NEE**-zhuh)	brady- = slow	slow movement

	-oma	tumor
hematoma (**hem**-ah-**TOH**-mah)	**hemat/o** = blood	accumulation of blood in a space, organ, or tissue due to a break in a blood vessel; examples are epidural and subdural hematomas. *NOTE:* Unlike other tumors, a hematoma is not an abnormal growth of tissue but an accumulation of blood in tissues after a hemorrhage.
glioma (glye-**OH**-mah)	**gli/o** = glue	tumor of neuroglial cells
meningioma (men-**in**-jee-**OH**-mah)	**mening/o** = meninges; membrane	benign tumor of meninges

	-phasia	speech
aphasia (ah-**FAY**-zee-ah)	a- = no; not	no speech
dysphasia (dis-**FAY**-zee-ah)	dys- = bad; difficult	difficult speech

	-plegia	paralysis (loss or impairment of motor function)
diplegia (dye-**PLEE**-jee-ah)	di- = two	paralysis of like extremities on both sides of the body

Term	Term Analysis	Definition
hemiplegia (**hem**-ee-**PLEE**-jee-ah)	hemi- = half	paralysis of either the right or the left half of the body
monoplegia (**mon**-oh-**PLEE**-jee-ah)	mono- = one	paralysis of one extremity
paraplegia (**par**-ah-**PLEE**-jee-ah)	para- = beside; near	paralysis of the lower part of the body and legs
quadriplegia (**kwad**-rih-**PLEE**-jee-ah	quadri- = four	paralysis of all four limbs

	-taxia	**order**
ataxia (ah-**TACK**-see-ah)	a- = no; not	no muscular coordination

PREFIXES

	de-	**lack of; removal**
Term	Term Analysis	Definition
demyelination (dee-**my**-eh-lih-**NAY**-shun)	-ion = process **myelin/o** = myelin sheath	lack of myelin sheath. *NOTE:* Demyelination occurs in a condition called multiple sclerosis (MS), in which loss of the myelin sheath results in a variety of disorders such as muscle weakness, paralysis, visual disturbances, and urinary dysfunction.

	pachy	**thick**
pachymeningitis (pack-ee-**men**-in-**JYE**-tis)	-itis = inflammation **mening/o** = meninges; membrane	inflammation of the pachymeninges. *NOTE:* Pachymeninges is another name for dura mater

9.9   Review of Terms

Define the terms in Tables 9-1 through 9-4 in the space provided.

TABLE 9-1

REVIEW OF ANATOMICAL TERMS

cerebellar	cerebral	cerebrospinal
cerebrovascular	cortical	corticospinal
epidural	myoneural	neurologist
neurology	subdural	thalamocortical

TABLE 9-2

REVIEW OF PATHOLOGIC TERMS

aphasia	ataxia	bradykinesia
cerebellitis	demyelination	diplegia
dysesthesia	dyskinesia	dysphasia
encephalitis	encephalomalacia	encephalopathy
glioma	hematoma	hemiplegia
hydrocephalus	hyperesthesia	hyperkinesis
hypoesthesia	meningioma	meningitis

continued on page 179

Table 9-2 *continued from page 178*

meningocele	meningoencephalitis	monoplegia
myelomeningocele	myeloradiculitis	myeloschisis
neuralgia	pachymeningitis	paraplegia
paresthesia	poliomyelitis	polyneuritis
quadriplegia		

TABLE 9-3

REVIEW OF DIAGNOSTIC TERMS

cerebral angiography	computed tomography	echoencephalography
electroencephalogram	electroencephalograph	electroencephalography
myelogram	myelography	magnetic resonance imaging

TABLE 9-4

REVIEW OF CLINICAL AND SURGICAL TERMS

anesthesia	neurolysis	spinal tap; lumbar puncture
ventriculostomy		

9.10   Abbreviations

Abbreviation	Meaning
ALS	amyotrophic lateral sclerosis (death of nerve cells in the brain and spinal cord results in muscular degeneration. Typically fatal within 3 to 5 years). Also known as Lou Gehrig's disease
BBB	blood-brain barrier
CNS	central nervous system
CSF	cerebrospinal fluid
CTS	carpal tunnel syndrome (pressure on a nerve in the lower forearm near the wrist results in pain and disuse of the hand)
CT	computed tomography
EEG	electroencephalography
HNP	herniated nucleus pulposus
LP	lumbar puncture
MRI	magnetic resonance imaging
MS	multiple sclerosis
PET	positron emission tomography (a type of radiographic procedure)
PNS	peripheral nervous system

9.11   Putting It All Together

Exercise 9-1   SHORT ANSWER

1. In what structure of the brain do the nerves cross?

2. Differentiate between the sensory and motor neurons.

_____

_____

_____

3. Name the meninges.

_____

4. Write the name and number of the spinal nerves in order from superior to inferior.

_____

_____

5. Describe the location of the cerebral cortex.

_____

Exercise 9-2   MATCHING

Match Column A with Column B.

Column A	Column B
_____ 1. cell body	A. divides the cerebrum into right and left hemispheres
_____ 2. axon	B. maintains homeostasis of appetite, thirst, and temperature
_____ 3. dendrites	C. part of neuron containing organelles
_____ 4. cerebral cortex	D. acts as a relay station for incoming sensory stimuli
_____ 5. neuroglia	E. part of neuron that transmits impulses
_____ 6. longitudinal fissure	F. part of neuron that looks like branches of a tree
_____ 7. thalamus	G. gray matter covering the cerebrum
_____ 8. hypothalamus	H. protects the nervous system

Exercise 9-3   WORD BUILDING

Build the word for each of the following definitions.

1. nerve pain   _____

2. a specialist in the study of the nervous system and its diseases   _____

3. nerve destruction   _____

4. inflammation of many nerves   _____

5. record of the electrical activity of the brain

    _____

6. hernia of the meninges

    _____

7. hernia of the spinal cord and meninges

    _____

8. loss of sensation

    _____

9. decreased sensation

    _____

10. increased sensation

    _____

11. irritating sensation in response to normal stimuli

    _____

12. abnormal sensation such as numbness and tingling

    _____

13. paralysis of like extremities on both sides of the body

    _____

14. paralysis of either the right half or the left half of the body

    _____

15. paralysis of one extremity

    _____

16. paralysis of the lower part of the body and legs

    _____

17. paralysis of all four limbs

    _____

18. inflammation of the brain

    _____

19. softening of the brain

    _____

20. any disease of the brain

    _____

Exercise 9-4   ADJECTIVAL FORMS

Give the adjectival form for the following.

1. cerebellum

    _____

2. cerebrum

    _____

3. cortex

    _____

4. nerve

    _____

5. dura

    _____

Exercise 9-5   DEFINITIONS

Write the meaning of the following terms.

1. hydrocephalus   _____

2. myeloradiculitis   _____

3. electroencephalograph _____

4. cerebral angiography   _____

5. echoencephalography   _____

6. hematoma   _____

7. demyelination   _____

8. pachymeningitis   _____

Exercise 9-6   SPELLING PRACTICE

Circle any misspelled words in the list below and correctly spell them in the space provided.

1. thalmus   _____

2. medula   _____

3. corpus callosum   _____

4. encephalomalasia   _____

5. cerrebelum   _____

6. epidurral space   _____

7. myeloschises   _____

8. ventricalostomy   _____

9. disphasia   _____

10. quadraplegia   _____

10 CHAPTER

The Eyes and Ears

CHAPTER OBJECTIVES

On completion of this chapter, you will be able to do the following:

1. Describe the structure, function, and location of the internal and external structures of the eye

2. Analyze, pronounce, define, and spell the medical terms common to the eye

3. Describe the structure, function, and location of the external, middle, and inner ear

4. Analyze, pronounce, define, and spell the medical terms common to the ear

5. Give meanings for abbreviations common to the eyes and ears

INTRODUCTION

Our eyes and ears are the windows that let in the light and sound of the outer world. Light waves and sound waves are transformed by these organs into nerve impulses. Impulses from the eye are sent to the occipital lobe of the brain for processing, and those from the ear are sent to the temporal lobe. The results are what we experience as vision and hearing.

10.1   The Eye

It is the job of the eye to let light in, focus it, transform it into nerve impulses, and send them on to the brain. Light enters the eye through an adjustable opening, the pupil, which regulates the amount of light allowed in. The lens, which lies behind the pupil, must focus the light much like the lens of eyeglasses. The difference is that the lens of the eye is not rigid like glass or plastic. It can adjust its shape in order to adapt to near and far objects. The light focused by the lens then goes to the back of the eyeball, where it strikes the retina. It is the retina that transforms the focused image into nerve impulses, which then travel along the optic nerve to the occipital lobe for processing.

The eye consists of the inner eye (the eyeball) and the outer eye (the facial structures and eye muscles surrounding the eye). As you read the following sections, refer to Figure 10-1, which illustrates the inner and outer eye.

INNER EYE

The inner eye consists of outer, middle, and inner layers. The outer layer consists of the **cornea** (**KOR**-nee-ah) and the **sclera** (**SKLEHR**-ah). The cornea is the transparent anterior portion, which allows light into the eye and participates in the focusing of light onto the back of the eye. The sclera is the white of the eye. It is a tough protective covering for most of the eyeball.

The middle layer is called the **uvea** (**YOU**-vee-ah), and consists of the **choroid** (**KOH**-roid), **ciliary body** (**SIL**-ee-ahr-ee), and **iris** (**EYE**-ris). The choroid is the inner lining of the sclera and contains blood vessels to nourish the eye. The ciliary body lies at the anterior edges of the choroid body and consists of the **ciliary muscles** and the **ciliary process**. The ciliary muscles adjust the shape of the lens for focusing. The ciliary process produces a watery substance, **aqueous humor**, which bathes the anterior region of the eye. The iris is the circular, colored portion of the eye. The central opening in the iris, called the **pupil**, regulates the amount of light that enters the eye. In bright light, certain muscle fibers of the iris that encircle the pupil contract, **constricting** the pupil. When these circular muscles relax in dimmer light, the pupil resumes normal size. Other muscles of the iris, called radial muscles, dilate (enlarge) the pupil beyond normal size when the person is stressed or excited.

The inner layer of the eye is the **retina** (**RET**-ih-nah). It has several layers of nervous tissue containing **cones** and **rods**, which are the cells that transform light into nerve impulses. The cones are responsible for central and bright-light vision and are concentrated in a small depression at the center of the retina called the **fovea centralis** (**FOH**-vee-ah sen-**TRAH**-lis), which lies within a small yellowish area called the **macula lutea** (**MACK**-you-lah **LOO**-tee-ah). The rods are responsible for peripheral and low-light vision and are

FIGURE 10-1
Structures of the eye: (A) inner eye, (B) anterior view of eye

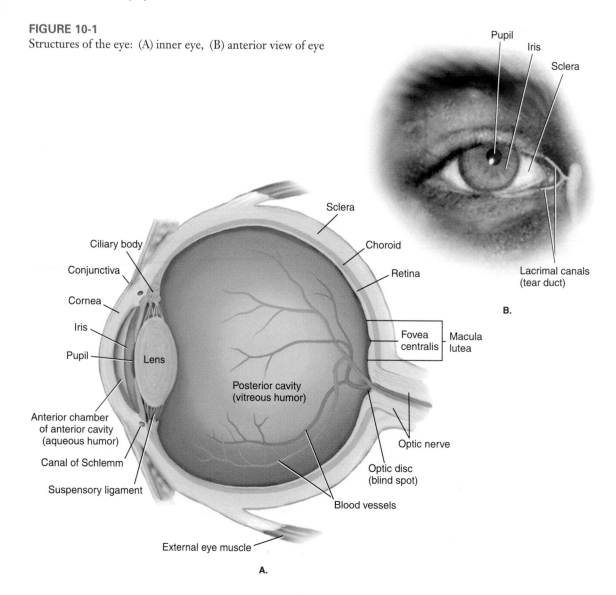

A.

B.

concentrated in the periphery of the retina, away from the macula lutea. One small area of the retina, medial to the fovea centralis, has no rods or cones, and thus does not produce a visual image. It is called the **optic disc**, or **blind spot**. It is the point at which the optic nerve begins, and the entry point for the major blood vessels of the eye. Ordinarily, you are not aware of the blind spot, but it is easy to observe. As you read this, close your left eye and place your index finger on the page. Move your finger to the right while keeping your eye focused on the left margin of the page. You may have to also move your finger up or down a little, but eventually you will find a spot where you cannot see the top of your finger, because it is in the blind spot of your visual field.

The **lens** is illustrated in Figure 10-2. It is not considered to be part of one of the layers of the eye. It is located posterior to the iris and is held in place by ligaments called **suspensory ligaments**. As light passes through the lens, it is bent. This is bending is called

FIGURE 10-2
Uvea (choroid, ciliary body, iris), lens, and other structures of the eye

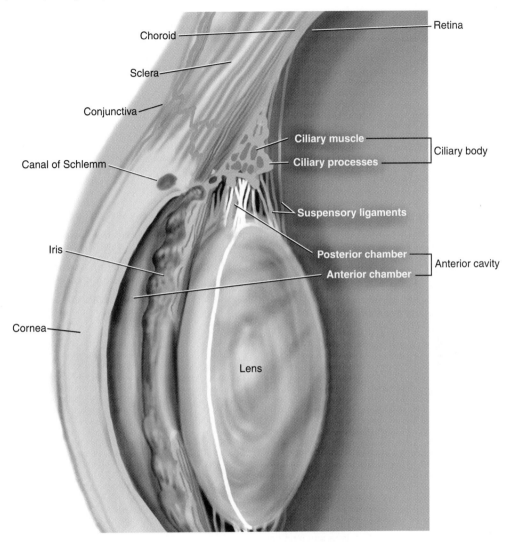

refraction (see Figure 10-9). The refracted light must be precisely focused on the retina for a clear image to be formed. In order to focus the light, the lens must change shape. The ciliary muscles change the shape of the lens to allow clear vision of near and far objects. This lens-shape changing is called **lens accommodation** (ah-**kom**-oh-**DAY**-shun). Light from distant objects does not need to be bent much to focus on the iris, whereas light from near objects does. As we reach our forties, the lenses lose some of their elasticity, and we have difficulty focusing light from near objects. Reading glasses furnish the additional refraction the lenses can no longer provide.

A common age-related eye condition is cataracts (Figure 10-3). With age, the lens loses its transparent quality. It becomes thick and dense, progressing to a lens that is opaque and

FIGURE 10-3

Cataract. *Courtesy of the National Eye Institute*

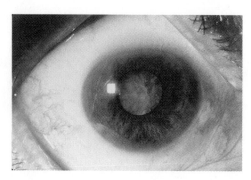

cloudy, thus interfering with the refraction of light rays. Cataracts were once a leading cause of serious vision loss but are now routinely removed surgically. One surgical technique is **extracapsular cataract extraction (ECCE)**, which is partial removal of the lens and lens capsule followed by insertion of a prosthetic (artificial) implant called an **intraocular** lens. A type of ECCE is **phacoemulsification (fack**-oh-ee-**MUL**-sih-fih-kay-shun), which destroys the cataract by means of ultrasonic sound waves. Any fragments left are removed by suction. Another technique is **intracapsular cataract extraction (ICCE)**, which is the removal of the entire lens and lens capsule (see Figure 10-4).

FIGURE 10-4

Types of cataract extraction

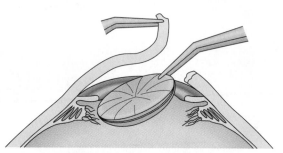

A. Intracapsular cataract extraction: Removal of the entire lens and lens capsule.

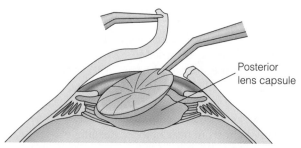

Posterior lens capsule

B. Extracapsular cataract extraction: Lens is removed with its anterior capsule, leaving posterior capsule intact.

Anterior and posterior to the lens are two cavities. The anterior cavity contains aqueous humor, produced by the ciliary processes. This watery fluid flows freely from the posterior chamber through the pupil to the anterior chamber. As this substance is produced and secreted, an equal amount is constantly drained through a lattice-type or meshwork structure called the **trabecula** (trah-**BECK**-you-lah) into the **canal of Schlemm** (shlem) and into the venous system (see Figure 10-2). Inability to drain aqueous humor causes increased intraocular pressure. This condition, called **glaucoma** (glaw-**KOH**-mah), can result in blindness because of damage to the retina and optic nerve caused by the extra pressure. The equality between production and drainage helps maintain the equilibrium of the **intraocular pressure (IOP)**.

The posterior cavity of the eye is filled with clear, jelly-like material called **vitreous** (**VIT**-ree-us) **humor**. It maintains the spherical shape of the eyeball, holds the retina firmly against the choroid, and transmits light.

Memory Key
- The inner eye consists of the
     outer layer (cornea and sclera)
     middle layer or uvea (choroid, ciliary body, and iris)
     inner layer (retina, containing rods and cones in the fovea centralis)
- The lens is not part of any of the layers. It is located posterior to the iris, held in place by suspensory ligaments. It refracts light in order to focus the image on the retina, through a process called lens accommodation.
- The pupil is an opening in the center of the iris. The pupil regulates the amount of light coming into the eye.
- The anterior cavity contains aqueous humor. The posterior cavity contains vitreous humor.

OUTER EYE

The outer eye is illustrated in Figure 10-5. It consists of the **orbital cavity, extrinsic ocular muscles, eyelids, conjunctival** (kon-junk-**TYE**-val) **membrane**, and **lacrimal** (**LACK**-rih-mal) **apparatus**. The orbital cavity is the bony depression into which the eyeball fits, providing protection. The six extrinsic ocular muscles attached to the sclera of each eye can move the eye in any direction. They are named according to their location and orientation: **rectus** means "straight," and **oblique** means "slanted." They are the superior rectus, inferior rectus, medial rectus, lateral rectus, superior oblique, and inferior oblique. The eyelids shield the eye from light, dust, and trauma. The conjunctival membrane is a thin mucous membrane lining the eyelids and the anterior part of the eye exposed to the air, providing protection and lubrication. The lacrimal apparatus produces, delivers, and drains tears from the eyes, thereby cleaning and lubricating them. The **lacrimal glands** produce the tears, which are continuously delivered to the eyes by the **lacrimal ducts**. Small openings called **punctae** (**PUNK**-tah) drain tears from the eyes into a system of canals in the nose. This is why your nose runs when you cry. Tears not only clean and lubricate the eyes; they also fight infectious microorganisms with an antibacterial enzyme called **lysozyme** (**LIGH**-so-zime).

Memory Key | The outer eye consists of the | orbital cavity | conjunctival membrane
| | extrinsic ocular muscles | lacrimal apparatus
| | eyelids |

FIGURE 10-5

External anatomy of the eye: (A) eyebrow, conjunctiva, orbit, ocular muscles, optic nerve; (B) lacrimal apparatus

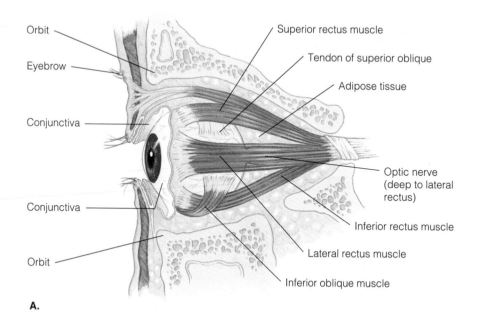

Orbit

Eyebrow

Conjunctiva

Conjunctiva

Orbit

Superior rectus muscle

Tendon of superior oblique

Adipose tissue

Optic nerve
(deep to lateral
rectus)

Inferior rectus muscle

Lateral rectus muscle

Inferior oblique muscle

A.

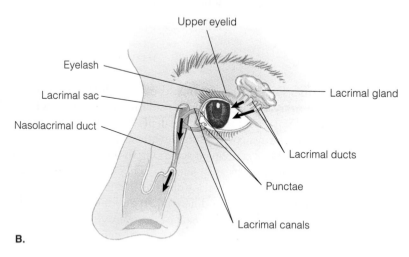

Upper eyelid

Eyelash

Lacrimal sac

Nasolacrimal duct

Lacrimal gland

Lacrimal ducts

Punctae

Lacrimal canals

B.

10.2   Additional Word Elements

Use these additional word elements when studying the terms in this chapter.

Root	Meaning
ambly/o	dull; dim
coagulati/o	to condense; to clot
dipl/o	double
emmetr/o	in proper measure
is/o	equal

Suffix	Meaning
-conus	cone-shaped
-edema	accumulation of fluid
-metrist	specialist in the measurement of
-ory	pertaining to
-schisis	splitting; cleft

Prefix	Meaning
myein-	to shut
presby-	old age
pseudo-	false

10.3   Term Analysis and Definition Pertaining to the Eye

	aque/o	water
Term	**Term Analysis**	**Definition**
aqueous humor (**AY**-kwee-us **HYOU**-mer)	-ous = pertaining to humor = body fluid	pertaining to a watery fluid found in the anterior cavity

	blephar/o	eyelid
blepharopexy (**blef**-ar-oh-**PECK**-see)	-pexy = surgical fixation	surgical fixation of the eyelid
blepharoplasty (**blef**-ah-roh-**PLAS**-tee)	-plasty = surgical reconstruction	surgical reconstruction of the eyelid
symblepharon (sim-**BLEF**-ah-ron)	sym- = together; with	adhesion of the eyeball to the eyelid

Memory Key	**Blephar/o** is most commonly used to indicate pathologic conditions of the eyelid.

	chori/o	choroid
chorioretinitis (**koh**-ree-oh-**ret**-in-**EYE**-tis)	-itis = inflammation **retin/o** = retina	inflammation of the choroid and retina

	choroid/o	choroid; membrane
choroiditis (**koh**-roid-**EYE**-tis)	-itis = inflammation	inflammation of the choroid

	conjunctiv/o	conjunctiva
conjunctivitis (kon-**junk**-tih-**VYE**-tis)	-itis = inflammation	inflammation of the conjunctiva

	core/o	**pupil**
Term	**Term Analysis**	**Definition**
anisocoria (**an**-ih-so-**KOH**-ree-ah)	-ia = condition an- = no; not **is/o** = equal	inequality in the size of the pupil
coreometer (**koh**-ree-**OM**-eh-ter)	-meter = instrument used to measure	instrument used to measure the pupil
	corne/o	**cornea**
corneal (**KOR**-nee-al)	-eal = pertaining to	pertaining to the cornea
	cycl/o	**ciliary body**
cycloplegia (**sigh**-kloh-**PLEE**-jee-ah)	-plegia = paralysis	pertaining to paralysis of the ciliary body
	dacry/o	**tear; lacrimal duct**
dacryostenosis (**dack**-ree-oh-steh-**NOH**-sis)	-stenosis = narrowing	narrowing of a lacrimal duct
	goni/o	**angle (of the anterior chamber)**
gonioscopy (**goh**-nee-**OS**-koh-pee)	-scopy = process of visual examination	process of visually examining the angle of the anterior chamber with the aid of a gonioscope. *NOTE:* A diagnostic tool for glaucoma
	irid/o; ir/o	**iris**
iridocyclitis (**ir**-ih-doh-seh-**KLYE**-tis)	-itis = inflammation **cycl/o** = ciliary body	inflammation of the iris and ciliary body
iritis (eye-**RYE**-tis)	-itis = inflammation	inflammation of the iris
iridectomy (**ir**-ih-**DECK**-toh-mee)	-ectomy = excision; surgical removal	excision of the iris

	kerat/o	cornea
Term	**Term Analysis**	**Definition**
keratoconjunctivitis (**ker**-ah-toh-kon-**junk**-tih-**VYE**-tis)	-itis = inflammation **conjunctiv/o** = conjunctiva	inflammation of the cornea and conjunctiva
keratoconus (**ker**-ah-toh-**KOH**-nus)	-conus = cone-shaped	abnormal, cone-shaped protrusion of the cornea. *NOTE:* Keratoconus is a degenerative disease causing blurred vision. It can be corrected by wearing glasses or contact lenses.
keratomycosis (**ker**-ah-toh-my-**KOH**-sis)	-osis = abnormal condition **myc/o** = fungus	fungal infection of the cornea
keratoplasty (**KER**-ah-toh-**plas**-tee)	-plasty = surgical reconstruction; surgical repair	surgical repair of the cornea; corneal transplant. *NOTE:* This operation, usually done under local anesthesia, includes the transplantation of a donor cornea from a cadaver into the eye of a recipient.

	lacrim/o	tears
nasolacrimal (**nay**-zoh-**LACK**-rih-mal)	-al = pertaining to **nas/o** = nose	pertaining to the nose and lacrimal apparatus

	mi/o	contraction; less
miosis (my-**OH**-sis)	-osis = abnormal condition	abnormal contraction of the pupil
miotic (my-**OT**-ick)	-tic = pertaining to	a drug used to constrict the pupil

	mydri/o	wide; dilation; dilatation
mydriasis (mih-**DRYE**-ah-sis)	-iasis = condition; process	dilation of the pupil
mydriatic (**mid**-ree-**AT**-ick)	-tic = pertaining to	pertaining to a drug used to dilate the pupil

	ocul/o	eye
Term	**Term Analysis**	**Definition**
extraocular (**ecks**-trah-**OCK**-you-lar)	-ar = pertaining to extra- = outside	pertaining to the outside of the eye
intraocular (**in**-trah-**OCK**-you-lar)	-ar = pertaining to intra- = within	pertaining to within the eye

	ophthalm/o	eye
exophthalmia (**eck**-sof-**THAL**-mee-ah)	-ia = condition ex- = outward	outward protrusion of the eyeball (see Figure 10-6)
ophthalmologist (**ahf**-thal-**MOL**-eh-jist)	-logist = specialist	a specialist in the study of the diagnosis and medical and surgical treatment of eye disorders
ophthalmology (**ahf**-thal-**MOL**-eh-jee)	-logy = study of	study of the eye including diseases and treatment
ophthalmoscopy (**ahf**-thal-**MOS**-koh-pee)	-scopy = process of visual examination with the aid of an instrument	process of visual examination of the eye. Also known as funduscopy or fundoscopy (see Figure 10-7)

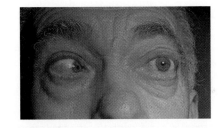

FIGURE 10-6
Exophthalmia. © *Phototake/CNRI/PNI*

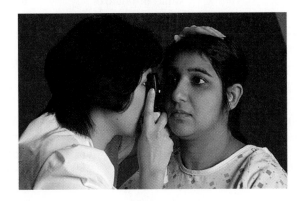

FIGURE 10-7
Ophthalmoscopy

	opt/o	vision; sight
Term	**Term Analysis**	**Definition**
optic (**OP**-tick)	-ic = pertaining to	pertaining to vision or sight
optician (op-**TISH**-an)	-ician = specialist; one who specializes; expert	expert who fills prescriptions for eyeglasses and contact lenses. *NOTE:* Opticians are not physicians and do not carry out medical and surgical treatment of eye conditions.
optometrist (op-**TOM**-eh-trist)	-metrist = specialist in the measurement of	specialist in the testing of visual function and in the diagnosis and nonsurgical treatment of eye conditions. *NOTE:* Optometrists prescribe eyeglasses and contact lenses and are licensed in some areas to prescribe medication. They do not have a degree in medicine.
	palpebr/o	**eyelid**
palpebral (**PAL**-peh-bral)	-al = pertaining to	pertaining to the eyelid
	papill/o	**optic disc**
papilledema (**pap**-ill-eh-**DEE**-mah)	-edema = accumulation of fluid	accumulation of fluid in the optic disc
	phac/o; phak/o	**lens**
aphakia (ah-**FAY**-kee-ah)	a- = no; not; lack of	absence of lens
phacomalacia (**fack**-oh-mah-**LAY**-shee-ah)	-malacia = softening	softening of the lens
pseudophakia (**soo**-doh-**FAY**-kee-ah)	-ia = condition pseudo- = false	condition characterized by replacement of the lens with connective tissue

	phot/o	light
Term	**Term Analysis**	**Definition**
cyclophotocoagulation (**sigh**-kloh-**foh**-toh-koh-**ag**-you-**LAY**-shun)	-ion = process **cycl/o** = ciliary body **coagulati/o** = to condense; to clot	destruction of a portion of the ciliary body using a laser
photocoagulation (**foh**-toh-koh-**ag**-you-**LAY**-shun)	-ion = process **coagulati/o** = to condense; to clot	a beam from a laser is aimed at the site of injury to condense the retinal tissue, thus repairing any retinal tears or detachment (see Figure 10-8 for a description of retinal detachment)
photophobia (**foh**-toh-**FOH**-bee-ah)	-phobia = fear	intolerance or sensitivity to light
	pupill/o	**pupil**
pupillary (**PYOU**-pih-lar-ee)	-ary = pertaining to	pertaining to the pupil

FIGURE 10-8
Retinal detachment

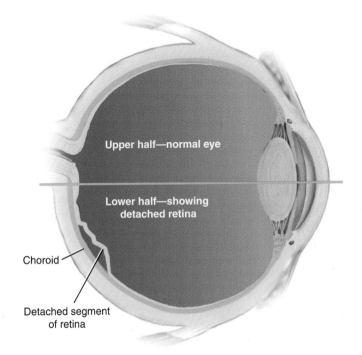

Upper half—normal eye

Lower half—showing detached retina

Choroid

Detached segment of retina

	retin/o	retina
Term	**Term Analysis**	**Definition**
retinal detachment (**RET**-ih-nal)	-al = pertaining to	separation of the retina from underlying tissue. *NOTE:* The detachment may develop as a result of diabetes or because the vitreous humor shrinks with age, pulling on and separating the retina from the underlying tissue (see Figure 10-8)
retinopathy (ret-ih-**NOP**-ah-thee)	-pathy = disease	any disease of the retina. *NOTE:* The most common retinopathy is due to diabetes.
retinopexy (**RET**-ih-noh-**peck**-see)	-pexy = surgical fixation	surgical fixation of the retina
retinoschisis (ret-ih-**NOS**-kih-sis)	-schisis = splitting; cleft	splitting of the retina

	scler/o	sclera
sclerectomy (skleh-**RECK**-toh-mee)	-ectomy = excision; surgical removal	excision of the sclera

	ton/o	tension
tonometry (toh-**NOM**-eh-tree)	-metry = process of measuring	measurement of intraocular pressure. *NOTE:* A diagnostic tool for glaucoma

	trabecul/o	meshwork; lattice
trabeculoplasty (trah-**BECK**-you-loh-**plas**-tee)	-plasty = surgical reconstruction; surgical repair	surgical reconstruction of the trabecular meshwork of the canal of Schlemm. *NOTE:* This operation is done by laser and increases the outflow of aqueous humor, thereby reducing intraocular pressure. Used in the treatment of glaucoma

		uve/o	**uvea (includes the choroid, ciliary body, and iris)**
Term		**Term Analysis**	**Definition**
uveitis (**you**-vee-**EYE**-tis)		-itis = inflammation	inflammation of the uvea
		vitre/o	**glasslike; gel-like**
vitrectomy (vih-**TRECK**-toh-mee)		-ectomy = surgical removal	removal of some or all of the vitreous humor and its replacement with a clear fluid. *NOTE:* This operation is necessary when there is an accumulation of scar tissue due to diabetic retinopathy.
vitreous humor (**VIT**-ree-us **HYOU**-mer)		-ous = pertaining to humor = body fluid	a gel-like, glassy substance in the posterior cavity

SUFFIXES

	-chalasis	relaxation
Term	**Term Analysis**	**Definition**
blepharochalasis (**blef**-ar-oh-**KAL**-ah-sis)	**blephar/o** = eyelid	relaxation of the eyelid
	-opia; -opsia	**visual condition; vision**
amblyopia (**am**-blee-**OH**-pee-ah)	**ambly/o** = dull; dim	dimness of vision
diplopia (dih-**PLOH**-pee-ah)	**dipl/o** = double	double vision
hemianopsia; hemianopia (**hem**-ee-an-**OP**-see-ah); (hem-ee-ah-**NOH**-pee-ah)	hemi- = half an- = no; not; lack of	lack of vision in half the visual field
presbyopia (**pres**-bee-**OH**-pee-ah)	presby- = old age	impaired vision due to advanced age

Term	Term Analysis	Definition
hyperopia (**high**-per-**OH**-pee-ah)	hyper- = above; beyond; excessive	light rays focus behind the retina; farsightedness (see Figure 10-9C)
myopia (my-**OH**-pee-ah)	myein- = to shut *NOTE: my* comes from the Greek word *myein*, which means "to shut."	light rays are focused in front of the retina; nearsightedness (see Figure 10-9B)

FIGURE 10-9
(A) Normal eye; (B) myopia (nearsightedness); (C) hyperopia (farsightedness)

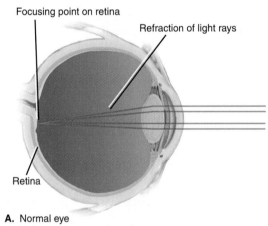

A. Normal eye
Light rays focus on the retina

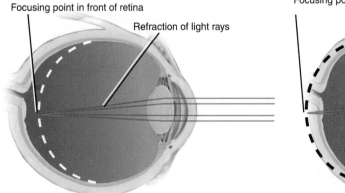

B. Myopia (nearsightedness)
Light rays focus in front of the retina

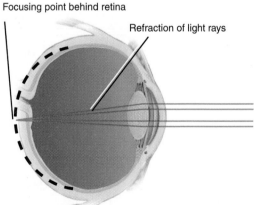

C. Hyperopia (farsightedness)
Light rays focus beyond the retina

	-tropia	turning
Term	**Term Analysis**	**Definition**
emmetropia (em-eh-**TROH**-pee-ah)	**emmetr/o** = in proper measure	normal vision
esotropia (es-oh-**TROH**-pee-ah)	eso- = inward	turning inward of the eyeball (see Figure 10-10B)
exotropia (**eck**-soh-**TROH**-pee-ah)	exo- = outward	turning outward of the eyeball (see Figure 10-10C)
hypertropia (**high**-per-**TROH**-pee-ah)	hyper- = above	upward turning of the eyeball
hypotropia (**high**-poh-**TROH**-pee-ah)	hypo- = below	downward turning of the eyeball

	-tropion	turning
ectropion (eck-**TROH**-pee-on)	ec- = out	outward turning of the eyelid
entropion (en-**TROH**-pee-on)	en- = inward	inward turning of the eyelid

FIGURE 10-10
Esotropia and exotropia

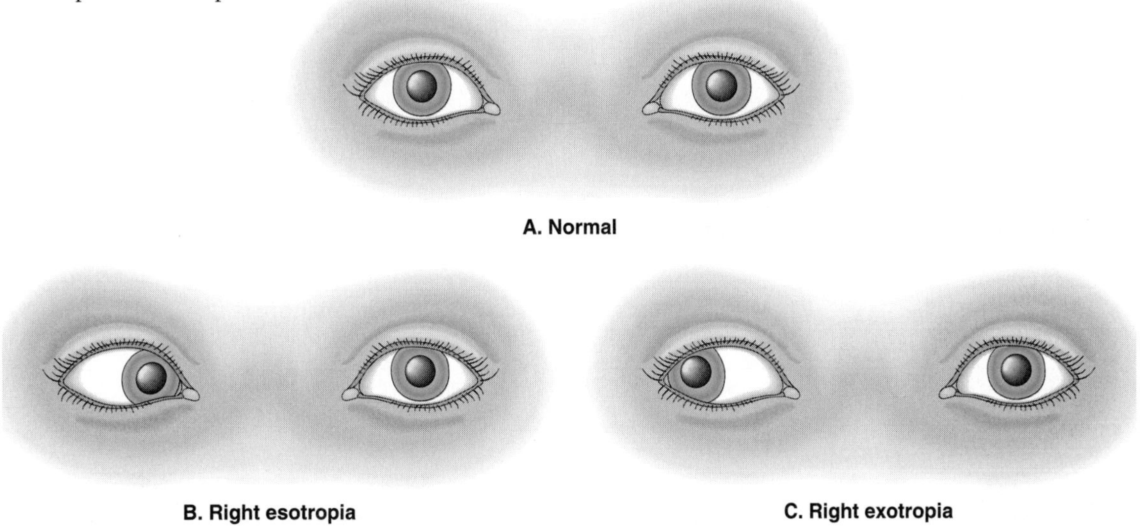

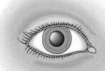

A. Normal

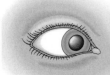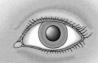

B. Right esotropia

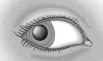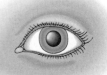

C. Right exotropia

10.4   Review of Terms Pertaining to the Eye

Define the following terms in Tables 10-1 through 10-4 in the space provided.

TABLE 10-1

REVIEW OF ANATOMICAL TERMS PERTAINING TO THE EYES

aqueous humor	corneal	emmetropia
extraocular	intraocular	nasolacrimal
ophthalmologist	ophthalmology	optic
optician	optometrist	palpebral
pupillary	vitreous humor	

TABLE 10-2

REVIEW OF PATHOLOGIC TERMS PERTAINING TO THE EYES

amblyopia	anisocoria	aphakia
blepharochalasis	blepharoptosis	blepharospasm
chorioretinitis	choroiditis	conjunctivitis
cycloplegia	dacryostenosis	diplopia
ectropion	entropion	esotropia
exophthalmia	exotropia	hemianopsia
hyperopia	hypertropia	hypotropia

continued on page 203

Table 10-2 *continued from page 202*

iridocyclitis	iritis	keratoconjunctivitis
keratoconus	keratomycosis	miosis
mydriasis	myopia	papilledema
phacomalacia	photophobia	presbyopia
pseudophakia	retinal detachment	retinopathy
retinoschisis	symblepharon	trabeculoplasty
uveitis	vitrectomy	

TABLE 10-3

REVIEW OF DIAGNOSTIC TERMS PERTAINING TO THE EYES

coreometer	gonioscopy	ophthalmoscopy
tonometry		

TABLE 10-4

REVIEW OF MEDICAL AND SURGICAL TERMS PERTAINING TO THE EYES

blepharopexy	cyclophotocoagulation	iridectomy
keratoplasty	miotic	mydriatic
photocoagulation	retinopexy	sclerectomy

10.5   Abbreviations Pertaining to the Eye

Abbreviation	Meaning
accom	accommodation
OD (oculus dextra)	right eye
OS (oculus sinistra)	left eye
OU (oculus unitas)	both eyes
PERLA	pupils equal, react to light and accommodation
PERRLA	pupils equal, round, regular, react to light and accommodation
EOM	extraocular movement
IOL	intraocular lens
IOP	intraocular pressure
VA	visual acuity
VF	visual field

10.6   The Ear

The ear consists of the external ear, the middle ear, and the inner ear, as illustrated in Figure 10-11. The ear is responsible for hearing and plays an important role in the maintenance of balance. The hearing process consists of detection and **transduction** (tranz-**DUCK**-shun). Detection involves receiving the sound stimulus. Transduction involves converting the detected sound into a nerve impulse, which is then sent on to the temporal lobe of the brain for processing. Balance is maintained through the interaction of visual signals and the balance mechanisms of the inner ear, discussed below.

Memory Key	The ear consists of the
	    external ear
	    middle ear
	    inner ear
	It is responsible for hearing and plays a prominent role in maintaining balance.

FIGURE 10-11
External, middle, and inner ear

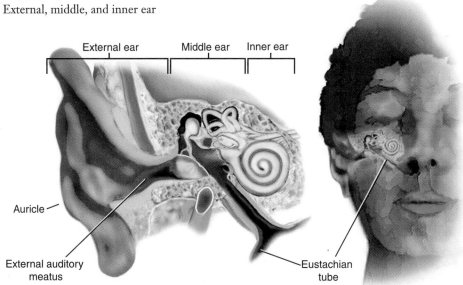

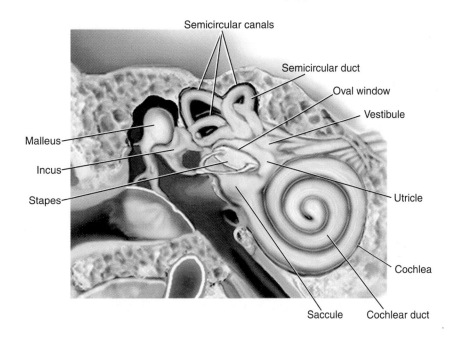

EXTERNAL EAR

The external ear is composed of the **auricle** (**AW**-rick-ul), or pinna, the **external auditory meatus** (mee-**AY**-tus), and the **eardrum** or **tympanic** (tim-**PAN**-ik) **membrane**. The auricle is the part of the ear external to the head. Sound travels down the external auditory meatus, which is the canal that leads to the eardrum. When sound reaches the eardrum, it vibrates. The waves from this vibration then travel into the middle ear.

The external ear is composed of the
auricle
external auditory meatus
eardrum (tympanic membrane)

MIDDLE EAR

The middle ear includes three tiny bones called the ossicles: the **malleus** (**MAL**-ee-us), the **incus** (**ING**-kus), and the **stapes** (**STAY**-peez), known also as the hammer, anvil, and stirrup, respectively. Sound is transmitted from the eardrum, to the malleus, to the incus, and then to the stapes. The stapes vibrates against the oval window (discussed further below), which transmits the amplified sound to the inner ear, where it is changed to electrical impulses that the brain can detect and interpret.

Air pressure on each side of the eardrum is equalized by the **eustachian tube** (you-**STAY**-shun), which connects the middle ear to the throat. When the eustachian tube is blocked, a sense of pressure is felt in the inner ear, and hearing ability is temporarily reduced. Often, pressure balance is restored with an audible popping sound. Sometimes, infectious material is transported up the eustachian tube from the throat, causing a middle ear infection (**otitis media**) (oh-**TYE**-tis **ME**-dee-ah), commonly seen in children.

The middle ear consists of three ossicles called the malleus, incus, and stapes.

INNER EAR (LABYRINTH)

If you have ever looked at a sponge, you will have a good image of what the inner ear is like: a twisting series of canals and larger spaces (**sacs**). The canals and sacs of the inner ear are encased in bone and are thus referred to as the **bony labyrinth** (**LAB**-ih-rinth). They are filled with fluid called **perilymph** (**PEAR**-ih-limf). Within the bony labyrinth are tubes called the membranous labyrinth, filled with a fluid called **endolymph** (**EN**-do-limf).

The bony labyrinth consists of the **vestibule** (**VES**-tib-youl), **semicircular canals**, and **cochlea** (**KOCK**-lee-ah). The vestibule consists of the **utricle** (**YOU**-trih-kul) and **saccule** (**SACK**-youl), which are membranous sacs that are important in maintaining balance. Behind the vestibule are the semicircular canals, which house the **semicircular ducts**, also involved in balance. The cochlea contains the **cochlear duct**, a membranous structure responsible for hearing. Figure 10-11 illustrates all of the structures of the inner ear.

Sound is transmitted to the inner ear by the action of the stapes vibrating against an opening on the inner ear called the **oval window**. Lying within the cochlear duct is the **organ of Corti** (**KOR**-tye). It contains sensitive hair cells that react to the vibrations of the stapes by moving, much as tall grass sways in the wind. The movement of the hair cells stimulates underlying nerve cell fibers that create nerve impulses, which travel to the temporal lobe of the brain.

• The inner ear contains the
bony labyrinth (vestibule, semicircular canals, and cochlea)
membranous labyrinth (utricle, saccule, semicircular ducts, and cochlear ducts)
• Sound is transmitted by the vibration of the stapes against the oval window, causing the hair cells in the organ of Corti to sway and stimulate the underlying nerve fibers that create nerve impulses, which travel to the temporal lobe of the brain.

DEAFNESS

Deafness is diminished or total loss of hearing. There are two types of deafness. **Conductive deafness** is caused by obstruction of the path traveled by sound waves from the external ear to the inner ear. Examples of obstruction are a buildup of earwax (cerumen) or a foreign body, such as popcorn, lodged in the external auditory meatus. The second type of deafness is **sensorineural deafness**, which results from damage to the auditory nerve or cochlea, causing failure of nerve stimuli to be sent to the brain from the inner ear. Sensorineural deafness can occur with age but also can be caused by loud noises from machinery or music, tumors, infections, and injury.

Conductive deafness is treated by removing the obstruction. If this treatment does not help, hearing aids may be used to amplify the sound; however, hearing aids will help only if the nerve and brain structures allowing the patient to hear function normally. Hearing aids may be helpful in treating sensorineural deafness; however, if a hearing aid is not successful, cochlear implants may be needed to have hearing restored.

Memory Key	The two types of deafness are conductive and sensorineural deafness.

10.7   Term Analysis and Definition Pertaining to the Ear

	audi/o	hearing
Term	**Term Analysis**	**Definition**
audiogram (**AW**-dee-oh-gram)	-gram = record	record of patient's hearing ability
audiometry (aw-dee-**OM**-eh-tree)	-metry = process of measuring	measurement of a patient's hearing ability
	audit/o	**hearing**
auditory (**AW**-dih-tor-ee)	-ory = pertaining to	pertaining to hearing
	aur/o	**ear**
aural (**AW**-ral)	-al = pertaining to	pertaining to the ear

	cochle/o	cochlea

Term	Term Analysis	Definition
cochlear (**KOCK**-lee-ar)	-ear = pertaining to	pertaining to the cochlea
electrocochleography (ee-**leck**-troh-**kock**-lee-**OG**-rah-fee)	-graphy = process of recording **electr/o** = electric	process of recording the electrical activity of the cochlea

	labyrinth/o	**inner ear; labyrinth**
labyrinthitis (**lab**-ih-rin-**THIGH**-tis)	-itis = inflammation	inflammation of the inner ear. *NOTE:* Often accompanied by **vertigo** (dizziness) and a loss of balance

	myring/o	**tympanic membrane; eardrum**
myringotomy (**mir**-in-**GOT**-oh-mee)	-tomy = process of cutting; to cut	process of cutting into the eardrum to remove fluid from the middle ear

	ossicul/o	**ossicles (malleus, incus, and stapes, collectively)**
ossiculoplasty (oss-**ICK**-you-loh-**plas**-tee)	-plasty = surgical repair; surgical reconstruction	surgical reconstruction of the ossicles

	ot/o	**ear**
otalgia (oh-**TAL**-gee-ah)	-algia = pain	earache
otitis media (oh-**TYE**-tis **ME**-dee-ah)	-itis = inflammation media = middle	inflammation of the middle ear. If the inflammation results in a buildup of watery fluid it is known as **serous** otitis media. If there is a buildup of pus, the condition is known as **purulent** (**PYOU**-roo-lent) otitis media (see Figure 10-12)
otorrhea (**oh**-toh-**REE**-ah)	-rrhea = discharge; flow	discharge from the ear

FIGURE 10-12
(A) Normal tympanic membrane is translucent, shiny, smooth, and pearly gray, with various landmarks, including malleus.
(B) Serous otitis media.
(C) Purulent otitis media.
NOTE: Hyperemic means increased blood in the blood vessels.

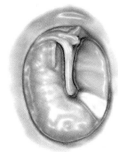

A. Normal tympanic membrane

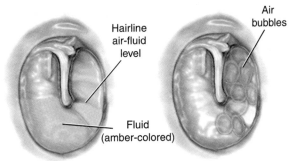

Hairline air-fluid level

Air bubbles

Fluid (amber-colored)

B. Serous otitis media

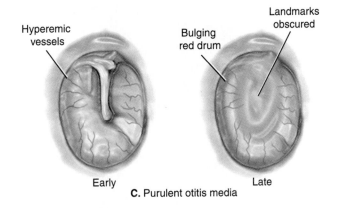

Landmarks obscured

Hyperemic vessels

Bulging red drum

Early

Late

C. Purulent otitis media

Term	Term Analysis	Definition
otosclerosis (**oh**-toh-skleh-**ROH**-sis)	-sclerosis = hardening	hardening of the ear. *NOTE:* A common disease of the middle ear. Otosclerosis results in conductive deafness because the stapes is immobilized owing to the buildup of excess bone. Treatment includes the placement of a middle-ear prosthesis to reconnect the ossicles.

Term	Term Analysis	Definition
otoscope (**OH**-toh-skope)	-scope = instrument used to visually examine	instrument used to visually examine the ear (see Figure 10-13)
	salping/o	**eustachian tube**
salpingoscope (sal-**PING**-goh-skohp)	-scope = instrument used to visually examine	instrument used to visually examine the eustachian tube

FIGURE 10-13

An otoscope is used to examine the ear canal and eardrum.

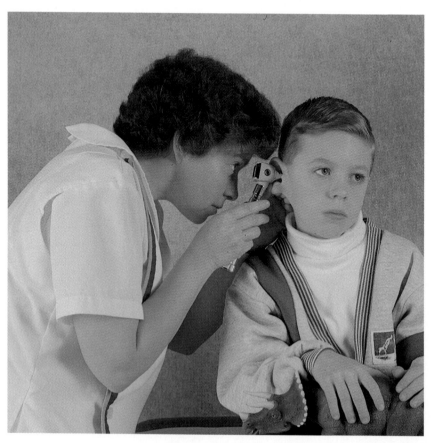

	staped/o	stapes
Term	**Term Analysis**	**Definition**
stapedectomy (stay-peh-**DECK**-toh-me)	-ectomy = excision; surgical removal	removal of the stapes

	tympan/o	**tympanic membrane; eardrum**
tympanoplasty (**tim**-pah-no-**PLAS**-tee)	-plasty = surgical repair; surgical reconstruction	surgical reconstruction of the eardrum; myringoplasty

SUFFIXES

	-cusis	hearing
Term	**Term Analysis**	**Definition**
presbycusis (**pres**-beh-**KOO**-sis)	presby- = old age	diminished hearing due to old age. *NOTE:* Presbycusis is often accompanied by **tinnitus**, a ringing in the ears.

10.8   Review of Terms Pertaining to the Ear

Define the following terms in Tables 10-5 through 10-8 in the space provided.

TABLE 10-5

REVIEW OF ANATOMICAL TERMS PERTAINING TO THE EARS

audiometer	auditory	aural
cochlear		

TABLE 10-6

REVIEW OF PATHOLOGIC TERMS PERTAINING TO THE EARS

labyrinthitis	otalgia	otitis media
otorrhea	presbycusis	

TABLE 10-7

REVIEW OF DIAGNOSTIC TERMS PERTAINING TO THE EARS

audiogram	audiometry	electrocochleography
otosclerosis	otoscope	salpingoscope

TABLE 10-8

REVIEW OF SURGICAL TERMS PERTAINING TO THE EARS

myringoplasty	myringotomy	stapedectomy
tympanoplasty		

10.9   Abbreviations Pertaining to the Ear

Abbreviation	Meaning
AC	air conduction
AD (auris dextra)	right ear
AS (auris sinistra)	left ear

continued on page 213

continued from page 212

Abbreviation	Meaning
AU (auris unitas)	both ears
BC	bone conduction
EENT	eyes, ears, nose, throat
ENT	ears, nose, throat
HD	hearing distance
NIHL	nerve-induced hearing loss
TM	tympanic membrane

10.10 Putting It All Together

Exercise 10-1   MATCHING

Match Column A with Column B.

Column A

_____ 1. cornea

_____ 2. iris

_____ 3. lens

_____ 4. tympanic membrane

_____ 5. sclera

_____ 6. malleus

_____ 7. pupil

_____ 8. utricle

_____ 9. ciliary process

_____ 10. uvea

Column B

A. white of the eye

B. regulates amount of light entering the eye

C. transmits sound waves

D. ciliary body, choroid, and iris

E. responsible for refraction and accommodation

F. colored portion of the eye

G. balance

H. produces aqueous humor

I. anterior portion of the eye refracting light rays

J. vibrates with sound waves

Exercise 10-2   ANALYSIS OF TERMS

Analyze the word into its component parts, then define the term.

Example: cycloplegia
            -plegia = paralysis
            cycl/o = ciliary body
            paralysis of the ciliary body

1. gonioscopy

_____

_____

_____

2. anisocoria

_____

_____

_____

3. miosis

_____

_____

_____

4. mydriatic

_____

_____

_____

5. optician

_____

_____

_____

6. tonometry

_____

_____

_____

7. retinoschisis

_____

_____

_____

8. hyperopia

_____

_____

_____

9. presbyopia

_____

_____

_____

10. entropion

_____

_____

_____

11. electrocochleography

_____

_____

_____

12. presbycusis

_____

_____

_____

13. otitis media

_____

_____

_____

14. audiometry

_____

_____

_____

15. aural

_____

_____

_____

Exercise 10-3   BUILDING MEDICAL TERMS

Build the medical term for the following definitions.

1. surgical fixation of the eyelid   _____

2. drooping of the eyelid   _____

3. sudden, involuntary contraction of
   the eyelid   _____

4. adhesion of the eyeball to the eyelid _____

5. inflammation of the iris
   and ciliary body   _____

6. excision of the iris   _____

7. inflammation of the cornea
   and conjunctiva   _____

8. abnormal, cone-shaped protrusion of
   the cornea   _____

9. fungal infection of the cornea   _____

10. surgical repair of the cornea   _____

11. earache   _____

12. discharge from the ear   _____

13. surgical repair of the eardrum   _____

14. process of cutting the eardrum   _____

15. removal of the stapes   _____

Exercise 10-4   DIFFERENCES IN TERMS

Distinguish between the following pairs.

1. amblyopia and diplopia

_____

2. esotropia and exotropia

_____

3. presbyopia, emmetropia, and presbycusis

_____

4. hypertropia and hypotropia

_____

5. ectropion and entropion

_____

6. optician, optometrist, and ophthalmologist

_____

_____

7. vertigo and tinnitus

_____

_____

Exercise 10-5   ADJECTIVAL FORMS

Write the adjectival form for the following. Use the dictionary if necessary.

1. cornea   _____
2. tears   _____
3. eye   _____
4. vision   _____
5. eyelid   _____
6. retina   _____
7. pupil   _____
8. ear   _____
9. hearing   _____
10. cochlea   _____

Exercise 10-6   SPELLING PRACTICE

Circle any misspelled words in the list below and correctly spell them in the space provided.

1. synblepharon   _____
2. goneoscopy   _____
3. miosis   _____

4. exopthalmia

   _____

5. papilledema

   _____

6. retinoschsis

   _____

7. uveitis

   _____

8. labyrinthitis

   _____

9. otalgia

   _____

10. presbycusis

   _____

Exercise 10-7   PLURALS

Write the plural form for the following terms. Use your dictionary if necessary.

1. iris

   _____

2. palpebra

   _____

3. retina

   _____

4. sclera

   _____

CHAPTER 11

The Endocrine System

CHAPTER ORGANIZATION

This chapter will help you learn the endocrine system. It is divided into the following sections:

CHAPTER OBJECTIVES

On completion of this chapter, you will be able to do the following:

1. Define hormones and homeostasis
2. Differentiate between exocrine and endocrine glands
3. Name the central and peripheral glands of the endocrine system
4. Define and name five trophic hormones
5. Name the hormones secreted by the anterior and posterior pituitary and describe their functions
6. Name the hormones secreted by the pancreas, thyroid, parathyroid, pineal, and adrenal glands and describe their functions
7. Analyze, pronounce, define, and spell terms related to the endocrine system
8. Define abbreviations common to the endocrine system

INTRODUCTION

When your body needs water, you feel a sense of thirst and take a drink. This is an example of one of the many ways in which the body maintains internal balance, or **homeostasis (hoh-mee-oh-STAY**-sis). The **endocrine (EN**-doh-krin) **system** is also involved with the maintenance of homeostasis. Endocrine glands secrete powerful substances called **hormones**, which are essential for the proper functioning of a variety of bodily processes. Just as your body tells you to drink when you are thirsty, these hormones are produced and secreted when the body signals a need for them. When proper levels within the blood have been reached, the signals cease, and hormone secretion stops. This is an example of a feedback mechanism.

The endocrine system consists of several glands: the **hypothalamus (high**-poh-**THAL**-ah-mus), **pituitary** (pih-**TOO**-ih-tar-ee), **thyroid** (**THIGH**-roid), **parathyroids** (par-ah-**THIGH**-roids), **adrenals** (ah-**DREE**-nalz), **pineal** (**PIN**-ee-al), and **pancreas** (**PAN**-kree-as). They secrete hormones into the bloodstream for delivery to the target organ. This distinguishes the endocrine glands from the **exocrine (ECK**-soh-krin) **glands** such as sweat glands (see Figure 11-1). Exocrine glands secrete chemicals into ducts, which then deliver the secretions to the target site. With the exception of the pancreas, which has both exocrine and endocrine functions, the endocrine glands have no ducts .

There are two categories of endocrine gland, the **central** and the **peripheral**. The central consists of two adjacent glands in the brain, the hypothalamus and pituitary, which coordinate to regulate body functions such as water and salt balance, growth, reproduction, and

FIGURE 11-1

Exocrine and endocrine glands

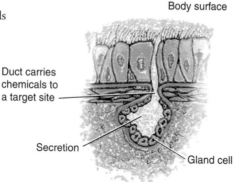

Body surface

Duct carries
chemicals to
a target site

Secretion

Gland cell

A. Exocrine gland
(has duct)

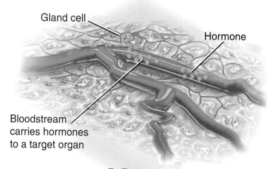

Gland cell

Hormone

Bloodstream
carries hormones
to a target organ

B. Endocrine gland
(ductless)

metabolism. The peripheral endocrine glands include the thyroid, parathyroids, adrenals, pineal, and pancreas. The first four have only one function, the production of hormones. The pancreas not only produces hormones, but also has important digestive system functions. In this way, the pancreas is similar to a host of mixed-function organs, such as the kidneys, small intestine, liver, heart, ovaries, testes, thymus, and placenta. In addition to their regular systemic functions, these organs secrete hormones. The function of these organs, except for the pancreas, will be taken up in their respective chapters. The endocrine glands are illustrated in Figure 11-2, the hypothalamus in Figure 11-3.

Memory Key	• The central endocrine glands are the hypothalamus and pituitary.

• The peripheral glands are the

thyroid	pineal
parathyroids	pancreas
adrenals	

• An endocrine function does not involve ducts. Hormones are secreted into the bloodstream, to be received by target organs.

• An exocrine function involves the secretion of fluids into ducts for delivery to a site.

FIGURE 11-2
The endocrine glands

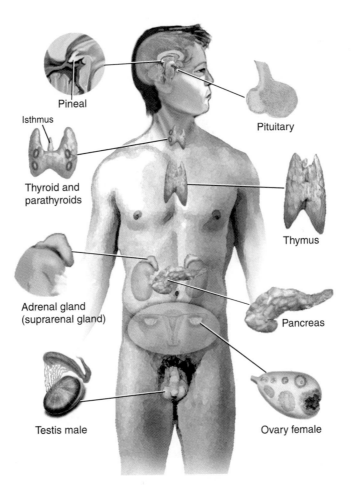

Pineal

Isthmus

Pituitary

Thyroid and parathyroids

Thymus

Adrenal gland
(suprarenal gland)

Pancreas

Testis male

Ovary female

FIGURE 11-3

The pituitary gland and its hormonal secretions

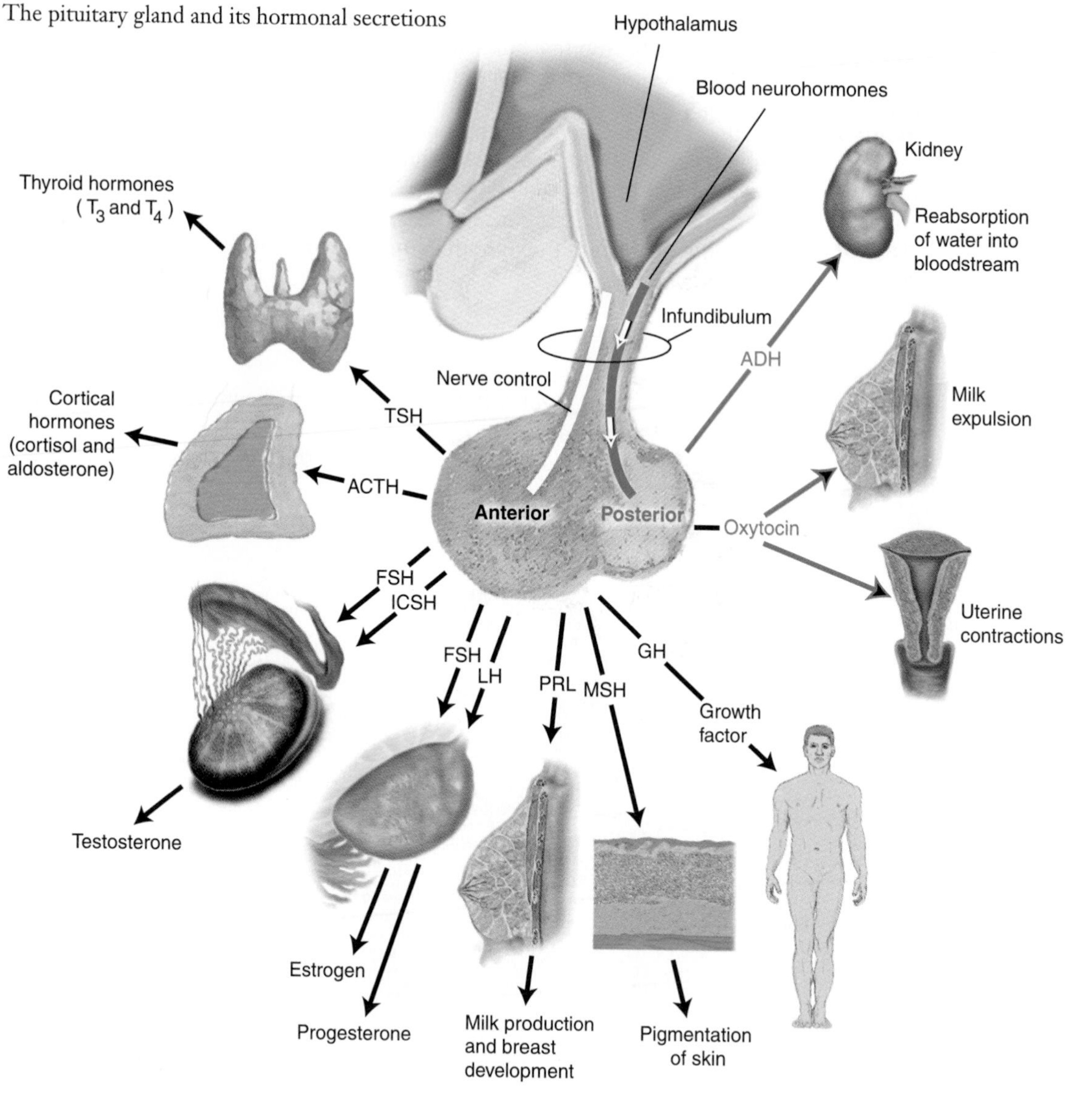

Hypothalamus

Blood neurohormones

Kidney

Reabsorption of water into bloodstream

Thyroid hormones (T_3 and T_4)

Infundibulum

ADH

Milk expulsion

Nerve control

Cortical hormones (cortisol and aldosterone)

TSH

ACTH

Anterior   **Posterior** — Oxytocin

Uterine contractions

FSH
ICSH

FSH
LH   PRL MSH   GH

Growth factor

Testosterone

Estrogen

Progesterone

Milk production and breast development

Pigmentation of skin

11.1   Central Endocrine Glands

HYPOTHALAMUS

The hypothalamus works in tandem with the pituitary. The location of the pituitary gland deep within the brain is illustrated in Figure 11-2. The hypothalamus secretes hormones that stimulate the pituitary to release other hormones. These are called **trophic** hormones because they stimulate the pituitary to secrete its own hormones. Often the suffixes -trophic

(-tropic) and -trophin (-tropin) are used in relation to substances that nourish or stimulate other organs to secrete hormones. The hypothalamus also produces **antidiuretic (an-tih-dye-you-RET-ick) hormone** and **oxytocin (ock-see-TOH-sin)**. These are neurohormones secreted by specialized neurons into the bloodstream (see Figure 11-3). These are not trophic hormones: they do not cause the pituitary to release other hormones. They are stored in the posterior pituitary and released when required.

Memory Key	• The hypothalamus secretes trophic hormones, which have an effect on pituitary activity.
	• The hypothalamus secretes two other hormones that are stored in the pituitary for later release.

PITUITARY GLAND

The pea-sized pituitary gland hangs from the hypothalamus by a stalk called the **infundibulum (in-fun-DIB-you-lum)**, as illustrated in Figure 11-3. The pituitary gland is divided into **anterior** and **posterior lobes**.

The **anterior** pituitary secretes seven hormones, triggered by hypothalamic-releasing hormones (see Figure 11-3). Five of the anterior pituitary hormones are stimulating (trophic) hormones, inducing other glands to release hormones. These five are:

1. **Adrenocorticotrophic (ah-dree-noh-kor-tih-koh-TROH-fik) hormone (ACTH)**, which stimulates the adrenal cortex to produce and secrete **cortisol (KOR-tih-sol)**, and **aldosterone (al-DOS-ter-own)**

2. **Growth hormone (GH)**, or **somatotrophin (so-ma-toh-TROH-fin)**, which stimulates growth in all body cells and controls the release of the hormone somatomedin from the liver

3. **Thyroid-stimulating hormone (TSH)**, or **thyrotrophin (thi-roh-TROH-fin)**, which stimulates the thyroid gland to produce and secrete its own hormones **thyroxine (thigh-ROCK-sin)** (T_4) and **triiodothyronine (try-eye-oh-doh-THIGH-roh-nen)** (T_3)

4. **Follicle-stimulating hormone (FSH)**, a **gonadotrophin (goh-na-doh-TROH-fin)**, which stimulates the development of the gonads (ovaries and testes). In males this hormone promotes sperm formation, and in females it promotes monthly development of the ovum (egg) and stimulates the secretion of the female hormone estrogen and progesterone.

5. **Luteinizing (LOO-tee-in-eye-zing) hormone (LH)**, another gonadotrophin that triggers ovulation in females. In males it regulates testosterone secretion and is called **interstitial cell stimulating hormone (ICSH)**.

Prolactin (pro-LACK-tin) (PRL) and **melanocyte-stimulating hormone (MSH)** are the sixth and seventh hormones produced by the anterior pituitary. These two hormones do not stimulate the production of other hormones and are therefore not trophic hormones. PRL stimulates breast development and milk production. MSH stimulates melanocytic activity in the skin.

The posterior pituitary stores and secretes two hormones produced by the hypothalamus. The first is antidiuretic hormone (ADH), also known as **vasopressin (vay-zoh-PRESS-in)**, and the second is oxytocin, produced by the hypothalamus. Antidiuretic hormone prevents excessive loss of water, and oxytocin stimulates uterine contractions to assist childbirth. Oxytocin also regulates the flow of milk from the mammary glands.

Figure 11-4 summarizes all of the anterior pituitary hormones.

Memory Key	• The anterior pituitary secretes several hormones critical to life: ACTH, GH, TSH, FSH, LH, PRL, and MSH. • The posterior pituitary stores and releases two hormones produced by the hypothalamus: antidiuretic hormone and oxytocin.

FIGURE 11-4

Summary of trophic hormones from the pituitary gland

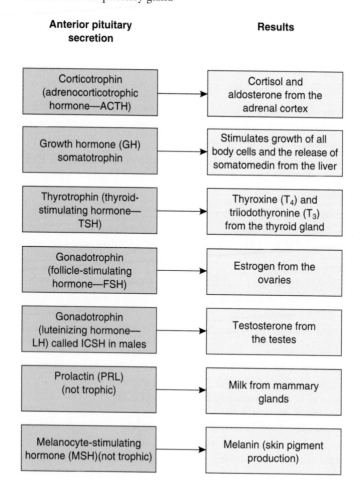

11.2   Peripheral Endocrine Glands

THYROID GLAND

Figure 11-2 illustrates the thyroid. It is located in the neck below the larynx and consists of right and left lobes connected by a structure called the **isthmus** (**ISS**-mus). The thyroid produces, stores, and secretes the two thyroid hormones: triiodothyronine (T_3) and thyroxine (T_4). These hormones regulate metabolic rate and increase the production of energy from food. Also produced by the thyroid is the hormone **calcitonin** (cal-sih-**TOH**-nin), which regulates blood calcium levels.

> **Memory Key**
> - The thyroid is in the throat area and produces T_3 and T_4, which regulate metabolic rate and increase energy production.
> - The thyroid also secretes calcitonin, which regulates blood calcium levels.

PARATHYROID GLANDS

As shown in Figure 11-2, there are four parathyroid glands, two on each of the thyroid lobes. These egg-shaped glands secrete **parathyroid** (par-ah-**THIGH**-roid) **hormone**, also called **parathormone** (par-ah-**THOR**-mohn). This hormone, referred to as **PTH**, contributes to the regulation of calcium and phosphorus.

> **Memory Key**
> - There are four parathyroids located on the thyroid.
> - The parathyroids secrete PTH, which regulates calcium and phosphorus levels.

ADRENAL GLANDS

The adrenal glands sit on top of the kidneys as shown in Figure 11-2. Functionally and structurally, there are two parts: the adrenal cortex and the adrenal medulla.

The adrenal cortex secretes three groups of hormones:

1. **Mineralocorticoids** (**min**-er-ahl-oh-**KOR**-tih-koidz), of which aldosterone is the most important. It plays a central role in the regulation of sodium and potassium levels.
2. **Glucocorticoids** (**gloo**-koh-**KOR**-tih-koidz), of which cortisol (hydrocortisone) is the most important. Cortisol is necessary for antibody production; plays a key role in the body's response to stress; and is necessary for the utilization of carbohydrates, fats, and proteins.
3. **Sex hormones**, called estrogens and androgens. Although these hormones are primarily secreted by the ovaries and testes, the adrenal cortex secretes small amounts, which play a role in the development of secondary sex characteristics such as the growth of pubic and facial hair and breast development.

The adrenal medulla produces **adrenaline** (ah-**DREN**-ah-len) and **noradrenaline** (nor-ah-**DREN**-ah-len), also respectively referred to as **epinephrine** (ep-ih-**NEF**-rin) and **norepinephrine** (nor-ep-ih-**NEF**-rin), and collectively as **catecholamines** (kat-eh-**KOHL**-ah-meenz).

These are the so-called fight or flight hormones, as they prepare the body for physical exertion during times of stress.

Memory Key	• The adrenals sit on top of the kidneys. • Each adrenal cortex secretes mineralocorticoids, glucocorticoids, and sex hormones. • Each adrenal medulla secretes the fight or flight hormones adrenaline (epinephrine) and noradrenaline (norepinephrine).

PINEAL GLAND

The **pineal** (**PIN**-ee-al) **gland** is shown in Figure 11-2. It looks like a pine cone and is located deep within the brain. It receives neural stimulation from the eye, which regulates its secretion of the hormone melatonin (**mel**-ah-**TOH**-nin). Light inhibits melatonin secretion; dark stimulates its production. Little is known about the role of the pineal gland, although there is evidence that the presence of melatonin increases the activity of the reproductive system.

Memory Key	The pineal gland is located deep in the brain and secretes melatonin, which may be involved with the activity of the reproductive system.

PANCREAS

The **pancreas** lies behind the stomach and secretes pancreatic juice, which travels along the pancreatic duct and into the duodenum. This is an exocrine function. The pancreas also secretes endocrine substances, the hormones **insulin** (**IN**-suh-lin) and **glucagon** (**GLOO**-kah-gon), which are important in the regulation of blood sugar. Insulin lowers blood sugar by stimulating the absorption of sugar by body cells. It also converts glucose into glycogen, which is the form in which sugar is stored in the liver. Glucagon increases blood sugar by converting glycogen back to glucose for use by the body when sugar is low.

Memory Key	• The pancreas lies near the stomach. • The pancreas has both exocrine and endocrine functions. • Its endocrine functions are to produce insulin and glucagon. • Insulin converts glucose into its storage form, glycogen, and stimulates the absorption of sugar by body cells. • Glucagon reconverts the glycogen into glucose when the body needs sugar.

Table 11-1 summarizes the endocrine glands, the hormones secreted, and their functions.

TABLE 11-1

SUMMARY OF ENDOCRINE GLANDS AND HORMONES

Gland	Hormone	Function
Anterior pituitary (adenohypophysis)	Somatotrophin: growth hormone (GH)	Stimulates growth in all body cells
	Thyrotrophin: thyroid-stimulating hormone (TSH)	Stimulates thyroid gland to produce T_3 and T_4
	Corticotrophin: adrenocorticotrophic hormone (ACTH)	Stimulates adrenal cortex to release cortisol and aldosterone
	Gonadotrophin: follicle-stimulating hormone (FSH)	Regulates development of ovaries and testes; promotes monthly growth of egg in females and sperm production in males
	Gonadotrophin: luteinizing hormone (LH) in females; interstitial cell stimulating hormone (ICSH) in males	Triggers ovulation in females; regulates sex hormone secretion in males
	Prolactin (PRL)	Stimulates production of milk in mammary gland
	Melanocyte-stimulating hormone (MSH)	Produces melanin for skin pigmentation
Posterior pituitary (neurohypophysis)	Antidiuretic hormone (ADH), also called vasopressin	Regulates water retention in the body
	Oxytocin	Regulates flow of milk in mammary glands and stimulates uterine contractions during childbirth
Thyroid	Thyroid hormones: thyroxine (T_4) and triiodothyronine (T_3)	Increases metabolic rate; stimulates growth
	Calcitonin	Regulates blood calcium
Parathyroids	Parathyroid hormone: parathormone (PTH)	Increases blood calcium; decreases blood phosphate

continued on page 228

Table 11-1 *continued from page 227*

Gland	Hormone	Function
Adrenal cortex	Glucocorticoid hormones, including cortisol, also called hydrocortisone	Antibody production; response to stress; metabolism of carbohydrates, fats, and proteins
	Mineralocorticoid hormones including aldosterone	Regulates sodium and potassium levels
	Sex hormones estrogen and testosterone	Development of secondary female and male characteristics
Adrenal medulla	Catecholamines: epinephrine (adrenaline) and norepinephrine (noradrenaline)	Help body respond to stress
Pineal gland	Melatonin	Function unknown in humans
Pancreas	Insulin, Glucagon	Insulin converts glucose to glycogen and stimulates the absorption of sugar. Glucagon converts glycogen to glucose.

11.3   Additional Word Elements

Use these additional word elements when studying the medical terms in this chapter.

Root	Meaning
immun/o	safe
radi/o	radioactive

Suffix	Meaning
-genesis	production
-gen	producing

Prefix	Meaning
eu-	normal

11.4   Term Analysis and Definition

	acr/o	extremity; top
Term acromegaly (**ack**-roh-**MEG**-ah-lee)	**Term Analysis** -megaly = enlargement	**Definition** enlargement of many skeletal structures including the extremities, nose, forehead, and jaw (see Figure 11-5)
	aden/o	**gland**
adenoma (**ad**-eh-**NO**-mah)	-oma = tumor; mass	benign tumor of a gland

FIGURE 11-5
Acromegaly. Notice the enlarged skeletal structures of nose, chin, and hands.
Courtesy of Matthew Leinung, MD, Albany Medical College, Albany, N.Y.

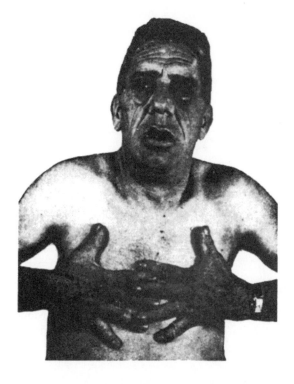

	adrenal/o; adren/o	**adrenal**
Term	**Term Analysis**	**Definition**
adrenalectomy (ah-**dree**-nal-**ECK**-toh-mee)	-ectomy = excision; surgical removal	excision of the adrenal gland
	andr/o	**male; man**
androgen (**AN**-droh-jen)	-gen = producing	substance producing male characteristics such as the hormone testosterone
	calc/o	**calcium**
hypercalcemia (**high**-per-kal-**SEE**-mee-ah)	-emia = blood condition hyper- = excessive; above normal	excessive amounts of calcium in the blood
	crin/o	**to secrete**
endocrinologist (**en**-doh-krih-**NOL**-oh-jist)	-logist = specialist endo- = within	specialist in endocrinology
endocrinology (**en**-doh-krih-**NOL**-oh-jee)	-logy = study of endo- = within	the study of the diagnosis and treatment of endocrine disorders
	estr/o	**female**
estrogen (**ES**-troh-jen)	-gen = producing	female sex hormones
	gluc/o	**sugar**
glucogenesis (**gloo**-koh-**JEN**-eh-sis)	-genesis = production	production of sugar
gluconeogenesis (**gloo**-koh-**nee**-oh-**JEN**-eh-sis)	-genesis = production neo- = new	production of sugar from fats and proteins

	glyc/o	**sugar**
Term	**Term Analysis**	**Definition**
glycolysis (glye-**KOL**-ih-sis)	-lysis = breakdown; separation; destruction	breakdown of sugars
hyperglycemia (**high**-per-glye-**SEE**-mee-ah)	-emia = blood condition hyper- = excessive; above normal	excessive amounts of sugar in the blood
hypoglycemia (**high**-poh-glye-**SEE**-mee-ah)	-emia = blood condition hypo- = deficient; below normal	deficient amounts of sugar in the blood
	glycogen/o	**glycogen (storage form of sugar)**
glycogenolysis (**glye**-koh-jen-**OL**-ih-sis)	-lysis = breakdown; separation; destruction	breakdown of glycogen to form glucose
	gonad/o	**gonads; sex glands (testes and ovaries)**
hypergonadism (**high**-per-**GO**-nad-izm)	-ism = condition; process; state of hyper- = excessive; above normal	condition characterized by excessive secretion of gonadal hormones resulting in early sexual development
	gynec/o	**woman**
gynecomastia (**guy**-neh-koh-**MAS**-tee-ah)	-ia = condition **mast/o** = breast	abnormal enlargement of the male breast
	home/o	**same**
homeostasis (**hoh**-mee-oh-**STAY**-sis)	-stasis = standing; stable; stopping; controlling	a balanced, yet sometimes varying state

	insulin/o	insulin
Term	**Term Analysis**	**Definition**
hypoinsulinism (**high**-poh-**IN**-suh-lin-izm)	-ism = condition; process; state of hypo- = deficient; below normal	condition characterized by decreased amounts of insulin secretion resulting in hyperglycemia
	kal/o	potassium
hyperkalemia (**high**-per-kah-**LEE**-mee-ah)	-emia = blood condition hyper- = excessive; above normal	excessive amounts of potassium in the blood
	natr/o	sodium
hyponatremia (**high**-poh-nah-**TREE**-mee-ah)	-emia = blood condition hypo- = deficient; below normal	deficient amounts of sodium in the blood
	pancreat/o	pancreas
pancreatogenic (**pan**-kree-ah-toh-**JEN**-ick)	-genic = produced by	produced by the pancreas
	parathyroid/o	parathyroid gland
hyperparathyroidism (**high**-per-**par**-ah-**THIGH**-roid-izm)	-ism = condition; process; state of hyper- = excessive; above normal	condition characterized by excessive secretion of parathormone resulting in loss of calcium from the bone
	pituitar/o	pituitary gland
panhypopituitarism (pan-**high**-poh-pih-**TOO**-ih-tar-izm)	-ism = condition; process; state of pan- = all hypo- = deficient; below normal	condition characterized by a deficiency of all pituitary hormones resulting in dwarfism and a deterioration of secondary sex characteristics

	thyr/o; thyroid/o	thyroid gland; shield
Term	**Term Analysis**	**Definition**
euthyroid (you-**THIGH**-roid)	-oid = resembling eu- = normal; good	normal thyroid gland
hyperthyroidism (**high**-per-**THIGH**-roid-izm)	-ism = condition; process; state of hyper- = excessive; above normal	condition characterized by excessive secretion of the thyroid hormones resulting in **goiter**, an enlarged thyroid gland, and **exophthalmos**, an abnormal protrusion of the eyes as seen in Figure 11-6
thyroiditis (thigh-roi-**DYE**-tis)	-itis = inflammation	inflammation of the thyroid gland
thyrotomy (thigh-**ROT**-oh-mee)	-tomy = to cut; incision	to cut into the thyroid gland

FIGURE 11-6
Hyperthyroidism

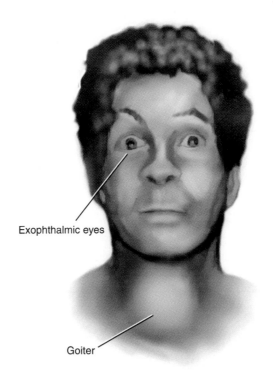

Exophthalmic eyes

Goiter

	ure/o	urea (end product of protein breakdown, found in urine)
Term	**Term Analysis**	**Definition**
antidiuretic hormone (**an**-tih-dye-you-**RET**-ick **HOR**-mohn)	-tic = pertaining to anti- = against dia- = through	a hormone that prevents the loss of excessive amounts of urine

Memory Key | The *a* in dia- is dropped because the word element **ure/o** begins with a vowel.

SUFFIXES

	-assay	analysis of a mixture to identify its contents
Term	**Term Analysis**	**Definition**
radioimmunoassay (RIA) (**ray**-dee-oh-**im**-you-no-**ASS**-ay)	**radi/o** = radioactive **immun/o** = safe	blood test used to identify hormone levels in blood plasma. The hormones are labeled with a radioactive substance.
	-crine	to secrete
endocrine hormones (**EN**-doh-krin)	endo- = within	hormones secreted by the endocrine glands into the bloodstream
exocrine glands (**ECK**-soh-krin)	exo- = outside; outward	glands that secrete chemicals into ducts
	-dipsia	thirst
polydipsia (**pol**-ee-**DIP**-see-ah)	poly- = many	excessive thirst

	-physis	to grow
Term	**Term Analysis**	**Definition**
adenohypophysis (**ad**-eh-noh-high-**POF**-ih-sis)	**aden/o** = gland hypo- = below; under	another name for anterior pituitary gland. So called because the anterior pituitary is made up of glandular tissue.
neurohypophysis (**new**-roh-high-**POF**-ih-is)	**neur/o** = nerve hypo- = below; under	another name for posterior pituitary gland. The root indicates that the posterior pituitary is made up of neural tissue.

	-trophic; tropic	**pertaining to nourishment**
adrenocorticotrophic hormone (ACTH) (ah-**dree**-noh-**kor**-tih-koh-**TROH**-fick)	**adren/o** = adrenal gland **cortic/o** = cortex; outer layer	pituitary hormone that stimulates the adrenal cortex to produce and secrete its own hormones
gonadotrophic hormone (**goh**-na-doh-**TROH**-fick)	**gonad/o** = gonads; sex glands (ovaries, testes)	pituitary hormone that stimulates the gonads to produce and secrete their own hormones
somatotrophic hormone (**soh**-ma-toh-**TROH**-fick)	**somat/o** = body	pituitary hormone that stimulates growth of body tissues

PREFIXES

	oxy-	**sharp; quick**
Term	**Term Analysis**	**Definition**
oxytocin (**ock**-see-**TOH**-sin)	-tocin = labor	pituitary hormone that quickens childbirth

11.5   Review of Terms

Define the terms in Tables 11-2 through 11-4 in the space provided.

TABLE 11-2

REVIEW OF ANATOMICAL TERMS

adenohypophysis	adrenocorticotrophic hormone	androgen
antidiuretic hormone	endocrine hormones	endocrinologist
endocrinology	estrogen	exocrine glands
glucogenesis	gluconeogenesis	glycogenolysis
glycolysis	gonadotrophic hormone	homeostasis
neurohypophysis	oxytocin	pancreatogenic
somatotrophic hormone		

TABLE 11-3

REVIEW OF PATHOLOGIC TERMS

acromegaly	adenoma	euthyroid
gynecomastia	hypercalcemia	hyperglycemia
hypergonadism	hyperkalemia	hyperparathyroidism
hyperthyroidism	hypoglycemia	hypoinsulinism
hyponatremia	panhypopituitarism	polydipsia
thyroiditis		

TABLE 11-4

REVIEW OF DIAGNOSTIC TESTS AND SURGICAL PROCEDURES

adrenalectomy	radioimmunoassay	thyrotomy

11.6   Abbreviations

Abbreviation	Meaning
ACTH	adrenocorticotrophic hormone
ADH	antidiuretic hormone
Ca	calcium; cancer
FSH	follicle-stimulating hormone
GH	growth hormone
K	potassium
LH	luteinizing hormone
MSH	melanocyte-stimulating hormone
Na	sodium
OT	oxytocin
P	phosphorus
PRL	prolactin
PTH	parathyroid hormone (parathormone)
RIA	radioimmunoassay
T_3	triiodothyronine
T_4	thyroxine
TFT	thyroid function tests
TRH	thyrotrophin-releasing hormone
TSH	thyroid-stimulating hormone

11.7   Putting It All Together

Exercise 11-1   IDENTIFICATION

Give alternative names for the following hormones.

1. growth hormone   _____

2. thyroid-stimulating hormone   _____

3. follicle-stimulating hormone   _____

4. luteinizing hormone   _____

5. hydrocortisone   _____

6. adrenaline   _____

Exercise 11-2   MATCHING

I. Match the gland in Column A with its hormonal secretion(s) in Column B.

Column A	Column B
_____ 1. anterior pituitary	A. growth hormone
_____ 2. posterior pituitary	B. calcitonin
_____ 3. thyroid gland	C. luteinizing hormone
_____ 4. parathyroid	D. oxytocin
_____ 5. adrenal cortex	E. melatonin
_____ 6. adrenal medulla	F. cortisol
_____ 7. pineal gland	G. adrenocorticotrophic
_____ 8. pancreas	H. insulin
	I. antidiuretic hormone
	J. glucagon
	K. prolactin
	L. parathormone
	M. aldosterone
	N. adrenaline

II. Match the hormone in Column A with its function in Column B.

Column A		**Column B**
_____	1. luteinizing hormone	A. stimulates milk production
_____	2. prolactin	B. stimulates osteoclast activity
_____	3. thyroxine	C. antibody production
_____	4. calcitonin	D. converts glucose to glycogen
_____	5. parathormone	E. triggers ovulation in females
_____	6. aldosterone	F. converts glycogen to glucose
_____	7. cortisol	G. regulates metabolic rate
_____	8. epinephrine	H. inhibits osteoclast activity
_____	9. insulin	I. regulates sodium and potassium
_____	10. glucagon	J. prepares the body for physical exertion during times of stress

Exercise 11-3   BUILDING TERMS

I. Using -trophic, build terms for the following definitions.

1. pituitary hormone that stimulates the adrenal cortex to secrete its own hormones _____

2. pituitary hormone that stimulates the gonads to secrete its own hormones _____

3. pituitary hormone that stimulates growth of body tissues _____

4. pituitary hormone that stimulates the thyroid to secrete its own hormones _____

II. Using -emia, build terms for the following definitions.

5. excessive amounts of sugar in the blood _____

6. deficient amounts of sugar in the blood _____

7. excessive amounts of potassium in the blood _____

8. deficient amounts of sodium in the blood _____

9. excessive amounts of calcium in the blood _____

III. Using -ism, build terms for the following definitions.

10. condition characterized by excessive secretions of gonadal hormones _____

11. decreased amounts of insulin secretion _____

12. condition characterized by excessive secretion of parathormone _____

13. condition characterized by a deficiency of all pituitary hormones _____

14. condition characterized by excessive secretion of the thyroid hormone _____

Exercise 11-4   DEFINITIONS

Define the following terms.

1. acromegaly _____

_____

2. androgen _____

_____

3. estrogen _____

_____

4. homeostasis _____

_____

5. pancreatogenic _____

_____

6. endocrinology _____

_____

7. polydipsia _____

_____

8. neurohypophysis _____

_____

9. exocrine glands _____

_____

10. endocrine glands _____

_____

Exercise 11-5   SPELLING

Circle any misspelled words in the list below and correctly spell them in the space provided.

1. pancrease   _____

2. gynecomastia   _____

3. epinephrine   _____

4. endocrene   _____

5. lutenizing   _____

6. oxytocin   _____

7. hypothalmus   _____

8. euthyroid   _____

9. adenohypophysis   _____

10. hypercalcimia   _____

CHAPTER

12

The Cardiovascular System

CHAPTER ORGANIZATION

This chapter will help you learn the cardiovascular system. It is divided into the following sections:

CHAPTER OBJECTIVES

On completion of this chapter, you will be able to do the following:

1. Name the major structures of the cardiovascular system
2. Define terms relating to the structure of the heart
3. Name and describe the walls of the heart
4. Identify the major structures of the heart on a diagram
5. Describe the pericardium
6. Describe the conduction system
7. Define common terminology used in an electrocardiogram
8. Describe blood pressure to include systole, diastole, systolic pressure, diastolic pressure, sphygmomanometer, hypertension, and hypotension
9. Differentiate between S_1 and S_2
10. Differentiate between the structure and function of arteries, veins, and capillaries
11. Describe the circulation of blood
12. Describe generally how arteries and veins are named
13. Pronounce, analyze, define, and spell the terms relating to the cardiovascular system
14. Define abbreviations common to the cardiovascular system

INTRODUCTION

The 70 to 80 trillion cells in the human body require a continuous supply of oxygen and nutrients. At the same time, body cells must get rid of their accumulated waste products. Waste is eliminated by the cardiovascular system (CVS) along with the blood and lymph discussed in Chapter 13. The cardiovascular system consists of the **heart** and **blood vessels**. Blood vessels are of three types: **arteries** (**AR**-ter-eez), **veins** (**VAYNZ**), and **capillaries** (ka-**PILL**-ah-reez). Arteries carry blood *away* from the heart. Veins carry blood *toward* the heart. Capillaries are tiny blood vessels that join the arterial and venous systems and carry blood to the organs.

As you study the cardiovascular system, keep in mind that the blood must travel to the lungs to become **oxygenated** (saturated with oxygen). Once oxygenated, the blood travels to the organs, where oxygen and nutrients are dropped off. **Deoxygenated blood** (blood released of oxygen) must travel through veins back to the heart, where it is pumped into the lungs to start the whole process over again. A more detailed discussion of blood circulation is in section 12.6.

Memory Key	• The cardiovascular system includes the

> **Memory Key**
> • The cardiovascular system includes the
>   heart
>   blood vessels (arteries, veins, and capillaries)
> • It delivers oxygen and nutrients to all of the body's cells, and carries away carbon dioxide and waste products.

12.1   Structure of the Heart

Your heart is about the same size as your fist. It is located in a fluid-filled sac called the **pericardium** (**per**-ih-**KAR**-dee-um), which lies within the thoracic cavity, posterior to the sternum and left of the midline. The heart is primarily composed of muscle tissue, which allows it to powerfully contract to pump blood throughout the body. As shown in Figure 12-1, the heart is connected to the aorta, the inferior and superior venae cavae, and the pulmonary veins and arteries.

> **Memory Key**
> • The heart lies within the pericardium, located in the thoracic cavity.
> • It is connected to the aorta, the inferior and superior venae cavae, and the pulmonary veins and arteries.

INTERIOR OF THE HEART

Figure 12-2 illustrates the interior of the heart. Note the four chambers: the right and left **atria** (**AY**-tree-ah) and the right and left **ventricles** (**VEN**-trick-ls). A structure called the **septum** (**SEP**-tum) separates the right and left sides of the heart.

The atria are separated from the ventricles by valves called **atrioventricular** (ay-tree-oh-ven-**TRICK**-you-lar) (**AV**) **valves**. They allow blood to flow only from the atrium into the ventricle. The right atrioventricular valve is also called the **tricuspid** (trigh-**KUS**-pid) **valve**, because it consists of three triangular flaps called **cusps**. The left atrioventricular valve has only two cusps and is therefore called the **bicuspid valve**. Another common name for it is the **mitral** (**MY**-tral) **valve**. The cusps of each atrioventricular valve are attached to the walls

FIGURE 12-1
Structures of the heart

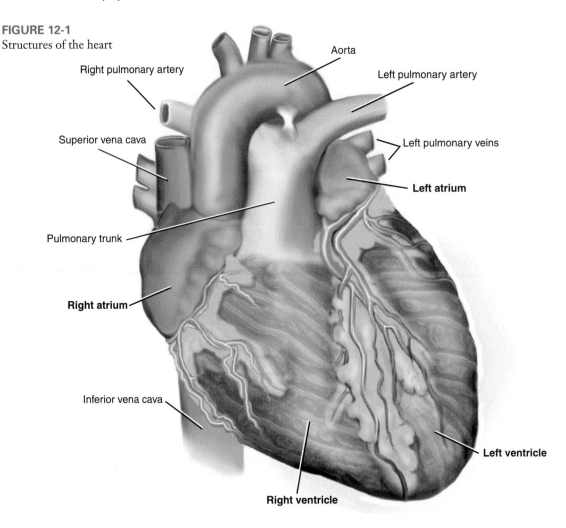

Aorta

Right pulmonary artery

Left pulmonary artery

Superior vena cava

Left pulmonary veins

Left atrium

Pulmonary trunk

Right atrium

Inferior vena cava

Left ventricle

Right ventricle

of the heart by strong, fibrous cords called the **chordae tendineae** (**KOR**-dee **TEN**-din-ee), which ensure that the valves close tightly, preventing backflow of blood (see Figure 12-2B).

Once blood has been pumped from the atria into the ventricles, it is pumped through half-moon–shaped valves called **semilunar valves**. The right ventricle pumps blood into the pulmonary artery through the **pulmonary semilunar valve**. The left ventricle pumps blood into the aorta through the **aortic semilunar valve**.

Memory Key	
• The heart has four chambers: right and left atria and right and left ventricles. • The septum separates the right and left sides of the heart. • The atrioventricular valves allow blood to flow from atria to ventricles. • The right atrioventricular valve is called the tricuspid valve. The left is called the bicuspid, or mitral, valve.	• The semilunar valves allow blood to flow from the ventricles to arteries. • The pulmonary semilunar valve allows blood to flow from the right ventricle into the pulmonary artery. • The aortic semilunar valve allows blood to flow from the left ventricle into the aorta.

FIGURE 12-2

Interior of the heart: (A) interior of the heart showing the chambers, valves, septum, and chordae tendineae; (B) photograph of chordae tendineae; (C) superior view of valves

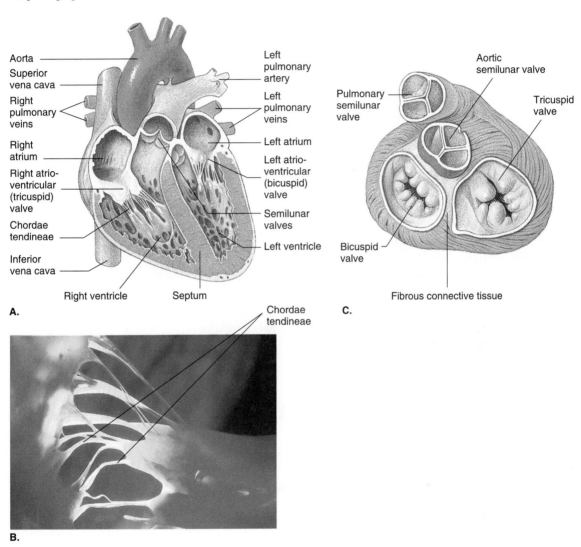

A.

B.

C.

WALLS OF THE HEART

The walls of the heart consist of three layers. The thick middle layer, the **myocardium** (**my**-oh-**KAR**-dee-um), consists of cardiac muscle tissue. The thin inside layer, the **endocardium** (**en**-do-**KAR**-dee-um), is epithelial tissue. The outer layer, the **epicardium** (**ep**-ih-**KAR**-dee-um), is connective and epithelial tissue. Each layer is illustrated in Figure 12-3.

Memory Key   From inside to out, the layers of the heart walls are endocardium, myocardium, and epicardium.

FIGURE 12-3
Heart walls

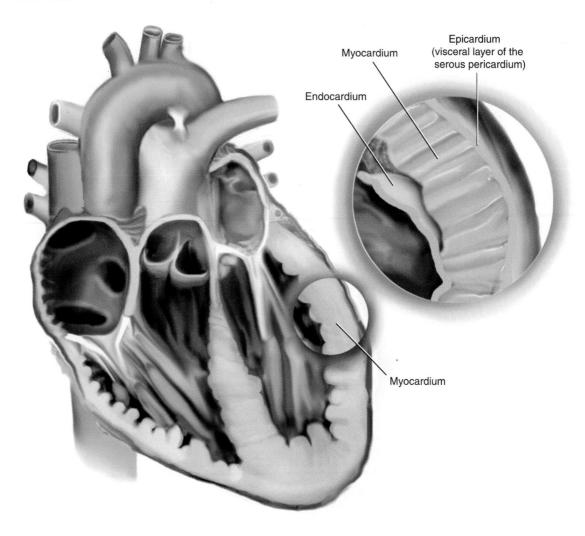

The heart is surrounded by the pericardium (Figure 12-4), which is a sac filled with **pericardial fluid**. Its outer covering is the **parietal** (pah-**RYE**-eh-tal) layer. The inner covering is the **visceral** (**VISS**-er-al) layer, which covers the heart and is another name for the epicardium referred to above.

Memory Key	• The pericardium is a sac filled with pericardial fluid.
	• The outer covering of the pericardium is the parietal layer.
	• The inner lining of the pericardium is the visceral layer, also called the epicardium.

FIGURE 12-4
Pericardium

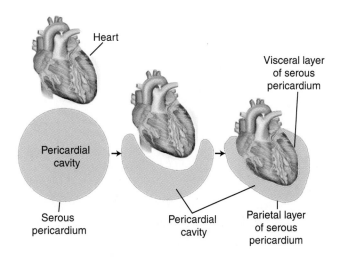

12.2   The Conduction System

If the heart is removed from the body, it will continue beating until it runs out of oxygen because it has its own electrical system, called the **conduction** (con-**DUCK**-shun) **system**. This system consists of the specialized network of muscle cells listed below and illustrated in Figure 12-5:

- **sinoatrial** (**sigh**-no-**AY**-tree-al) **node** (**SA node**, or pacemaker)
- **atrioventricular node** (**AV node**)
- **atrioventricular bundle** (**AV bundle**, or **bundle of His**)
- **right** and **left bundle branches**
- **Purkinje** (per-**KIN**-jee) **fibers**

The SA node spontaneously initiates electrical impulses that cause the heart to contract at regular intervals (60 to 95 beats per minute is a normal range). Because the SA node sets the rhythm for the heart, it is referred to as the **pacemaker**. The impulses from the SA node are transmitted to the AV node, which, like the SA node, is situated in the wall of the right atrium. The AV node causes both the right and left atria to contract simultaneously. For the next beat, the AV node sends an impulse to the AV bundle, which in turn sends the signal on to the Purkinje fibers. Because these fibers reach deep into the myocardium, they are able to stimulate the simultaneous contraction of the ventricles.

Memory Key	• The conduction system is the heart's electrical system. • The SA node (the pacemaker) initiates an impulse, which is sent to the AV node, causing the atria to contract, and then to the AV bundle and Purkinje fibers, causing the ventricles to contract.

FIGURE 12-5
Conduction system

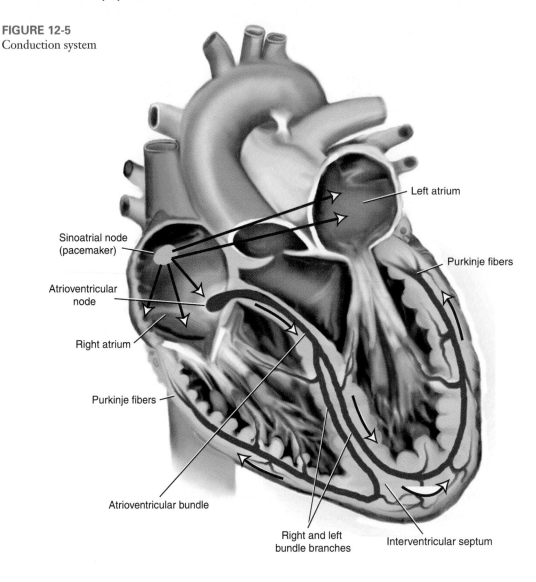

Left atrium

Sinoatrial node
(pacemaker)

Purkinje fibers

Atrioventricular
node

Right atrium

Purkinje fibers

Atrioventricular bundle

Right and left
bundle branches

Interventricular septum

An instrument called an **electrocardiograph** (ee-**leck**-troh-**KAR**-dee-oh-graff) can monitor and produce a written record of the electrical activity of the heart, called an electrocardiogram or ECG (EKG). This record consists of a series of waves, as illustrated in Figure 12-6. The P wave registers the atrial contraction, the QRS wave registers the ventricular contraction, and the T wave registers the recovery or repolarization of the ventricles. A measurement of the interval between P and R (the P-R interval) indicates how long it takes for impulses sent from the SA and AV nodes to reach the Purkinje fibers.

Memory Key	An ECG shows	P waves (atrial contraction)
		QRS waves (ventricular contraction)
		T waves (ventricular recovery)

FIGURE 12-6

Electrocardiogram: (A) the heart's function is monitored during exercise; (B) normal electrocardiogram showing P waves, QRS wave, T wave, P-R interval

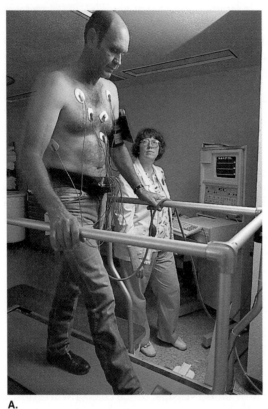

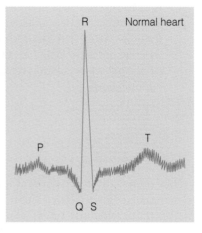

P = strength of atrial contraction

QRS = strength of ventricular contraction

T = resting state of ventricles

P-R interval = time required for impulses to travel from SA node to Purkinje fibers.

A.

B.

12.3   Blood Pressure

When the atria contract, the ventricles are at rest so that they can receive the blood pumped into them from the atria. Likewise, the atria are at rest when the ventricles are contracting. A heartbeat consists of one contraction phase of the ventricles, called the **systole** (**SIS**-toh-lee), and one resting phase, called the **diastole** (dye-**AS**-toh-lee). During the systole, blood is being forced under pressure out of the ventricles and into the arterial system. The arteries dilate, and this dilation is felt as a **pulse** at certain points in the body. The pressure of the blood against the arterial walls is called **blood pressure**. The pressure during systolic and diastolic phases is measured and expressed as two numbers by an instrument called a **sphygmomanometer** (**sfig**-moh-man-**OM**-eh-ter). **Systolic pressure** is the first number. It is higher because the ventricles are contracting during this phase. **Diastolic pressure**, the second number, is lower because it is a measure of pressure during the ventricular resting phase. A normal blood pressure measurement would range from

100/60 to 120/80. High blood pressure is called **hypertension**, and low blood pressure is called **hypotension**.

Memory Key	• A heartbeat consists of the systole (contraction phase) and diastole (resting phase).
	• The dilation of the arteries during the systolic phase is felt as a pulse.
	• Blood pressure is measured with a sphygmomanometer.
	• Systolic pressure is higher; diastolic pressure is lower.
	• Abnormally high blood pressure is called hypertension; low blood pressure is hypotension.

12.4 Heart Sounds

The sounds the heart makes as it beats come from the closing of the valves. When the atrioventricular valves close, a "lupp" sound is heard. This is called the **first heart sound**, or S_1. When the semilunar valves close, a "dubb" sound is heard. This is called the **second heart sound**, or S_2. A complete heartbeat, or a single cardiac cycle, consists of one "lupp-dubb." A **murmur** is a blowing sound indicative of abnormal blood flow.

Memory Key	• "Lupp" (S_1) is the sound of the atrioventricular valves closing.
	• "Dubb" (S_2) is the sound of the semilunar valves closing.

12.5 Blood Vessels

Blood is carried throughout the body by **blood vessels**, which consist of **arteries**, **arterioles** (ar-**TEE**-ree-ohlz), **veins**, **venules** (**VEN**-youlz), and **capillaries**.

Arteries are thick, muscular, and elastic, capable of expanding to accommodate the surge of blood when the heart contracts. Arteries branch off into smaller vessels called arterioles, which then lead into the capillaries, which are discussed later (see Figure 12-8). The arterial walls dilate and contract in unison with the heartbeat. These movements, known as a pulse, can be readily detected at certain sites. Pulses can be felt at the following arteries: temporal, carotid, brachial, radial, femoral, popliteal, and dorsalis pedis (see Figure 12-7).

Veins have the same composition as arteries, except that they are less elastic and muscular. Blood pressure in the veins is too low to push blood to the heart from areas such as the legs. Assistance is needed to overcome gravity. Skeletal muscle contraction helps, as does a system of tiny valves that prevent backflow of blood. If these valves are faulty, blood tends to pool in the veins of the legs, resulting in the condition known as varicose veins.

Capillaries are extremely tiny and have very thin walls, only one cell in thickness, composed of endothelium. They are embedded in the various organs of the body in **capillary beds**, which are large concentrations of capillaries. The capillary beds are the connection between the arterial and venous systems. The thin walls of the capillaries make the transfer of oxygen to the organs and carbon dioxide from the organs possible. It is the capillaries that feed the walls of the arteries and veins. As discussed in the next section, blood from capillaries empties into small veins called venules, which then lead to the veins.

Figure 12-8 illustrates the capillary, arterial, and venous relationship.

FIGURE 12-7
Pulse points of the body

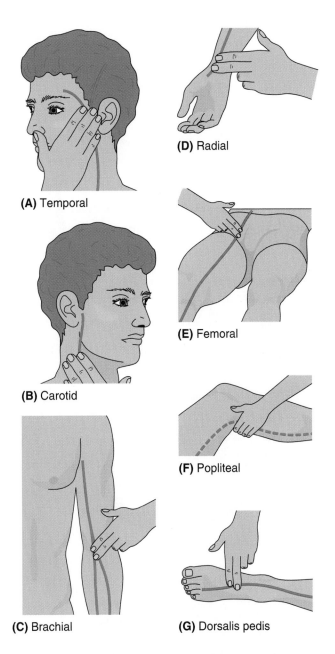

(A) Temporal

(B) Carotid

(C) Brachial

(D) Radial

(E) Femoral

(F) Popliteal

(G) Dorsalis pedis

Memory Key	• Blood vessels consist of

• Blood vessels consist of

    arteries   venules

    arterioles   capillaries

    veins

• Capillary beds are embedded in the organs.

• Capillaries feed the cells, take away waste, and connect the arterial and venous systems.

FIGURE 12-8
Schematic drawing of circulation through the lungs and body

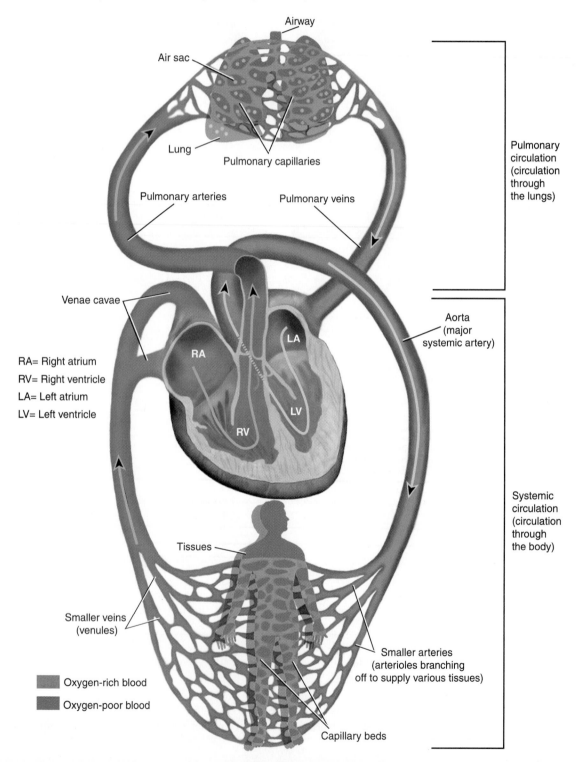

Airway

Air sac

Lung

Pulmonary capillaries

Pulmonary arteries

Pulmonary veins

Pulmonary circulation (circulation through the lungs)

Venae cavae

Aorta (major systemic artery)

LA

RA

LV

RV

RA= Right atrium
RV= Right ventricle
LA= Left atrium
LV= Left ventricle

Systemic circulation (circulation through the body)

Tissues

Smaller veins (venules)

Smaller arteries (arterioles branching off to supply various tissues)

Oxygen-rich blood

Oxygen-poor blood

Capillary beds

12.6   Circulation

Arteries (and arterioles) carry blood away from the heart, while veins (and venules) carry blood toward the heart. Although very tiny, capillaries are the most important vessels of all. Oxygenated blood is fed into them from the arterioles, and because they are located within the organs and have very thin walls (only one cell in thickness), they give off the oxygen to the organs. They then pick up carbon dioxide. The capillaries connect the arterial and venous systems, so that once the oxygen is distributed to the organs and carbon dioxide is picked up, the blood enters the venous system to begin its journey back to the heart.

Veins in the head and arms drain into the **superior vena cava**. Veins in the rest of the body drain into the **inferior vena cava**. Each of these major veins returns blood to the **right atrium**, where it is pumped into the **right ventricle** through the **tricuspid valve**. From there, it is pumped into the **pulmonary trunk**, through the **pulmonary semilunar valve** and through the **pulmonary arteries** to the **lungs**, where carbon dioxide in the blood is exchanged for oxygen, thus oxygenating the blood once again. The oxygenated blood returns through the **pulmonary veins** to the **left atrium** and is then pumped through the **bicuspid valve** into the **left ventricle**. Oxygenated blood is pumped out of the left ventricle, through the **aortic semilunar valve** into the **aorta**. It is then distributed to smaller arteries, branching out into the arterioles and ultimately reaching the capillaries, where oxygen and carbon dioxide transfer take place.

As you can see, all arteries except the pulmonary arteries carry oxygenated blood. Likewise, all veins except the pulmonary veins carry deoxygenated blood.

A simple illustration of the circulatory system appears in Figure 12-8.

> **Memory Key** • Circulation: superior and inferior venae cavae > right atrium > tricuspid valve > right ventricle > pulmonary semilunar valve > pulmonary arteries > lungs > pulmonary veins > left atrium > bicuspid valve > left ventricle > aortic semilunar valve > aorta > arteries > arterioles > capillaries > venules > veins.
> • All arteries except the pulmonaries carry oxygenated blood.
> • All veins except the pulmonaries carry deoxygenated blood.

The heart cannot feed itself from the blood that flows through it. Its walls are far too thick and muscular to absorb oxygen and give off carbon dioxide. It therefore requires its own system of capillaries to feed it, just as any other organ does, and this system of capillaries needs a system of arteries and veins to furnish oxygenated blood and carry away deoxygenated blood. These are the **coronary** arteries and veins (see Figure 12-9). A heart attack, or myocardial infarction (MI), is simply a blockage in one of the coronary arteries. Because oxygenated blood can no longer reach this part of the heart muscle, the muscle is damaged.

The risk of blockage in any of the arteries is minimized by the fact that the entire circulatory system has built-in parallel routes. Imagine it as a network of roads in a city. There is always more than one way to get somewhere. If one road is blocked off for repair, you just take another route. This is called **collateral** circulation.

Although there are some exceptions, arteries and veins are usually named after the organs through which they pass. For example, the kidneys have **renal** arteries and veins; the stomach has **gastric** arteries and veins. Capillaries are not named.

> **Memory Key** • The heart is fed by the coronary arteries.
> • The arterial system has parallel routes to allow for blockages.
> • Arteries and veins are usually named after the organ through which they pass.

FIGURE 12-9

Major coronary arteries: right coronary artery, left coronary artery, circumflex artery, right marginal branch, anterior and posterior interventricular arteries

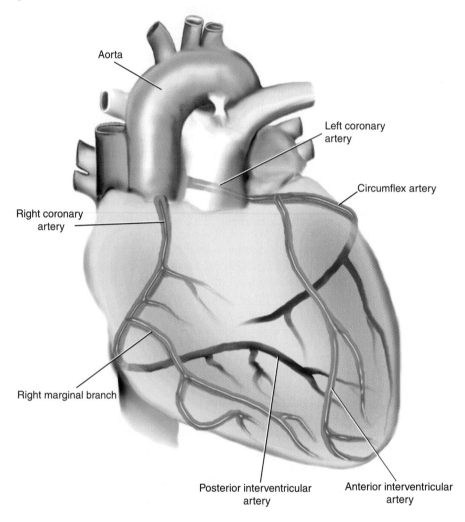

Aorta

Left coronary artery

Circumflex artery

Right coronary artery

Right marginal branch

Posterior interventricular artery

Anterior interventricular artery

12.7   Additional Word Elements

Use these additional word elements when studying the medical terms in this chapter.

Root	Meaning
constrict/o	to draw together
dilat/o	to expand

12.8   Term Analysis and Definition

	angi/o	vessel
Term	**Term Analysis**	**Definition**
angiography (**an**-jee-**OG**-rah-fee)	-graphy = process of recording	process of recording a blood vessel using x-rays following injection of a contrast medium (see Figure 12-10). *NOTE:* A contrast medium highlights internal structures, which are otherwise difficult to observe on an x-ray film.

FIGURE 12-10

An angiogram showing the femoral arteries

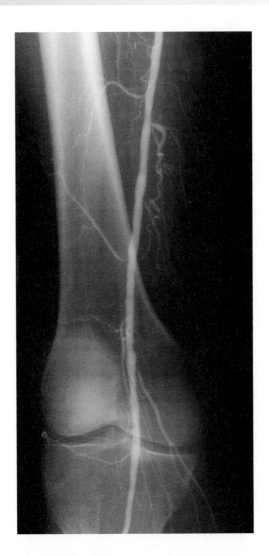

Term	Term Analysis	Definition
angioplasty (**AN**-jee-oh-**plas**-tee)	-plasty = surgical repair; surgical reconstruction	surgical repair of stenosed (narrowed) blood vessels. *NOTE:* Stenosis is caused by the accumulation of fatty debris on the artery wall. Balloon angioplasty flattens the fatty deposits against the walls of the artery, thereby increasing blood flow. In one type, percutaneous transluminal coronary angioplasty (PTCA) shown in Figure 12-11, a balloon-tipped catheter flattens the fatty plaque. A tiny support structure called a **stent** may be placed inside the artery to keep the artery open. Cells quickly grow over the stent, providing a smooth inner lining.

FIGURE 12-11
Percutaneous transluminal coronary angioplasty

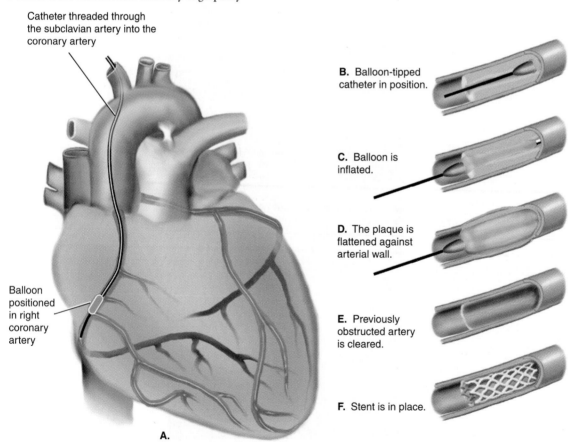

Catheter threaded through the subclavian artery into the coronary artery

Balloon positioned in right coronary artery

B. Balloon-tipped catheter in position.

C. Balloon is inflated.

D. The plaque is flattened against arterial wall.

E. Previously obstructed artery is cleared.

F. Stent is in place.

A.

Term	Term Analysis	Definition
angiospasm (**AN**-jee-oh-spazm)	-spasm = sudden, involuntary contraction	sudden, involuntary contraction of a blood vessel; vasospasm
	aort/o	**aorta**
aortostenosis (ay-**or**-toh-sten-**OH**-sis)	-stenosis = narrowing	narrowing of the aorta
	arteri/o	**artery**
arteriography (**ar**-tee-ree-**OG**-rah-fee)	-graphy = process of recording	process of recording the arteries using x-rays and following injection of a contrast medium
arteriole (ar-**TEE**-ree-ohl)	-ole = small	small arteries
arteriosclerosis (ar-**tee**-ree-oh-skleh-**ROH**-sis)	-sclerosis = hardening	hardening of the arteries due to the loss of elasticity of the arterial walls
arteriostenosis (ar-**tee**-ree-oh-steh-**NOH**-sis)	-stenosis = narrowing	narrowing of an artery
endarterectomy (**end**-ar-ter-**ECK**-toh-mee)	-ectomy = surgical removal; excision endo- = within	removal of the inner lining of the arterial wall. A surgical procedure used to treat atherosclerosis (see atherosclerosis below)
	ather/o	**fatty debris; fatty plaque**
atheroma (**ath**-er-**OH**-mah)	-oma = mass; tumor	fatty mass or debris (see Figure 12-12)
atherosclerosis (**ath**-er-oh-skleh-**ROH**-sis)	-sclerosis = hardening	accumulation of fatty debris on the inner arterial wall. A type of arteriosclerosis (see Figure 12-12)

	atri/o	**atrium (upper chamber of the heart)**
Term	**Term Analysis**	**Definition**
interatrial septum (**in**-ter-**AY**-tree-al)	-al = pertaining to inter- = between septum = wall	wall between the atria

	cardi/o	**heart**
cardiologist (**kar**-dee-**OL**-oh-jist)	-logist = specialist	specialist in the study of cardiology
cardiology (**kar**-dee-**OL**-oh-jee)	-logy = study of	the study of the heart, including the diagnosis and treatment of heart disorders
cardiomegaly (**kar**-dee-oh-**MEG**-ah-lee)	-megaly = enlargement	enlarged heart
electrocardiogram (ee-**leck**-troh-**KAR**-dee-oh-**gram**)	-gram = record **electr/o** = electric	record of the electrical activity of the heart
myocardial (**my**-oh-**KAR**-dee-al)	-al = pertaining to **my/o** = muscle	pertaining to the heart muscle
myocardiopathy (**my**-oh-**kar**-dee-**OP**-ah-thee)	-pathy = disease **my/o** = muscle	disease of the heart muscle
pancarditis (**pan**-kar-**DYE**-tis)	-itis = inflammation pan- = all	inflammation of all the walls of the heart, including the epicardium, myocardium, and endocardium
pericarditis (**per**-ih-kar-**DYE**-tis)	-itis = inflammation peri- = around	inflammation of the pericardium
pericardium (**per**-ih-**KAR**-dee-um)	-um = structure peri- = around	structure around the heart

	coron/o	**crown**
coronary arteries (**KOR**-uh-**nerr**-ee)	-ary = pertaining to	the arteries that supply the heart with blood. *NOTE:* The coronary arteries sit on top of the heart like a crown.

	ech/o	sound
Term	**Term Analysis**	**Definition**
echocardiogram (**eck**-oh-**KAR**-dee-oh-**gram**)	-gram = record **cardi/o** = heart	record of the heart produced by sound waves
	embol/o	**plug**
embolus (**EM**-boh-lus)	-us = condition; thing	a plug of clotted blood that is transported through the bloodstream by the blood current. *NOTE:* An embolus can cause arterial obstruction, resulting in loss of blood to a part. It may be fatal.
	isch/o	**hold back**
myocardial ischemia (**my**-oh-**KAR**-dee-al iss-**KEE**-me-ah)	-emia = blood condition -al = pertaining to **my/o** = muscle **cardi/o** = heart	a hold back of blood to the heart muscle. *NOTE:* Myocardial ischemia leads to **myocardial infarction**, which is the area of tissue that has undergone necrosis (death) due to a lack of blood supply to the heart (see Figure 12-12). A common symptom of myocardial ischemia is **angina pectoris**, which is defined as severe chest pain.
	phleb/o	**vein**
phlebothrombosis (**fleb**-oh-throm-**BOH**-sis)	-osis = abnormal condition **thromb/o** = clot	abnormal condition of clots in a vein
thrombophlebitis (**throm**-boh-fleh-**BYE**-tis)	-itis = inflammation **thromb/o** = clot	inflammation of a vein with clot formation
	rhythm/o	**rhythm**
arrhythmia (ah-**RITH**-mee-ah)	-ia = state of; condition; process a(n)- = no; not	deviation from the normal heart rhythm

FIGURE 12-12
Ischemia

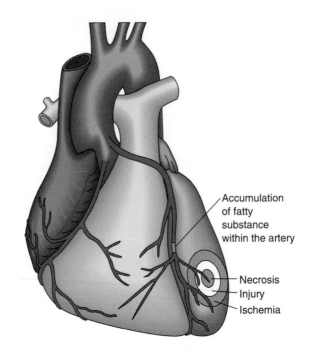

Accumulation
of fatty
substance
within the artery

Necrosis
Injury
Ischemia

	scler/o	hardening
Term	**Term Analysis**	**Definition**
sclerotherapy (**skleh**-roh-**THER**-ah-pee)	-therapy = treatment	injection of a solution into a vein for the purpose of destroying the vein's inner lining by sclerosis. *NOTE:* Sclerotherapy is very effective in treating varicose veins (see below) and requires no hospitalization.
	thromb/o	**clot**
thrombus (**THROM**-bus)	-us = condition; thing	a blood clot that obstructs a blood vessel
	valvul/o	**valve**
valvuloplasty (**VAL**-view-loh-**plas**-tee)	-plasty = surgical repair; surgical reconstruction	surgical repair of a valve

	varic/o	**twisted and swollen**
Term varicose veins (**VAR**-ih-kohs)	**Term Analysis** -ose = pertaining to	**Definition** twisted, swollen superficial veins, typically of the **saphenous** vein of the lower leg (see Figure 12-13). *NOTE:* Varicose veins occur when incompetent valves in the vein fail to push the blood forward, causing backflow of blood. Veins become dilated, and blood stagnates, creating unsightly clusters of protruding veins.
	vascul/o	**vessel**
avascular (a-**VAS**-kyou-lar)	a- = not -ar = pertaining to	pertaining to no blood vessels

FIGURE 12-13

(A) Schematic drawing of normal veins with normal valves, (B) schematic drawing of varicose veins and abnormal valves, (C) photograph of varicose veins

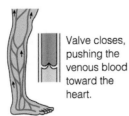 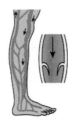 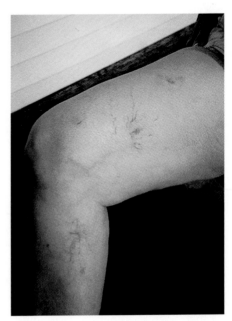

Valve closes, pushing the venous blood toward the heart.

A. Normal veins

Valves remain open, pooling the blood in the veins.

B. Varicose veins

C.

Term	Term Analysis	Definition
cerebrovascular accident (CVA) (**ser**-eh-broh-**VAS**-kyou-lar)	-ar = pertaining to **cerebr/o** = brain	disturbance in the flow of blood to one or more parts of the brain; commonly known as a stroke
	vas/o	**vein**
extravasation (ecks-**trav**-ah-**SAY**-shun)	-ion = process extra- = outside	escape of fluid into the surrounding tissue; for example, the escape of blood from a blood vessel into the surrounding tissue
vasoconstriction (**vas**-oh-kon-**STRICK**-shun)	-ion = process **constrict/o** = to draw together	process of drawing together the walls of a vessel; narrowing of the lumen; vasospasm
vasodilation (**vas**-oh-dye-**LAY**-shun)	-ion = process **dilat/o** = to expand	process of vessel expansion; widening of the vessel
	ven/o	**vein**
venous (**VEE**-nus)	-ous = pertaining to	pertaining to a vein
venule (**VEN**-youl)	-ule = small	small vein
	ventricul/o	**ventricle (lower chamber of the heart)**
interventricular septum (**in**-ter-ven-**TRICK**-you-lar)	-ar = pertaining to inter- = between septum = wall	pertaining to the wall between the ventricles

SUFFIXES

	-ectasis	**dilation; dilatation; stretching**
Term	**Term Analysis**	**Definition**
angiectasis (**an**-jee-**ECK**-tah-sis)	**angi/o** = vessel	dilation of a blood vessel

PREFIXES

	-brady	slow
Term	**Term Analysis**	**Definition**
bradycardia (**brad**-ee-**KAR**-dee-uh)	-ia = condition; state of **cardi/o** = heart	slow heartbeat
	-tachy	**fast**
tachycardia (**tack**-ee-**KAR**-dee-ah)	-ia = condition; state of **cardi/o** = heart	fast heartbeat

Memory Key   In *bradycardia* and *tachycardia*, both the *i* and the *o* are dropped from **cardi/o**; the suffix is -ia, meaning "condition" or "state of."

12.9   Review of Terms

Define the terms in Tables 12-1 through 12-4 in the space provided.

TABLE 12-1

REVIEW OF ANATOMICAL TERMS

arteriole	cardiologist	cardiology
coronary arteries	interatrial septum	interventricular septum
myocardial	pericardium	vascular
venous	venule	

TABLE 12-2

REVIEW OF PATHOLOGIC TERMS

angiectasis	angiospasm	aortostenosis
arrhythmia	arteriosclerosis	arteriostenosis
atheroma	atherosclerosis	bradycardia
cardiomegaly	cerebrovascular accident	embolus
extravasation	myocardial ischemia	myocardiopathy
pancarditis	pericarditis	phlebothrombosis
tachycardia	thrombophlebitis	thrombus
vasoconstriction	vasodilation	varicose veins

TABLE 12-3

REVIEW OF DIAGNOSTIC TERMS

angiography	arteriography	echocardiogram
electrocardiogram		

TABLE 12-4

REVIEW OF SURGICAL PROCEDURES

angioplasty	endarterectomy	sclerotherapy
valvuloplasty		

12.10 Abbreviations

Abbreviation	Meaning
AV	atrioventricular
ASHD	arteriosclerotic heart disease (damage to the heart due to the obstruction of a coronary artery)
BP	blood pressure
CABG	coronary artery bypass graft (a procedure performed to reestablish adequate circulation to one or more segments of the heart when coronary artery disease diminishes blood flow. A section of vein is removed from the leg or breast and used as a graft to reroute the blood around the blockage.)
CAD	coronary artery disease
CCU	cardiac/coronary care unit
CHF	congestive heart failure (myocardial disease results in the failure of the heart to pump blood effectively through the blood vessels, resulting in congestion or pooling of blood in the veins)
CPR	cardiopulmonary resuscitation
CV	cardiovascular
CVA	cerebrovascular accident
ECG; EKG	electrocardiogram
HHD	hypertensive heart disease (with long-term high blood pressure, the heart needs to work harder to pump the blood through the blood vessels; over time this extra work damages the heart)
IVC	inferior vena cava
LA	left atrium

continued on page 266

continued from page 265

Abbreviation	Meaning
LV	left ventricle
MI	myocardial infarction
MVP	mitral valve prolapse (incomplete closure of the mitral valve resulting in the backflow of blood into the left atrium from the left ventricle)
PVC	premature ventricular contraction
RA	right atrium
RV	right ventricle
SA	sinoatrial
SVC	superior vena cava

12.11 Putting It All Together

Exercise 12-1   SHORT ANSWER

1. List the structures through which blood passes in the oxygenation of tissues. Start with the right atrium and end with the superior and inferior venae cavae.

_____

_____

_____

2. Differentiate between the pericardium, myocardium, endocardium, and epicardium. Which structure is the same as the visceral pericardium?

_____

_____

_____

3. What is the function of the conduction system? List five structures of the conduction system. Which structure is known as the pacemaker? Why?

_____

_____

_____

_____

_____

_____

4. Define:

a. systolic pressure   _____

b. diastolic pressure   _____

c. sphygmomanometer   _____

d. P wave   _____

e. P-R interval   _____

5. How are arteries and veins named?

_____

Exercise 12-2   OPPOSITES

Give the opposite of the following terms.

1. vasodilation   _____

2. hypertension   _____

3. bradycardia   _____

4. diastole   _____

Exercise 12-3   ROOTS AND DEFINITIONS

Underline the root(s) and give the definition of the following terms.

1. endarterectomy   _____

2. interatrial   _____

3. pancarditis   _____

4. echocardiogram   _____

5. phlebothrombosis _____

6. cerebrovascular accident _____

7. atheroma _____

Exercise 12-4   BUILDING MEDICAL TERMS

Build the medical term for the following definitions.

1. dilation of a blood vessel _____

2. process of recording a blood vessel _____

3. surgical repair of a stenosed blood vessel _____

4. sudden, involuntary contraction of blood vessels _____

5. process of recording arteries _____

6. small arteries _____

7. hardening of the artery _____

8. pertaining to a vein _____

9. small vein _____

10. specialist in the study of the heart _____

Exercise 12-5   DEFINITIONS

Define the following terms.

1. atherosclerosis _____

2. myocardial ischemia _____

3. thrombophlebitis _____

4. extravasation _____

5. electrocardiogram _____

Exercise 12-6   SPELLING

Circle any misspelled words in the list below and correctly spell them in the space provided.

1. paricardium _____

2. ventrical _____

3. atrium _____

4. myocardeum _____

5. capillaries _____

6. Purkinje _____

7. sfigmomanometer _____

8. extravasashun _____

9. bicuspit _____

10. lumen _____

Exercise 12-7   ADJECTIVAL FORMS

Give the adjectival form for the following.

1. vessel _____

2. aorta _____

3. artery _____

4. atrium _____

5. heart _____

6. valve _____

7. vein _____

8. ventricle _____

CHAPTER

13

Blood and the Immune and Lymphatic Systems

CHAPTER ORGANIZATION

This chapter will help you learn about blood and the immune and lymphatic systems. It is divided into the following sections:

CHAPTER OBJECTIVES

On completion of this chapter, you will be able to do the following:

1. Name and describe the components of the blood

2. Define terms relating to the immune system

3. Locate and describe the organs of the lymphatic system

4. Analyze, define, pronounce, and spell terms related to the blood and the immune and lymphatic systems

5. Define common abbreviations related to the blood and the immune and lymphatic systems

INTRODUCTION

In the chapter on the skeletal system, you learned that blood cells are formed in the red bone marrow. When you studied the cardiovascular system, you learned about the veins and arteries that transport blood throughout the body and how blood functions to provide oxygen and nutrients to the organs and carry away wastes. In this chapter, you will learn about the makeup of the blood, and the important role it plays in fighting disease. You will also learn about the body's other circulatory system, the lymphatic system, and how it functions together with the circulatory (blood) system to protect us from infection.

13.1   The Blood

Whole blood is about 55% liquid and 45% solid, as illustrated in Figure 13-1. The liquid is called **plasma** (**PLAZ**-mah). The solid portion is referred to as **formed elements** and consists of three types of blood cell: **red blood cells** (**RBCs**), or **erythrocytes** (eh-**RITH**-roh-sights); **white blood cells** (**WBCs**), or **leukocytes** (**LOO**-koh-sights); and **platelets** (**PLAYT**-lets), or **thrombocytes** (**THROM**-boh-sights). Because plasma is more than 90% water, it is thin and almost colorless when it is separated from the blood cells.

Memory Key	Blood consists of plasma and the following formed elements: erythrocytes (RBCs), leukocytes (WBCs), and thrombocytes (platelets).

In addition to carrying the blood cells, plasma transports fats, proteins, gases, salts, and hormones to their various destinations throughout the body and picks up waste materials from organ cells. The fats, such as **triglyceride** (try-**GLIS**-er-eyed), **phospholipid** (fos-foh-**LIP**-id), and **cholesterol** (koh-**LES**-ter-ol), are transported to tissues by attaching to proteins. The plasma proteins are **albumin** (al-**BYOU**-min), **globulin** (**GLOB**-you-lin), and **fibrinogen** (figh-**BRIN**-oh-jen). Fibrinogen is the blood-clotting agent. When fibrinogen and other clotting factors are removed, the plasma is called **serum** (**SEER**-um).

Memory Key	• Plasma carries the	
	blood cells	gases
	fats (triglyceride, phospholipid, and cholesterol)	salts
	proteins (albumin, globulin, and fibrinogen)	hormones
	• Serum is plasma with fibrinogen and other clotting factors removed.	

Blood cells start out as undifferentiated cells called **hemocytoblasts** (hee-moh-**SIGHT**-oh-blasts), also called **stem cells**. The general process of their development into specialized blood cells is called **hematopoiesis** (hee-mah-toh-poi-**EE**-sis). The specific process for the development of erythrocytes is called **erythropoiesis** (eh-**rith**-roh-poi-**EE**-sis); for leukocytes, it is **leukopoiesis** (**loo**-koh-poi-**EE**-sis); and for thrombocytes it is **thrombopoiesis** (**throm**-boh-poi-**EE**-sis).

Memory Key	• Hemocytoblasts develop into blood cells by hematopoiesis.
	• The specific processes are erythropoiesis, leukopoiesis, and thrombopoiesis.

FIGURE 13-1
Plasma, formed elements, erythrocytes, leukocytes, and thrombocytes

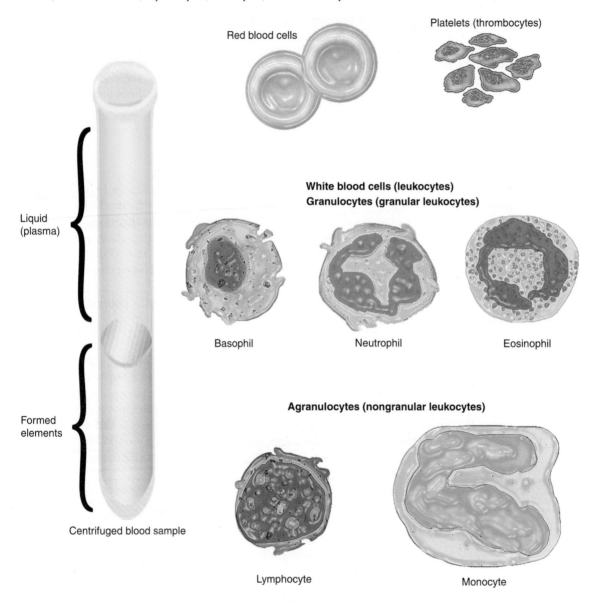

Red blood cells

Platelets (thrombocytes)

White blood cells (leukocytes)
Granulocytes (granular leukocytes)

Basophil   Neutrophil   Eosinophil

Agranulocytes (nongranular leukocytes)

Liquid
(plasma)

Formed
elements

Centrifuged blood sample

Lymphocyte   Monocyte

Erythrocytes (RBCs) are shaped like biconcave discs. They contain **hemoglobin** (Hgb) (**hee**-moh-**GLOH**-bin), a protein that contains iron and has the ability to bind with oxygen and carbon dioxide. This ability enables the blood to transport oxygen to the organ cells and carbon dioxide away from them. Erythropoiesis, the maturation process for red blood cells, involves several stages. In the second-to-last stage, the cell is called a **reticulocyte** (reh-**TICK**-you-loh-**sight**). Once the reticulocyte becomes an erythrocyte, it leaves the red bone marrow and enters the bloodstream, where it can be measured in a laboratory test called a

reticulocyte count. This test is a direct indication of the bone marrow's production of red blood cells. After approximately 120 days, the erythrocyte ruptures and dies, releasing hemoglobin, which eventually finds its way back to the bone marrow to be recycled.

Memory Key	• RBCs (erythrocytes) contain hemoglobin, which transports oxygen and carbon dioxide. • Reticulocytes develop into RBCs. • RBCs live about 120 days, then rupture.

Leukocytes (white blood cells) fight infections. They have the ability to migrate from the bloodstream into the tissues to the site of infection. They are classified as either **granular** or **agranular** (see Figure 13-1). The granular leukocytes are further classified as either **eosinophils** (ee-oh-**SIN**-oh-fills), **basophils** (**BAY**-soh-fills), or **neutrophils** (**NEW**-troh-fills). The eosinophils release chemicals into the bloodstream that can neutralize toxic substances. The basophils release **histamine**, a natural toxin that initiates the inflammatory process by dilating the blood vessels. This dilation increases blood flow into the site of the infection, thereby speeding recovery. Neutrophils, also known as **polymorphonuclear** (**poly**-more-foh-**NEW**-klee-ar) leukocytes, ingest bacteria and other harmful matter through a process called phagocytosis (**fag**-oh-sigh-**TOH**-sis). The agranular leukocytes are classified as either **monocytes** (**MON**-oh-sights) or **lymphocytes** (**LIM**-foh-sights). Monocytes act much like neutrophils, ingesting harmful microorganisms. Lymphocytes are important in the immune system, discussed below.

Memory Key	WBCs (leukocytes) fight infection and are either granular (eosinophils, basophils, and neutrophils) or agranular (monocytes and lymphocytes).

Thrombocytes (or platelets, because of their platelike appearance) initiate blood clotting when bleeding occurs. Through the release of clotting agents such as **prothrombin** (pro-**THROM**-bin) and fibrinogen, a platelet plug is formed where a vessel wall has ruptured, thus halting bleeding.

Memory Key	Platelets (thrombocytes) release prothrombin and fibrinogen for blood clotting.

Any substance that stimulates the body's immune response (bacteria, viruses, and pollens, for example) is referred to as an **antigen** (**AN**-tih-jen), which is an abbreviation for the term "antibody generator." Specific to our discussion on blood cells, there are two types of proteins on the surface of the red blood cells that are antigens. They are referred to as type A and type B antigens. Blood is classified as type **A, B, AB,** or **O,** depending on the presence or absence of these antigens. Type A blood has only type A antigens, type B has only type B antigens; AB has both, and O has neither. The type of blood a person receives in a transfusion depends on the presence or absence of the A, B, AB, and O antigens. If a person receives the wrong type of blood, blood that does not match his or her own blood type, **antibodies** will be formed against the specific antigen as they recognize the antigen to be foreign to the body. This is an antigen-antibody reaction. Persons with type A blood generate antibodies if type B blood is injected into them. Those with type B blood generate antibodies if type A blood is injected into them. Persons with AB blood can accept any type. Type O persons require type O blood but can donate to all others. The antigen-antibody reaction may cause a clumping of red blood cells, or **agglutination**. It is for this reason that the blood must be **cross-matched** before it is transfused into a patient. In cross-matching, the donor's blood is mixed with the recipient's blood and analyzed for agglutination.

> **Memory Key** | Type A blood has only type A antigens; type B blood has only type B antigens; type AB has both; and type O has neither.

There are several other blood antigens. The most important is the **Rh antigen**, which was first discovered by examining the blood of Rhesus monkeys. Most people are **Rh positive**, meaning they have the Rh antigen. Those who lack it are Rh negative.

> **Memory Key** | Most people are Rh positive (have Rh antigen).

13.2   Additional Word Elements

Use these additional word elements when studying the medical terms in this chapter.

Root	Meaning
anis/o	unequal
bilirubin/o	bilirubin (a bile pigment)
cholesterol/o	cholesterol
granul/o	granules
lipid/o	fat
norm/o	normal
poikil/o	variation; irregular

Suffix	Meaning
-edema	accumulation of fluid

13.3   Term Analysis and Definition Pertaining to the Blood

	chrom/o	color
Term	**Term Analysis**	**Definition**
hyperchromia (**high**-per-**KROH**-mee-ah)	-ia = condition; state of hyper- = excessive; above normal	excessively pigmented red blood cells
hypochromia (**high**-poh-**KROH**-mee-ah)	-ia = condition; state of hypo- = below; deficient	underpigmented red blood cells
normochromia (**nor**-moh-**KROH**-mee-ah)	-ia = condition; state of **norm/o** = normal	normally pigmented red blood cells

	erythr/o	red
erythrocyte (eh-**RITH**-roh-sight)	-cyte = cell	red blood cell

	hemat/o; hem/o	blood
hemolysis (hee-**MOL**-ih-sis)	-lysis = breakdown separation; destruction	breakdown of blood
hematologist (**hee**-mah-**TOL**-oh-jist)	-logist = specialist	specialist in the study of blood and blood disorders
hematology (**hee**-mah-**TOL**-oh-jee)	-logy = study of	study of blood and blood disorders

	leuk/o	white
leukocyte (**LOO**-koh-sight)	-cyte = cell	white blood cell

	myel/o	bone marrow
Term	**Term Analysis**	**Definition**
myelogenous (**my**-eh-**LOJ**-en-us)	-genous = produced by	produced by the bone marrow
myeloid (**MY**-eh-loid)	-oid = resembling	resembling bone marrow

	reticul/o	network
reticulocyte (reh-**TICK**-you-loh-sight)	-cyte = cell	a young red blood cell characterized by a network of granules within the cell membrane

	thromb/o	clot
thrombocyte (**THROM**-boh-sight)	-cyte = cell	clotting cell; platelet
thrombolysis (throm-**BOL**-ih-sis)	-lysis = destruction; breakdown; separation	breakdown of a clot that has formed in the blood
thrombosis (throm-**BOH**-sis)	-osis = abnormal condition	blood clot; abnormal condition of clot formation

SUFFIXES

	-blast	**immature, growing thing**
Term	**Term Analysis**	**Definition**
hemocytoblast (**hee**-moh-**SIGHT**-oh-blast)	**hem/o** = blood **cyt/o** = cell	immature blood cell
lymphoblast (**LIM**-foh-blast)	**lymph/o** = lymph	immature lymphocyte
monoblast (**MON**-oh-blast)	**mon/o** = one	immature monocyte

	-crit	**separate**
hematocrit (HCT) (he-**MAT**-oh-krit)	**hemat/o** = blood	a laboratory test that determines the percentage of erythrocytes in a blood sample

	-cytosis	**increase in the number of cells**

Term	**Term Analysis**	**Definition**
anisocytosis (an-**eye**-soh-sigh-**TOH**-sis)	**anis/o** = unequal	increased variation in the size of cells, particularly red blood cells
leukocytosis (**loo**-koh-sigh-**TOH**-sis)	**leuk/o** = white	marked increase in the number of white blood cells
poikilocytosis (**poi**-kil-oh-sigh-**TOH**-sis)	**poikil/o** = variation; irregular	increased variation in the shape of cells, particularly red blood cells

	-emia	**blood condition**
anemia (ah-**NEE**-mee-ah)	an- = no; not; lack of	lack of red blood cells or hemoglobin content in the blood
erythremia (er-ih-**THREE**-mee-ah)	**erythr/o** = red	abnormal increase in the number of red blood cells. *NOTE:* Erythremia is a chronic, life-threatening condition, cause unknown. Also called polycythemia vera.
hyperbilirubinemia (**high**-per-**bil**-ih-**roo**-bih-**NEE**-mee-ah)	hyper- = excessive; above normal **bilirubin/o** = bilirubin (a bile pigment)	excessive amounts of bilirubin in the blood
hypercholesterolemia (**high**-per-koh-**les**-ter-ol-**EE**-mee-ah)	hyper- = excessive; above normal **cholesterol/o** = cholesterol	excessive amounts of cholesterol in the blood
hyperlipidemia (**high**-per-**lip**-ih-**DEE**-mee-ah)	hyper- = excessive; above normal **lipid/o** = fat	excessive amounts of fats in the blood
leukemia (loo-**KEE**-mee-ah)	**leuk/o** = white	malignant increase in the number of white blood cells in the blood; considered a form of cancer

	-penia	**deficient; decrease**
Term	**Term Analysis**	**Definition**
erythrocytopenia (eh-**rith**-roh-**sigh**-toh-**PEE**-nee-ah)	**erythr/o** = red **cyt/o** = cell	decrease in the number of red blood cells
leukocytopenia (**loo**-koh-**sigh**-toh-**PEE**-nee-ah)	**leuk/o** = white **cyt/o** = cell	decrease in the number of white blood cells
pancytopenia (**pan**-sigh-toh-**PEE**-nee-ah)	pan- = all **cyt/o** = cell	decrease in the number of all blood cells
thrombocytopenia (**throm**-boh-**sigh**-toh-**PEE**-nee-ah)	**thromb/o** = clot **cyt/o** = cell	decrease in the number of clotting cells
	-phoresis	**transmission; carry**
electrophoresis (ee-**leck**-troh-for-**EE**-sis)	**electr/o** = electric	a laboratory test in which substances in a mixture, usually proteins, are separated by an electrical current
	-poiesis	**production; manufacture; formation**
erythropoiesis (eh-**rith**-roh-poi-**EE**-sis)	**erythr/o** = red	production of red blood cells
hematopoiesis (**hee**-mah-toh-poi-**EE**-sis)	**hemat/o** = blood	production of blood cells
	-poietin	**hormones regulating the production of blood cells**
erythropoietin (eh-**rith**-roh-**POI**-eh-tin)	**erythr/o** = red	a hormone in the kidney that stimulates the production of red blood cells
	-stasis	**stopping; controlling**
hemostasis (**hee**-moh-**STAY**-sis)	**hem/o** = blood	stoppage of blood

13.4   Review of Terms Pertaining to the Blood

Define the terms in Tables 13-1 through 13-3 in the space provided.

TABLE 13-1

REVIEW OF ANATOMICAL TERMS

erythrocyte	erythropoiesis	erythropoietin
hematologist	hematology	hematopoiesis
hemocytoblast	leukocyte	lymphoblast
monoblast	myelogenous	myeloid
normochromia	reticulocyte	thrombocyte

TABLE 13-2

REVIEW OF PATHOLOGIC TERMS

agranulocytosis	anemia	anisocytosis
erythremia	erythrocytopenia	hemolysis
hyperbilirubinemia	hypercholesterolemia	hyperchromia
hyperlipidemia	hypochromia	leukemia
leukocytopenia	leukocytosis	pancytopenia
poikilocytosis	thrombocytopenia	thrombolysis
thrombosis		

TABLE 13-3

REVIEW OF DIAGNOSTIC TESTS AND CLINICAL PROCEDURES

electrophoresis	hematocrit	hemostasis

13.5   Abbreviations Pertaining to the Blood

Abbreviation	Meaning
ABO	three main blood groups
CBC	complete blood count
diff	differential count (laboratory test to determine the number of different types of white blood cells)
eos	eosinophil
ESR	erythrocyte sedimentation rate
Hb; Hgb	hemoglobin
HCT; HcT	hematocrit
lymphs	lymphocytes
mono	monocyte
PMN	polymorphonuclear
polys	polymorphonuclear leukocytes
RBC; rbc	red blood cell
segs	segmented polymorphonuclear leukocytes
WBC; wbc	white blood cell

13.6   The Immune System

As mentioned above, lymphocytes are one of the two types of agranular leukocytes and are responsible for initiating the immune response. Two types of lymphocytes are involved: **T lymphocytes (T cells)**, which are produced in the red bone marrow but mature in the thymus, and **B lymphocytes (B cells)**, which develop and mature in the red bone marrow.

Memory Key	Lymphocytes are agranular leukocytes. They are of two types: T lymphocytes (T cells) and B lymphocytes (B cells).

T cells protect us through a process called **cellular immunity**. These cells have the ability to recognize viral invasion of the body's cells. The T cell attacks and kills the infected cell, and the virus is unable to replicate itself. When enough infected cells have been killed, the viral infection abates. T cells also recognize and kill cancerous cells. Because T cells will detect and kill foreign cells, their activity will lead to rejection of transplanted organs unless drugs are administered to prevent their doing so.

Memory Key	T cells provide cellular immunity by killing virus-infected cells. They also kill cancerous cells and foreign cells.

B cells utilize a different process called **humoral** (**HEW**-moh-ral) **immunity**. They produce **antibodies** called immunoglobulins (Igs). **Immunoglobulins** (im-you-no-**GLOB**-you-lins) are proteins that travel through the circulatory system and have the ability to attach to foreign cells, labeling them for destruction by bacteria-eating white blood cells called **phagocytes** (**FAG**-oh-sights). B cells are particularly effective against bacterial infections. **Humoral** refers to body fluids or substances contained in them. Antibodies, which play a significant part in humoral immunity, are substances found in the blood.

Memory Key	B cells provide humoral immunity by producing antibodies that attach to foreign cells, such as bacteria, labeling them for destruction by phagocytes.

T cells and B cells create memory cells that remember how a particular invader was killed. These memory cells are permanently stored in the **lymphoid** (**LIM**-foid) tissue. When the same invader comes along again, the memory cells know precisely how to deal with it and dispatch it much more quickly than the first time, so quickly in fact, that we are usually unaware of these subsequent infections.

Memory Key	T cells and B cells create memory cells that remember how an invader was killed, thus allowing the body to readily deal with a new infection of that type.

13.7   The Lymphatic System

The **lymphatic** (lim-**FAH**-tick) **system** consists of a vascular system, fluid called **lymph** (**LIMF**), the lymph nodes, the **thymus** (**THIGH**-mus) **gland**, the **spleen**, the **tonsils**, and **Peyer's** (**PIE**-erz) **patches**. It is illustrated in Figure 13-2. The lymphatic system serves a number of important functions in the body. Of primary importance is the task of draining excess fluids away from body tissues into the bloodstream. It also carries nutrients, hormones, and oxygen to body tissues and transports lipids (fat cells) from the digestive system. Because of the presence of lymphocytes and monocytes, this system also plays an important role in the body's defense against infection.

Memory Key	
• The lymphatic system consists of	

    a vascular system   thymus gland   Peyer's patches

    lymph   spleen

    lymph nodes   tonsils

• This system drains fluids; carries nutrients, hormones, oxygen, and fats; and fights infection.

The vascular system consists of three types of vessels. The smallest are the **lymphatic capillaries**, which are present in all body tissue and originate in capillary beds with those of the circulatory system (see Figure 13-3). Plasma routinely seeps out of arterial capillaries into body tissues. This fluid, called interstitial fluid, picks up bacteria and cellular wastes and seeps back into the arterial system or into the lymphatic capillaries, in which case it is called lymph. The lymph drains from the lymphatic capillaries into larger vessels called **lymphatics**, which ultimately drain into the largest vessels of the lymphatic system, the **right** and **left lymph ducts**. The right lymph duct receives lymph from the right side of the head, neck, and chest and the right arm. Lymph from the rest of the body drains into the left duct, also known as the thoracic duct. Both of the lymph ducts drain into the bloodstream (see Figure 13-4).

Memory Key	
• The vascular system consists of	

    lymphatic capillaries

    lymphatics

    two lymph ducts

• The right lymph duct drains the right side of the head, neck, and chest and the right arm.
• The left thoracic lymph duct drains the rest of the body.

As illustrated in Figures 13-3 and 13-4, some lymphatics drain into **lymph nodes**. They are concentrated at various sites in the body. The lymph nodes act as filtration devices for lymph and contain great concentrations of phagocytes, which consume bacteria. This process is called **phagocytosis** (**fag**-oh-sigh-**TOH**-sis). With bacterial infections, the lymph nodes can become swollen and tender because of the huge concentration of bacteria in them. This condition is referred to as **lymphadenopathy** (lim-**fad**-eh-**NOP**-ah-thee). The principal clusters of nodes are the **cervical**, **submandibular**, **axillary**, and **inguinal**, as illustrated in Figure 13-4.

Memory Key	
• Lymph nodes contain phagocytes, which consume bacteria (phagocytosis).	

• The nodes are clustered as follows: cervical, submandibular, axillary, and inguinal.
• Lymphadenopathy is swollen lymph nodes.

FIGURE 13-2
The lymphatic system

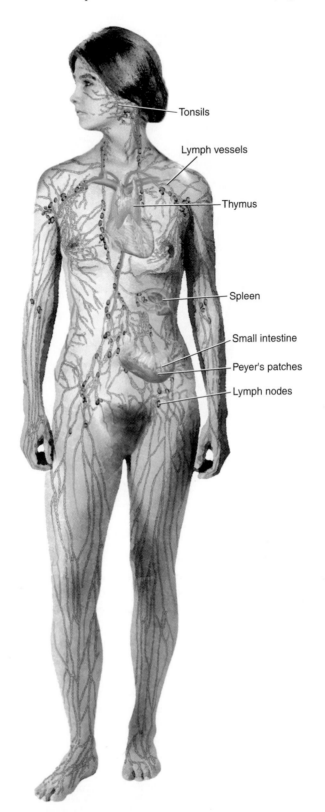

Tonsils

Lymph vessels

Thymus

Spleen

Small intestine

Peyer's patches

Lymph nodes

FIGURE 13-3
Lymph vessels

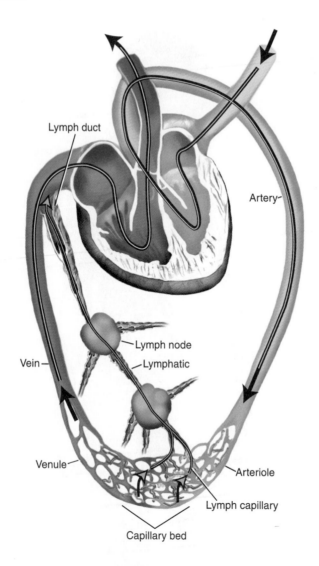

The **thymus gland**, located near the heart in the thoracic cavity, is both a lymph organ and an endocrine gland. It secretes a hormone called **thymosin** (thigh-**MOH**-sin), which stimulates red bone marrow to produce T cells. The T cells mature in the thymus.

Memory Key	The thymus gland secretes thymosin, which stimulates red bone marrow to produce T cells.

The **spleen** is located in the left side of the abdominal cavity. It is a storehouse for red blood cells, releasing them when the body requires them. It also contains a great many phagocytes and thus plays a role in ridding the body of cellular debris, old red blood cells, and bacteria. In the adult, if the bone marrow is damaged, the spleen can function to produce red blood cells.

Memory Key	The spleen stores blood and contains many phagocytes.

FIGURE 13-4
Body areas served by the two lymph ducts

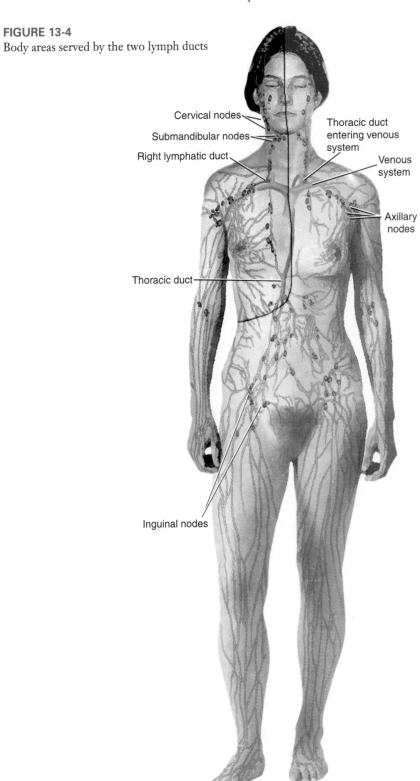

Tonsils are filters for bacteria and are made of lymphatic tissue. Three pairs are located in the throat. The **palatine** (**PAL**-ah-tine) tonsils, normally referred to simply as tonsils, are at the back of the oral cavity. The **pharyngeal** (far-**IN**-jee-al) tonsils, also called the **adenoids** (**AD**-eh-noids), are in the nasopharynx. The **lingual** (**LING**-gwal) tonsils are near the base of the tongue. Peyer's patches are lymphatic filters located in the small intestine.

Memory Key	• Tonsils are made of lymphatic tissue.
	• Tonsils filter bacteria and consist of the palatine, pharyngeal (adenoids), and lingual tonsils.
	• Peyer's patches are lymphatic filters located in the small intestine.

13.8 Term Analysis and Definition Pertaining to the Immune and Lymphatic Systems

	immun/o	**immunity; safe**
Term	**Term Analysis**	**Definition**
immunodeficiency (**im**-you-no-dee-**FISH**-en-see)	deficiency = lacking	inadequate immune response
immunology (**im**-you-**NOL**-oh-jee)	-logy = study of	study of the immune system; study of how the body responds to foreign substances
	lymphaden/o	**lymph node**
lymphadenitis (lim-**fad**-eh-**NIGH**-tis)	-itis = inflammation	inflammation of the lymph nodes
lymphadenopathy (lim-**fad**-eh-**NOP**-ah-thee)	-pathy = disease	disease (particularly enlargement) of the lymph nodes
	lymphangi/o	**lymph vessels**
lymphangiography (lim-**fan**-jee-**OG**-rah-fee)	-graphy = process of recording; producing images	process of recording the lymph vessels by the use of x-rays following injection of a contrast medium

Term	Term Analysis	Definition
lymphangitis (**lim**-fan-**JIGH**-tis)	-itis = inflammation	inflammation of the lymph vessels
	lymph/o	**lymph**
lymphedema (lim-feh-**DEE**-mah)	-edema = accumulation of fluid	accumulation of fluid due to obstruction of lymphatic structures
lymphoma (lim-**FOH**-mah)	-oma = tumor; mass	tumor of the lymphatic structures
	splen/o	**spleen**
splenomegaly (**splee**-noh-**MEG**-ah-lee)	-megaly = enlargement	enlargement of the spleen
splenorrhagia (**splee**-noh-**RAY**-jee-ah)	-rrhagia = bursting forth	hemorrhage from the spleen
splenorrhaphy (splee-**NOR**-ah-fee)	-rrhaphy = suture	suture of the spleen
	thym/o	**thymus gland**
thymectomy (thigh-**MECK**-toh-mee)	-ectomy = excision; surgical removal	excision of the thymus gland

SUFFIXES

	-immune	**immunity; safe**
Term	**Term Analysis**	**Definition**
autoimmune disease (**aw**-toh-ih-**MYOUN**)	auto- = self	an immune response to one's own body tissue; destruction of one's own cells by the immune system

13.9   Abbreviations Pertaining to the Immune and Lymphatic Systems

Abbreviation	Meaning
Ab	antibody (a protein substance, formed by lymphocytes, that is stimulated by the presence of antigens in the body. An antibody then helps neutralize or inactivate the antigen that stimulated its formation.)
Ag	antigen (a foreign substance that stimulates the production of an antibody)
AIDS	acquired immune deficiency syndrome
HIV-I	human immunodeficiency virus (the agent attacking the immune system and causing AIDS)
Ig	immunoglobulin (antibody occurring naturally in the body)

13.10 Review of Terms Pertaining to the Immune and Lymphatic Systems

Define the terms in Tables 13-4 through 13-7 in the space provided.

TABLE 13-4

REVIEW OF ANATOMICAL TERMS

immunology

TABLE 13-5

REVIEW OF PATHOLOGIC TERMS

autoimmune disease	immunodeficiency	lymphadenitis
lymphadenopathy	lymphangitis	lymphedema
lymphoma	splenorrhagia	

TABLE 13-6

REVIEW OF DIAGNOSTIC TERMS

lymphangiography

TABLE 13-7

REVIEW OF SURGICAL PROCEDURES

splenomegaly	splenorrhaphy	thymectomy

13.11 Putting It All Together

Exercise 13-1 SHORT ANSWER

1. Name three plasma proteins found in the blood.

2. Differentiate between:

   (a) plasma and serum

(b) eosinophils, basophils, and neutrophils

_____

_____

_____

(c) A, B, AB, and O type blood

_____

_____

_____

3. List three functions of the lymphatic system.

_____

_____

_____

4. Define:

(a) phagocytes

_____

_____

(b) thymosin

_____

_____

(c) pharyngeal tonsils

_____

_____

(d) T lymphocytes

_____

_____

(e) B lymphocytes

_____

_____

5. Name four groups of lymph nodes.

_____

_____

Exercise 13-2   IDENTIFICATION

Give the meaning for the following component parts.

1. chrom/o _____

2. reticul/o _____

3. immun/o _____

4. lymphaden/o _____

5. lymphangi/o _____

6. thromb/o _____

7. -crit _____

8. -phoresis _____

9. -poiesis _____

10. -stasis _____

Exercise 13-3   BUILDING MEDICAL TERMS

I. Use -penia to build terms for the following definitions.

1. decrease in the number of red blood cells _____

2. decrease in the number of white blood cells _____

3. decrease in the number of clotting cells _____

4. decrease in the number of all blood cells _____

II. Use -cytosis to build terms for the following definitions.

5. increased variation in the size of cells _____

6. marked increase in the number of white blood cells _____

7. increased variation in the shape of cells _____

III. Use -emia to build terms for the following definitions.

8. lack of red blood cells or hemoglobin _____

9. abnormal increase in the number of red blood cells _____

10. excessive amounts of bilirubin in the blood _____

11. excessive amounts of cholesterol in the blood _____

12. excessive amounts of fats in the blood _____

Exercise 13-4   BUILDING MEDICAL TERMS

Build the medical term for each of the following definitions.

1. excessively pigmented red blood cells _____

2. process of recording the lymph vessels _____

3. accumulation of fluid due to obstruction
   of lymphatic structures _____

4. resembling bone marrow _____

5. suturing of the spleen _____

6. abnormal condition of clot formation _____

7. production of red blood cells _____

8. stoppage of blood _____

9. immunity against one's own body tissue _____

10. produced by the bone marrow _____

Exercise 13-5   DEFINITIONS

Define the following terms.

1. hypochromia _____

2. hematology _____

3. immunodeficiency _____

4. lymphadenopathy _____

5. hematocrit _____

6. hemoglobin _____

7. electrophoresis _____

8. erythropoietin _____

C H A P T E R

The Respiratory System

14

CHAPTER ORGANIZATION

This chapter will help you learn the respiratory system. It is divided into the following sections:

CHAPTER OBJECTIVES

On completion of this chapter, you will be able to do the following:

1. Differentiate between inhalation and expiration

2. Name, locate, and describe the functions of the respiratory structures

3. Define Adams's apple, epiglottis, cilia, bronchial tree, paranasal sinuses

4. Define the terms that describe the structures of the lung

5. Pronounce, analyze, define, and spell terms relating to the respiratory system

6. Define abbreviations common to the respiratory system

INTRODUCTION

As we learned in the chapter on the cardiovascular system, the body's trillions of cells need to take in oxygen and eliminate carbon dioxide on a continuous basis. This interchange of gases, called **respiration**, or **breathing**, occurs when oxygen is inhaled into the lungs from the air and passes into the blood and when carbon dioxide moves from the blood to the lungs and is exhaled into the air. The breathing in of air is called **inhalation** or **inspiration**. The breathing out of air is called **exhalation** or **expiration**.

Figure 14-1 illustrates all of the structures of the respiratory system: the **nose, nasal cavity, pharynx (FAR-inks), larynx (LAR-inks), trachea (TRAY-kee-ah), bronchi (BRONG-kye), and lungs**. Each of these structures is described in the following sections.

Memory Key	The structures of the respiratory system are
	nose and nasal cavity
	pharynx
	larynx
	trachea
	bronchi
	lungs

FIGURE 14-1
Structures of the respiratory system

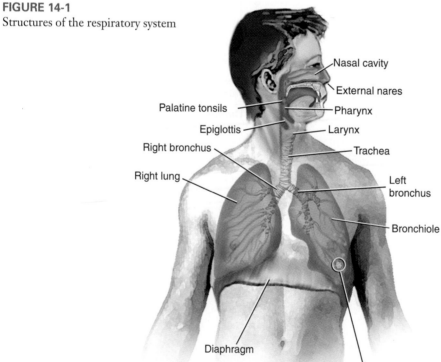

14.1   The Nose, Nasal Cavities, and Paranasal Sinuses

The **external nares** (**NAH**-reez), or nostrils, allow both inspiration and expiration of air. The hairs, or **cilia** (**SIL**-ee-ah), in the nares filter out dust particles in the air. The **nasal cavity** extends from the external nares to the pharynx. It is divided into right and left cavities by the **nasal septum** (**SEP**-tum). The nasal cavity warms and moistens air and provides us with our sense of smell through **olfactory** (ol-**FACK**-toh-ree) **neurons** in the lining of the nasal tract. Hollow spaces within the skull called **paranasal sinuses** lighten the skull. Because they are lined with mucous membrane, the paranasal sinuses also play a role in respiration by moistening air. They lie above, between, and under the eyes in pairs and are called the frontal, ethmoid, sphenoid, and maxillary sinuses (see Figure 14-2).

Memory Key	• The nostrils are called external nares.
	• The nasal cavity extends from the external nares to the pharynx, divided by the nasal septum.
	• The paranasal sinuses are the frontal, ethmoid, sphenoid, and maxillary.

FIGURE 14-2
Paranasal sinuses

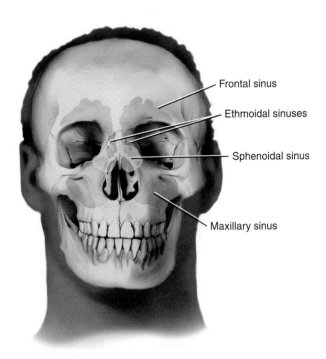

Frontal sinus

Ethmoidal sinuses

Sphenoidal sinus

Maxillary sinus

14.2   The Pharynx, Larynx, and Trachea

THE PHARYNX

The pharynx is the throat. It consists of the **nasopharynx** (nay-zo-**FAR**-inks), the **oropharynx** (or-oh-**FAR**-inks), and the **laryngopharynx** (lar-**ING**-oh-**FAR**-inks). The nasopharynx is posterior to the nasal cavity. It has two openings called **internal nares** that open into the nasal cavity and two others that open into the **eustachian** (you-**STAY**-shun) tube. It also contains the adenoids, or pharyngeal tonsils. The oropharynx is posterior to the oral cavity and contains the **palatine** (**PAL**-ah-tine) **tonsils** and the **lingual** (**LING**-gwal) **tonsils**. Chapter 13 discusses the functions of these organs. The laryngopharynx opens into the larynx and esophagus.

Memory Key	• The nasopharynx contains internal nares opening into the nasal cavity and openings into the eustachian tube. • The oropharynx contains the tonsils. • The laryngopharynx opens into the larynx and esophagus.

THE LARYNX

The larynx (Figure 14-3) is the voice box. A portion of the larynx is the **Adam's apple**, a large shield of cartilage protecting inner structures. Another structure of the larynx is the **epiglottis** (ep-ih-**GLOT**-is), which swings up and down like a lid, covering the opening of the larynx during swallowing so that the air passage is sealed. The **vocal cords**, responsible for sound, are folds of mucous membrane. The slit between them is the **glottis**. Sound is produced as air moves out of the lungs through the glottis, causing vibrations in the vocal cords. Voice pitch is determined by the length and tension of the vocal cords.

Memory Key	• The larynx is the voice box. • The Adam's apple is a shield of cartilage. • The epiglottis is a flap that swings up and down to close off air passage during swallowing. • The vocal cords are mucous membrane containing a slit called the glottis. • Vibration of vocal cords produces sound.

THE TRACHEA

The trachea (see Figure 14-3) is the windpipe. It extends from the larynx to the bronchi. It is lined with mucous membrane and **cilia** (**SIL**-ee-ah), which filter the air. The trachea is composed mostly of muscle fibers. It also contains C-shaped cartilage, which prevents the trachea from collapsing.

Memory Key	The trachea is the windpipe, connecting to the bronchi. It consists of muscle and C-shaped cartilage, lined with mucous membrane and cilia.

FIGURE 14-3
Larynx, trachea, and bronchial tree

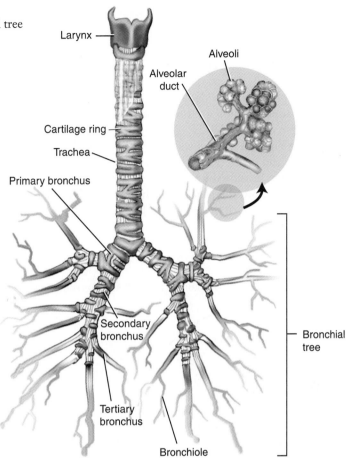

14.3   The Bronchi and Lungs

THE BRONCHI

The trachea divides into two **primary bronchi**, each of which leads to a lung. The primary bronchi split off into smaller bronchi, the **secondary** and **tertiary bronchi**, within the lungs. The tertiary bronchi connect to **bronchioles** (**BRONG**-kee-ohlz). Because of its resemblance to an inverted tree, the bronchial system is referred to as the **bronchial tree** (see Figure 14-3).

A common condition of the bronchus is **bronchial asthma**, in which the bronchus goes into spasm, cutting off the patient's air supply. The patient then experiences **paroxysmal dyspnea** (**par**-ox-**SYS**-mal **DISP**-nee-ah), which is difficulty in breathing of an off-and-on nature. These attacks are recurrent and often allergic in nature.

Memory Key   In the lungs, the two primary bronchi divide into secondary and tertiary bronchi, which connect to bronchioles.

THE LUNGS

The lungs lie in the thoracic cavity and attach to the body at the **root**, which consists of blood vessels, nerves, bronchi, and lymph vessels. The structures forming the root pass through an area called the **hilum** (**HIGH**-lum). The top of each lung is called the **apex**, and the bottom is the **base**.

The right lung is divided into three **lobes**, the **superior**, **middle**, and **inferior**. The left has only superior and inferior lobes. Inside each lung are approximately 300 million microscopic **alveoli** (al-**VEE**-oh-lye), which are connected to the bronchioles by **alveolar ducts** (see Figure 14-3). The alveoli are like tiny balloons, expanding and contracting with inspiration and expiration. The alveoli are surrounded by **pulmonary capillaries**, which deliver carbon dioxide to the alveoli and absorb oxygen from them. The carbon dioxide is then expelled from the lungs, and the oxygenated blood continues on to the heart, to be pumped to the cells of the body (see Figure 14-4).

FIGURE 14-4
The lungs: (A) structures of the lung; (B) pulmonary capillaries surrounding the alveoli for the exchange of gases

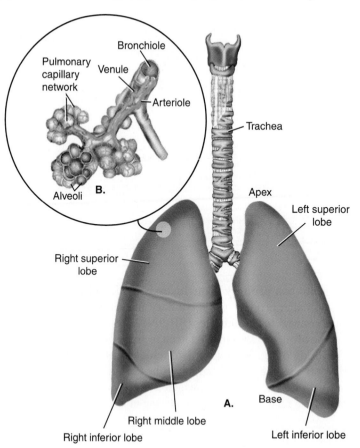

Memory Key
- The lungs lie in the thoracic cavity.
- The top of the lung is the apex; the bottom, the base.
- Blood vessels, nerves, bronchi, and lymph vessels form the root and enter at the hilum.
- The right lung has superior, middle, and inferior lobes; the left, superior and inferior.
- The respiratory bronchioles connect by alveolar ducts with the alveoli, which are tiny balloons responsible for gas exchange with the pulmonary capillaries.

THE PLEURAL AND MEDIASTINAL CAVITIES

The thoracic cavity contains two smaller cavities: the **pleural** (**PLOOR**-al) and **mediastinal** (**me**-dee-as-**TYE**-nal) cavities. The pleural cavity surrounds the lungs (Figure 14-5). Its outer layer is the parietal pleura. The inner layer is the visceral pleura. Between these two layers is the pleural cavity, filled with pleural fluid. The mediastinal cavity lies between the lungs (see Figure 14-5) and contains the heart, aorta, trachea, and esophagus.

Memory Key
- The pleural cavity surrounds the lungs.
- The mediastinal cavity is between the lungs.

FIGURE 14-5
Pleural cavities (pleura) and mediastinal cavity (mediastinum)

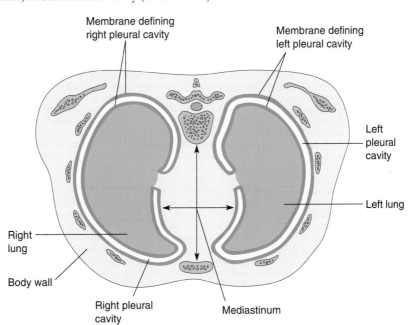

14.4   Additional Word Elements

Use these additional word elements when studying the medical terms in this chapter.

Root	Meaning
coni/o	dust

Prefix	Meaning
oligo-	scanty; few

14.5   Term Analysis and Definition

	adenoid/o	**adenoids**
Term	**Term Analysis**	**Definition**
adenoidectomy (**ad**-eh-noid-**ECK**-toh-mee)	-ectomy = excision	excision of the adenoids. *NOTE:* If the adenoids become enlarged, airflow is obstructed, necessitating adenoidectomy.
	alveol/o	**alveolus; air sacs**
alveolar (al-**VEE**-oh-lar)	-ar = pertaining to	pertaining to the alveolus
alveolitis (**al**-vee-oh-**LYE**-tis)	-itis = inflammation	inflammation of the alveolus
	bronchi/o; bronch/o	**bronchus**
bronchiectasis (**brong**-kee-**ECK**-tah-sis)	-ectasis = dilation; stretching	dilation of the bronchus. *NOTE:* Types of dilations are named according to the shape of the bronchi and include: saccular, cylindrical, and fusiform (see Figure 14-6).
bronchitis (brong-**KYE**-tis)	-itis = inflammation	inflammation of the bronchus

FIGURE 14-6
Bronchiectasis

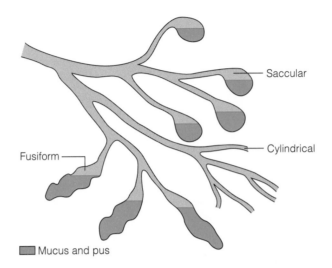

Saccular

Cylindrical

Fusiform

▉ Mucus and pus

Term	Term Analysis	Definition
bronchodilator (**brong**-koh-**DYE**-lay-tor)	-or = person or thing that does something **dilat/o** = dilation; widening	drugs used to dilate the bronchus to relieve bronchospasm (see Figure 14-7)
bronchoscopy (brong-**KOS**-koh-pee)	-scopy = process of visual examination	process of visually examining the bronchus
bronchospasm (**BRONG**-koh-spazm)	-spasm = sudden, involuntary contraction	sudden, involuntary contraction of the bronchus

FIGURE 14-7
Patient using bronchodilator

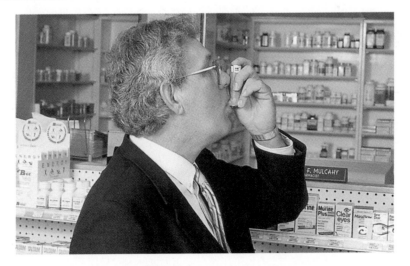

Term	Term Analysis	Definition
bronchogenic carcinoma (**BRONG**-koh-gen-ic)	-genic = produced by carcinoma = malignant tumor	a malignant tumor of the lung that originates in the bronchi. *NOTE:* Bronchogenic carcinoma is the most common form of lung cancer. It metastasizes (spreads) rapidly to other body parts such as the liver, kidney, and bones. Smoking is the leading cause of lung cancer.
	bronchiol/o	**bronchioles; little bronchi**
bronchiolitis (**brong**-kee-oh-**LYE**-tis)	-itis = inflammation	inflammation of the bronchioles
	laryng/o	**larynx; voice box**
laryngeal (lar-**INN**-jee-al)	-eal = pertaining to	pertaining to the voice box
laryngospasm (lar-**ING**-oh-spazm)	-spasm = sudden, involuntary contraction	sudden, involuntary contraction of the voice box
	lob/o	**lobe**
lobar (**LOH**-bar)	-ar = pertaining to	pertaining to the lobe of the lung
lobectomy (loh-**BECK**-toh-mee)	-ectomy = excision; surgical removal	excision of a lobe of the lung
	muc/o	**mucus (a sticky, thick secretion of mucous membrane)**
mucolytic (**myou**-koh-**LIH**-tick)	-lytic = breakdown; destruction; separate	drugs used to break down thick mucus so it can be coughed up

Memory Key	• Mucus is the noun.
	• Mucous is the adjective, as in mucous membrane.

	nas/o	nose
Term	**Term Analysis**	**Definition**
nasolacrimal (**nay**-zoh-**LACK**-rih-mal)	-al = pertaining to **lacrim/o** = lacrimal apparatus; tears	pertaining to the nose and lacrimal apparatus
nasopharyngeal (**nay**-zoh-far-**INN**-jee-al)	-eal = pertaining to **pharyng/o** = pharynx; throat	pertaining to the nasopharynx (the portion of the pharynx located behind the nose)

	ox/o	oxygen
anoxia (ah-**NOCK**-see-ah)	-ia = state of; condition a(n)- = no; not; lack of	lack of oxygen. *NOTE: Anoxia is often used interchangeably with hypoxia.*

Memory Key | An- is used instead of a- before component parts beginning with a vowel.

hypoxia (high-**POCK**-see-ah)	-ia = state of; condition hypo- = deficient; abnormal decrease	deficiency of oxygen

	pector/o	chest
pectoral (**PECK**-toh-rahl)	-al = pertaining to	pertaining to the chest

	pharyng/o	pharynx; throat
pharyngoglossal (far-**IN**-goh-**GLOS**-al)	-al = pertaining to **gloss/o** = tongue	pertaining to the pharynx and tongue

	phren/o	diaphragm
phrenic (**FREN**-ick)	-ic = pertaining to	pertaining to the diaphragm
phrenotomy (fren-**OT**-oh-mee)	-tomy = process of cutting	process of cutting into the diaphragm

	pleur/a; pleur/o	**pleura; pleural cavity**
Term	**Term Analysis**	**Definition**
pleuralgia (ploor-**AL**-jee-ah)	-algia = pain	pain in the pleura

	pneumat/o; pneum/o	**air; respiration; lungs**
pneumatic (new-**MAT**-ick)	-ic = pertaining to	pertaining to air or respiration
pneumoconiosis (**new**-moh-**koh**-nee-**OH**-sis)	-osis = abnormal condition **coni/o** = dust	abnormal condition of dust in the lungs; black lung
pneumopleuritis (**new**-moh-ploo-**RYE**-tis)	-itis = inflammation **pleur/o** = pleura	inflammation of the lungs and pleura

	pneumon/o; pulmon/o	**lungs**
pneumonia (new-**MOH**-nee-ah)	-ia = condition; state of	inflammation of the lung; also known as pneumonitis (see Figure 14-8)
pulmonary (**PUL**-moh-neh-ree)	-ary = pertaining to	pertaining to the lungs

FIGURE 14-8
Types of pneumonia

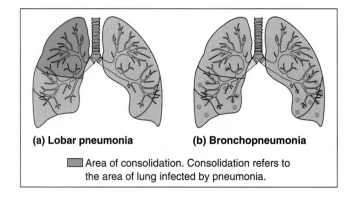

(a) Lobar pneumonia   **(b) Bronchopneumonia**

Area of consolidation. Consolidation refers to the area of lung infected by pneumonia.

	rhin/o	**nose**
Term	**Term Analysis**	**Definition**
otorhinolaryngologist (**oh**-toh-**rye**-no-**lar**-in-**GOL**-oh-jist)	-logist = specialist **ot/o** = ear **laryng/o** = voice box; larynx	a specialist in the study of the structure, function, diseases, and treatment of the ears, nose, and throat
otorhinolaryngology (**oh**-toh-**rye**-no-**lar**-in-**GOL**-oh-jee)	-logy = study of **ot/o** = ear **laryng/o** = voice box; larynx	the study of the ear, nose, and throat, including their structure, function, and diseases; also known as ENT (ears, nose, and throat)
rhinitis (rye-**NIGH**-tis)	-itis = inflammation	inflammation of the mucous membrane of the nose
rhinorrhea (**rih**-noh-**REE**-ah)	-rrhea = discharge	discharge from the nose
rhinoplasty (**RYE**-noh-**plas**-tee)	-plasty = surgical reconstruction; surgical repair	surgical repair of the nose; plastic surgery on the nose for cosmetic or reconstructive purposes; a nose job

	sinus/o	**sinuses**
pansinusitis (**pan**-sigh-nuhs-**EYE**-tis)	-itis = inflammation pan- = all	inflammation of all the paranasal sinuses
sinusotomy (**sigh**-nuhs-**OT**-oh-mee)	-tomy = process of cutting	process of cutting into the sinus

	spir/o	**breathing**
spirometer (spye-**ROM**-et-er)	-meter = instrument used to measure	instrument used to measure airflow and volume into and out of the lungs
spirometry (spye-**ROM**-eh-tree)	-metry = process of measuring	process of measuring airflow and volume into and out of the lungs (see Figure 14-9)

	steth/o	**chest**
stethoscope (**STETH**-oh-skope)	-scope = instrument used to examine	instrument used to listen to chest sounds

FIGURE 14-9
Spirometry

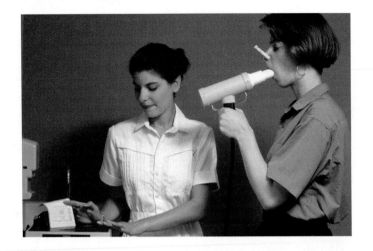

	thorac/o	chest
Term	**Term Analysis**	**Definition**
thoracocentesis (**thoh**-rah-koh-sen-**TEE**-sis)	-centesis = surgical puncture	surgical puncture to remove fluid from the pleural cavity; also known as thoracentesis, pleurocentesis, and pleuracentesis (see Figure 14-10)
thoracodynia (**thor**-ack-oh-**DIN**-ee-ah)	-dynia = pain	chest pain
thoracoplasty (**thor**-ah-koh-**PLAS**-tee)	-plasty = surgical reconstruction; surgical repair	surgical reconstruction of the thorax
thoracotomy (**thor**-ah-**KOT**-toh-mee)	-tomy = process of cutting	process of cutting into the chest

FIGURE 14-10
Thoracocentesis

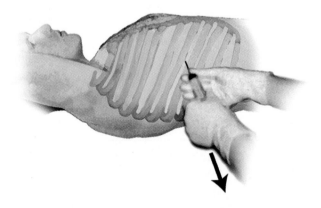

Chapter 14   The Respiratory System   **307**

	tonsill/o	tonsils
Term	**Term Analysis**	**Definition**
tonsillar (**TON**-sih-lar)	-ar = pertaining to	pertaining to the tonsils
tonsillectomy (**ton**-sih-**LECK**-toh-mee)	-ectomy = surgical excision; removal	excision of the tonsils
tonsillitis (**ton**-sih-**LYE**-tis)	-itis = inflammation	inflammation of the tonsils
tonsillotome (ton-**SIL**-oh-tohm)	-tome = instrument used to cut	instrument used to cut the tonsils

	trache/o	trachea; windpipe
endotracheal (**en**-doh-**TRAY**-kee-al)	-eal = pertaining to endo- = within	pertaining to within the trachea
laryngotracheobronchitis (lah-**ring**-goh-**tray**-kee-oh-brong-**KYE**-tis)	-itis = inflammation **laryng/o** = larynx; voice box **bronch/o** = bronchus	inflammation of the larynx, trachea, and bronchus; also known as **croup**
tracheoesophageal (**tray**-kee-oh-ee-**sof**-ah-**JEE**-al)	-eal = pertaining to **esophag/o** = esophagus	pertaining to the trachea and esophagus
tracheostomy (**tray**-kee-**OS**-toh-mee)	-stomy = new opening	new opening into the trachea is created through the neck and a tube is inserted to assist breathing. The tracheostomy tube may be temporary or permanent (see Figure 14-11B)
tracheotomy (**tray**-kee-**OT**-oh-mee)	-tomy = process of cutting	process of cutting into the trachea (see Figure 14-11A)

SUFFIXES

	-capnia	carbon dioxide
Term	**Term Analysis**	**Definition**
hypercapnia (**high**-per-**KAP**-nee-ah)	hyper- = abnormal increase; excessive	excessive amounts of carbon dioxide in the blood
hypocapnia (**high**-poh-**KAP**-nee-ah)	hypo- = below normal; decrease	decreased amounts of carbon dioxide in the blood

FIGURE 14-11
(A) Tracheotomy, (B) tracheostomy

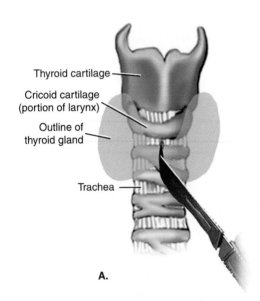

Thyroid cartilage

Cricoid cartilage
(portion of larynx)

Outline of
thyroid gland

Trachea

A.

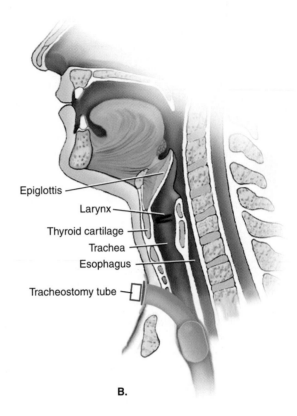

Epiglottis

Larynx

Thyroid cartilage

Trachea

Esophagus

Tracheostomy tube

B.

	-graphy	process of recording; producing images
Term	**Term Analysis**	**Definition**
bronchography (brong-**KOG**-rah-fee)	**bronch/o** = bronchus	process of producing an image of the bronchi following injection of contrast medium
pulmonary angiography (**PUL**-moh-**nar**-ee **an**-jee-**OG**-rah-fee)	**angi/o** = vessel -ary = pertaining to **pulmon/o** = lungs	process of producing an image of the blood vessels of the lung following injection of contrast medium
	-phonia	**voice**
aphonia (ah-**FOH**-nee-ah)	a- = no; not; lack of	loss of voice
dysphonia (dis-**FOH**-nee-ah)	dys- = difficult bad; painful	difficulty in speaking

	-pnea	breathing
Term	**Term Analysis**	**Definition**
apnea (ap-**NEE**-ah)	a- = no; not; lack of	no breathing
bradypnea (**brad**-ihp-**NEE**-ah)	brady- = slow	slow breathing
dyspnea (**DISP**-nee-ah)	dys- = painful; difficult; bad	painful breathing
eupnea (youp-**NEE**-ah)	eu- = normal	normal breathing
hyperpnea (**high**-perp-**NEE**-ah)	hyper- = abnormal increase; excessive	abnormal increase in depth and rate of breathing
oligopnea (ol-ih-**GOP**-nee-ah)	oligo- = scanty; few	infrequent breathing resulting in a reduction of air entering the lungs
orthopnea (**or**-thop-**NEE**-ah)	ortho- = straight	breathing only in the upright position
tachypnea (**tack**-ihp-**NEE**-ah)	tachy- = fast	fast breathing

	-ptysis	spitting
hemoptysis (he-**MOP**-tih-sis)	**hem/o** = blood	spitting up of blood

	-thorax	chest
hemothorax (**he**-moh-**THOR**-acks)	**hem/o** = blood	blood in the pleural cavity
hydrothorax (**high**-droh-**THOR**-acks)	**hydr/o** = water	fluid in the pleural cavity
pneumothorax (**new**-moh-**THOR**-acks)	**pneum/o** = air	collection of air in the pleural cavity (see Figure 14-12)
pyothorax (**pye**-oh-**THOR**-acks)	**py/o** = pus	pus in the pleural cavity; also known as **empyema** (see Figure 14-12)

FIGURE 14-12
Pneumothorax, pyothorax

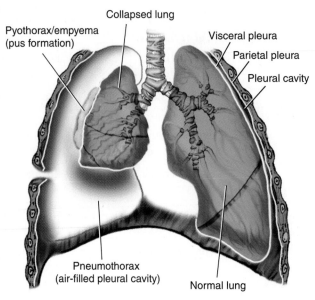

Collapsed lung

Pyothorax/empyema
(pus formation)

Visceral pleura

Parietal pleura

Pleural cavity

Pneumothorax
(air-filled pleural cavity)

Normal lung

14.6   Review of Terms

Define the terms in Tables 14-1 through 14-5 in the space provided.

TABLE 14-1

REVIEW OF ANATOMICAL TERMS

alveolar	endotracheal	laryngeal
lobar	nasolacrimal	nasopharyngeal
otorhinolaryngologist	otorhinolaryngology	pectoral
pharyngoglossal	phrenic	pneumatic
pulmonary	tonsillar	tracheoesophageal

TABLE 14-2

REVIEW OF PATHOLOGIC TERMS

alveolitis	anoxia	aphonia
apnea	bradypnea	bronchiectasis
bronchiolitis	bronchitis	bronchogenic carcinoma
bronchospasm	dysphonia	dyspnea
eupnea	hemoptysis	hemothorax
hydrothorax	hypercapnia	hyperpnea
hypocapnia	hypoxia	laryngospasm
laryngotracheobronchitis	oliopnea	orthopnea
pansinusitis	pleuralgia	pneumoconiosis
pneumonia	pneumopleuritis	pneumothorax
pyothorax	rhinitis	rhinorrhea
tachypnea	thoracodynia	tonsillitis

TABLE 14-3

REVIEW OF DIAGNOSTIC TERMS

bronchography	bronchoscopy	pulmonary angiography
spirometer	spirometry	stethoscope

TABLE 14-4

REVIEW CLINICAL PROCEDURES, SURGICAL PROCEDURES, AND SURGICAL INSTRUMENTS

adenoidectomy	lobectomy	phrenotomy
pneumonectomy	rhinoplasty	sinusotomy
thoracocentesis	thoracoplasty	thoracotomy
tonsillectomy	tonsillotome	tracheostomy
tracheotomy		

TABLE 14-5

REVIEW OF TERMS USED IN TREATMENT

bronchodilator	mucolytic	

14.7   Abbreviations

Abbreviation	Meaning
AP	anteroposterior
CO_2	carbon dioxide
CXR	chest x-ray
ERV	expiratory reserve volume (test of pulmonary function)

continued on page 313

continued from page 312

Abbreviation	Meaning
IRV	inspiratory reserve volume (test of pulmonary function)
O_2	oxygen
PA	posteroanterior
PFT	pulmonary function tests (various tests of lung performance using a spirometer) *NOTE:* Pulmonary function tests include tidal volume (TV or V_T), inspiratory reserve volume (IRV), expiratory reserve volume (ERV), residual volume (RV).
R	respiration
RV	residual volume (test of pulmonary function)
SOA	shortness of air
SOB	shortness of breath
T&A	tonsillectomy and adenoidectomy
TV, V_T	tidal volume (test of pulmonary function)
URI	upper respiratory infection
URT	upper respiratory tract

14.8   Putting It All Together

Exercise 14-1   SHORT ANSWER

1. Differentiate between inhalation and expiration.

_____

_____

2. Name and locate the respiratory structures. Describe their functions.

_____

_____

_____

_____

_____

_____

_____

3. Define: a. Adam's apple _____

b. epiglottis _____

c. cilia _____

d. bronchial tree _____

e. paranasal sinuses _____

4. Define the following terms describing the structures of the lung: root, hilum, apex, base, lobes, alveoli.

_____

_____

_____

_____

_____

_____

_____

Exercise 14-2   ADJECTIVAL FORMS

Give the adjectival form for each of the following.

1. alveolus _____   6. larynx _____

2. bronchus _____   7. diaphragm _____

3. lobe _____   8. pleura _____

4. nose _____   9. lungs _____

5. pharynx _____   10. chest _____

Exercise 14-3   IDENTIFICATION

Place an **X** beside the terms that indicate treatment.

1. bronchodilator _____

2. bronchiectasis _____

3. laryngospasm _____

4. lobectomy _____

5. mucolytic _____

6. pneumoconiosis _____

7. phrenotomy _____

8. rhinorrhea _____

9. thoracocentesis _____

10. thoracodynia _____

11. thoracoplasty _____

12. tracheoesophageal _____

13. dysphonia _____

14. hemoptysis _____

Exercise 14-4   BUILDING MEDICAL TERMS

Build the medical terms for the following definitions.

1. no breathing _____

2. slow breathing _____

3. painful breathing _____

4. normal breathing _____

5. abnormal increase in depth and rate of breathing _____

6. infrequent breathing _____

7. breathing in only the upright position _____

8. fast breathing _____

9. excessive amounts of carbon dioxide in the blood _____

10. decreased amounts of carbon dioxide in the blood _____

11. blood in the pleural cavity _____

12. water in the pleural cavity _____

13. collection of air in the pleural cavity _____

14. pus in the pleural cavity _____

15. instrument used to listen to chest sounds _____

Exercise 14-5   DEFINITIONS

Define the following terms.

1. alveolitis _____

2. nasolacrimal _____

3. anoxia _____

4. pharyngoglossal _____

5. pleuralgia _____

6. pneumonia _____

7. pneumorrhagia _____

8. pansinusitis _____

9. tonsillotome _____

10. laryngotracheo-
    bronchitis _____

Exercise 14-6   ALTERNATIVE TERMS

Give an alternative term for each of the following.

1. pleuracentesis _____

2. laryngotracheobronchitis _____

Exercise 14-7   PLURALS

Give the plural of the following terms. Use your medical dictionary if necessary.

1. alveolus _____

2. bronchus _____

3. larynx _____

4. tonsil _____

5. trachea _____

Exercise 14-8   SPELLING

Circle any misspelled words in the list below and correctly spell them in the space provided.

1. alveolor _____

2. pulmonary _____

3. bronchiolitis _____

4. mucolytic _____

5. diaphram _____

6. pneumoconioses _____

7. pneumopluritis _____

8. sperometer _____

9. rhinorrhea _____

10. dispnea _____

11. oligopnea _____

12. bronchography _____

13. bronhectasis _____

14. tonsilar _____

15. adenoidectomy _____

15 CHAPTER

The Digestive System

CHAPTER ORGANIZATION

This chapter will help you understand the digestive system. It is divided into the following sections:

CHAPTER OBJECTIVES

On completion of this chapter, you will be able to do the following:

1. Name, locate, and describe the functions of the six major organs of the digestive system

2. Name, locate, and describe the functions of the accessory organs of the digestive system

3. Name the three portions of the small intestine

4. Name the three regions of the large intestine

5. Describe the peritoneum

6. State the major functions of the digestive system

7. Pronounce, analyze, define, and spell terms relating to the digestive system

8. Define abbreviations common to the digestive system

INTRODUCTION

Figure 15-1 is an overview of the digestive system. You can see that it is essentially a long tube, plus four accessory organs described below. The tube is called the **digestive tract** or **gastrointestinal tract** (GIT). It is approximately 16 feet (5 m) long and extends from the mouth to the anus. Its functions are to take in food, break it down into simpler molecules that may be utilized by the body, and eliminate wastes. The process of breaking food down is called **digestion**. Once the food is broken down, the molecules move through the wall of the digestive tract into the blood and lymph for distribution throughout the body. This process is called **absorption**.

Six regions along the digestive tract perform specialized functions. They are the **oral cavity**, or mouth; the **pharynx** (**FAR**-inks), or throat; the **esophagus** (eh-**SOF**-ah-gus); the **stomach**; the **small intestine**; and the **large intestine**.

The accessory organs are the **salivary glands**, **pancreas** (**PAN**-kree-as), **liver**, and **gallbladder**. They are connected to the digestive tract by ducts and secrete substances into the tract that aid the processes of digestion and absorption.

FIGURE 15-1
Structures of the digestive system

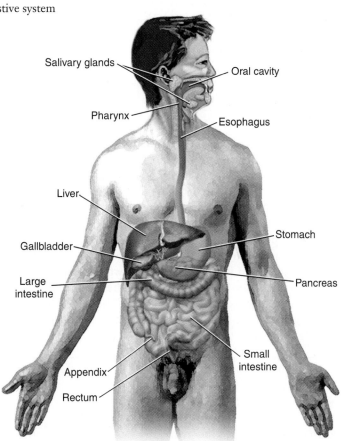

15.1 The Oral Cavity

All of the structures of the mouth are considered to be part of the oral cavity. The only external structure is the lips, which are muscular folds. The inside lining of the cheeks (bucca) is mucous membrane called **buccal mucosa** (**BUK**-ahl myou-**KOH**-sa). The **palate** (**PAL**-at), the roof of the mouth, separates the mouth from the nasal cavity. Its anterior portion (the **hard palate**) is bony; the posterior portion (the **soft palate**) consists of muscle and connective tissue. At the back of the palate is the **uvula** (**YOU**-view-lah), a saclike structure that hangs into the throat and closes off the nasal passage during swallowing.

Memory Key	• Cheeks are lined with buccal mucosa.
	• The hard and soft palates separate the mouth from the nasal cavity.
	• The uvula closes off the nasal passage during swallowing.

The **tongue** is the most versatile muscle in the body. It is tremendously important in the production of speech; yet its primary functions are to provide a sense of taste and to assist in swallowing. The tongue is connected to the bottom of the mouth by a mucous membrane cord called the **frenulum** (**FREN**-you-lum). Projections on the surface of the tongue called **papillae** (pah-**PIL**-ee) add roughness to aid licking and contain taste buds for sensing sweetness, sourness, saltiness, and bitterness.

Memory Key	The tongue is for talk, taste, and swallowing. Its roughness comes from papillae, which sense sweet, sour, salt, and bitter.

There are four types of teeth. **Incisors** and **canines** (**cuspids**) are located toward the front of the mouth, and **bicuspids** (**premolars**) and **molars** are located toward the back of the mouth. The two main parts of the tooth are the crown, located above the gums, and the root, below the gums.

Between the ages of 6 months and 2 years, children get 20 temporary or **deciduous** (deh-**SID**-you-us) teeth, which are replaced with 32 permanent teeth. At the core of each tooth is a cavity containing **pulp** made up of blood vessels and nerves, which extend into the root through the **root canal**. Covering the pulp cavity is a layer of **dentin**. The portion of the tooth lying above the gum is covered by hard, white **enamel**, and the root is covered by an outer layer of **cementum** (seh-**MEN**-tum). The root is anchored in a bony socket called the **alveolus** (al-vee-**OH**-lus) (see Figure 15-2). The teeth are ideally made for the simple tasks required of them. The front teeth slice or tear, and the back teeth chew or **masticate** (**MAS**-tih-kate) food.

Memory Key	• Temporary teeth are called deciduous.
	• Types of teeth are
	incisors bicuspids
	canines molars
	• The crown is located above the gums; the root, below the gums.
	• From inside out, teeth consist of pulp, enamel, dentin, and cementum
	• Front teeth tear food, and back teeth masticate it.

FIGURE 15-2
Structures of a Tooth

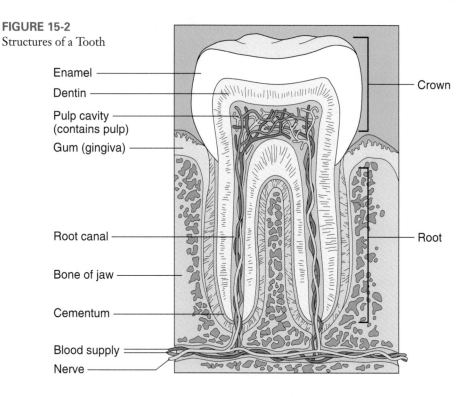

Enamel

Dentin

Pulp cavity
(contains pulp)

Gum (gingiva)

Root canal

Bone of jaw

Cementum

Blood supply

Nerve

Crown

Root

15.2   The Pharnyx

During mastication, the food is mixed with saliva, producing a softened ball of food called a **bolus** (**BO**-lus), which is pushed by the tongue into the throat, or **pharynx**. This pushing commences the process of swallowing, also called **deglutition** (**deg**-loo-**TISH**-un). Since the pharynx opens to both the respiratory system via the **trachea** (**TRAY**-kee-ah) and to the digestive system via the **esophagus**, swallowing must be neatly coordinated to avoid aspirating food (taking it into the lungs). A small flap of tissue on the voice box called the **epiglottis** (**ep**-ih-**GLOT**-is) performs this function by reflexively covering the trachea during swallowing.

Memory Key	Swallowing is deglutition. The food (bolus) passes through the pharynx to the esophagus.

15.3   The Esophagus

The esophagus is a 10-inch (25 cm) tube. It begins at the pharynx and passes through an opening in the diaphragm called the **esophageal hiatus** (high-**AYE**-tus) before reaching the stomach. It contains muscles that create wavelike contractions called **peristaltic** (**per**-ih-**STAL**-tik) **waves** to push the bolus down to the stomach. At the proximal end is a circular muscle called the **upper esophageal** or **pharyngoesophageal sphincter** (far-ing-goh-ee-sof-ah-**JEE**-al **SFINK**-ter), which opens to allow food in and closes to prevent air from entering the esophagus. At the junction between the esophagus and the stomach is a second circular muscle, the **lower esophageal sphincter**, also known as the **gastroesophageal** or **cardiac sphincter**, which opens to allow food into the stomach and then closes to prevent stomach contents from reentering.

Memory Key	The bolus moves down the esophagus by peristalsis and into the stomach through the lower esophageal sphincter.

15.4   The Stomach

During the process of eating, the taste and smell of food initiate the secretion of gastric juices in the stomach. Once the bolus passes through the lower esophageal sphincter into the stomach, muscle action causes churning, mixing the bolus with the gastric juices (mucus, hydrochloric acid, enzymes, and other chemicals) into a semiliquid called **chyme** (**KYM**).

Figure 15-3 is a cut-away illustration of the stomach. Note the inner lining of the stomach. It consists of a series of folds called **rugae** (**ROO**-jee), which stretch to accommodate food. Structurally, the stomach is J-shaped, with four regions: the **cardia** (**KAR**-dee-ah), **fundus** (**FUN**-dus), **body**, and **antrum**. The medial curve is called the **lesser curvature**, and the lateral curve is called the **greater curvature**. Food leaves the stomach for the small intestine through another circular muscle called the **pyloric** (pie-**LOR**-ik) **sphincter**.

FIGURE 15-3
Stomach

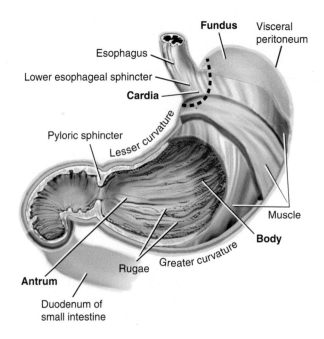

Memory Key	• Food enters the stomach through the lower esophageal sphincter and leaves through the pyloric sphincter.
	• The bolus is mixed with gastric juices to form chyme.
	• The folds of the stomach walls are rugae.
	• The regions are cardia, fundus, body, and antrum.
	• The curves are called lesser and greater.

15.5   The Small Intestine

Figure 15-4 illustrates the small intestine. Coiled within the abdominopelvic cavity, the 21-foot-long (7 m) small intestine has three regions: the **duodenum** (**dew**-oh-**DEE**-num), the **jejunum** (jeh-**JOO**-num), and the **ileum** (**ILL**-ee-um). Although the diameter is only about 1 inch (2.54 cm), the inner surface area is greatly increased by folds called **plicae circulares** (**PLYE**-kee **sir**-kyou-**LAR**-eez), illustrated in Figure 15-5. Many fingerlike projections called **villi** (**VIL**-eye) protrude from the plicae circulares. Each villus has a

FIGURE 15-4
Small intestine

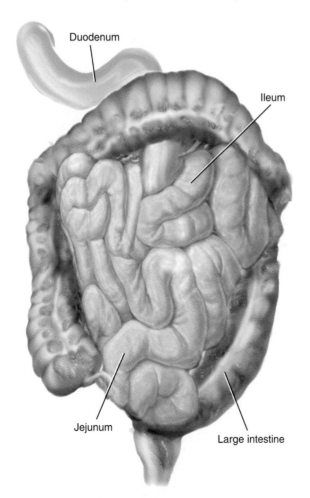

Duodenum

Ileum

Jejunum

Large intestine

network of capillaries that permit the absorption of nutrients from digested food into the bloodstream. The remaining waste product enters the large intestine through a valve at the end of the ileum called the **ileocecal** (**ill-ee-oh-SEE**-kal) **valve**.

Memory Key
- The small intestine is 1 inch in diameter and 21 feet long.
- Its three regions are the duodenum, jejunum, and ileum.
- Nutrients are absorbed by villi, which protrude from the plicae circulares.
- Waste leaves through the ileocecal valve.

FIGURE 15-5

Structures of absorption in the small intestine: (A) plicae circulares, (B) villi, (C) capillaries

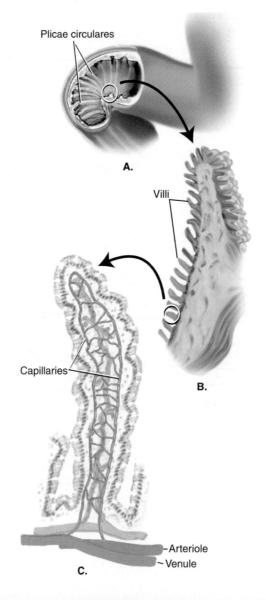

Plicae circulares

A.

Villi

B.

Capillaries

Arteriole

Venule

C.

15.6   The Large Intestine

The large intestine is about 5 feet (1.8 m) long and 2.4 inches (6 cm) in diameter. Its functions are to absorb water, vitamin K, and some B vitamins and to eliminate waste by **defecation (def-eh-KAY-shun)**. It has three regions, as illustrated in Figure 15-6: a pouch called the **cecum (SEE-kum)**, the **colon**, and the **rectum**. The colon forms a long, square arch consisting of the **ascending colon, transverse colon, descending colon,** and **sigmoid colon**. The rectum is about 8 inches long and is lined with mucous folds. The final segment of the rectum is the **anal canal**. It is surrounded by the **internal** and **external sphincters**, circular muscles that regulate the evacuation of feces through the anus. The **appendix**, which has no known function, hangs down from the cecum.

Memory Key	• The large intestine is 5 feet long and 2.4 inches in diameter.

- The large intestine is 5 feet long and 2.4 inches in diameter.
- It absorbs water, vitamin K, and some B vitamins and eliminates waste.
- The regions of the large intestine are

  cecum   rectum

  colon
- The regions of the colon are

  ascending   descending

  transverse   sigmoid
- The rectum includes

  anal canal   external and internal sphincters

  anus

FIGURE 15-6
The large intestine

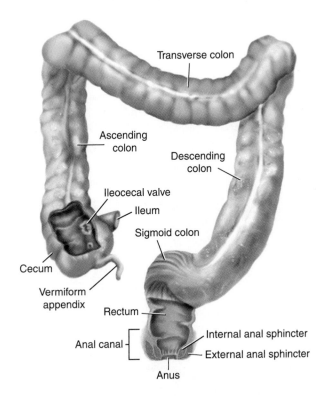

15.7   Accessory Organs

THE SALIVARY GLANDS

There are three pairs of **salivary glands**: the **parotid** (pah-**ROT**-id), the **submandibular** (**sub**-man-**DIB**-you-lar), and **sublingual** (sub-**LING**-gwal). They are located outside the mouth and drain saliva into the oral cavity via salivary ducts. Saliva contains an important enzyme, **salivary amylase** (**AM**-ih-lays), which begins the digestion of carbohydrates.

Memory Key	• The salivary glands are the

• The salivary glands are the
  parotid
  submandibular
  sublingual
• Saliva contains salivary amylase, which begins the digestion of carbohydrates.

THE LIVER AND BILIARY TRACT

The liver is the largest organ in the body, weighing on the average 4 pounds (1.75 kg). It is located below the diaphragm, in the right upper quadrant (RUQ) of the abdomen. As illustrated in Figure 15-7, the liver is divided into right and left lobes, which in turn divide into smaller lobes. The liver performs the following functions:

1. Production of bile for the breakdown of fat in the duodenum
2. Breakdown of carbohydrates, fats, and proteins so that they can be absorbed or stored for later use

FIGURE 15-7
Liver, gallbladder, and pancreas

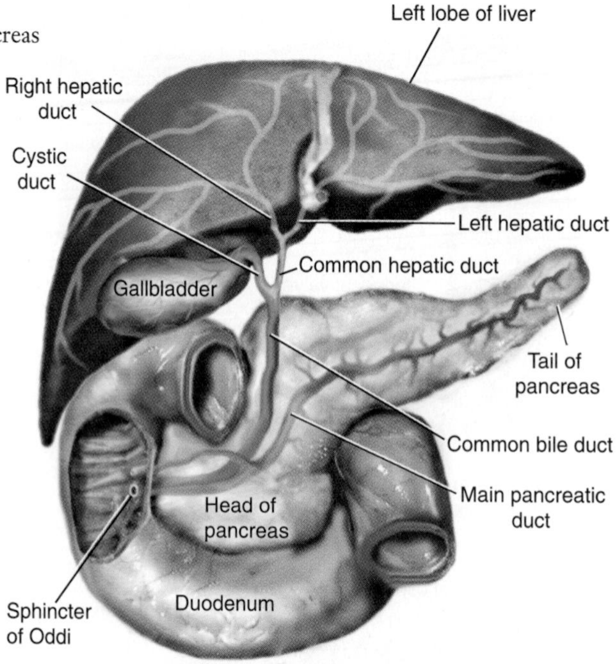

Left lobe of liver
Right hepatic duct
Cystic duct
Left hepatic duct
Common hepatic duct
Gallbladder
Tail of pancreas
Common bile duct
Main pancreatic duct
Head of pancreas
Sphincter of Oddi
Duodenum

3. Storage of excess sugar as glycogen
4. Storage of vitamins A, D, E, and K; iron; and copper
5. Detoxification of harmful substances by the action of cells called **Kupffer's** (**KOOP**-ferz) cells
6. Production of blood proteins such as **prothrombin** (pro-**THROM**-bin) and **fibrinogen** (figh-**BRIN**-oh-jen), which are necessary for blood clotting

The **biliary tract** includes the **gallbladder** (**GB**), the **hepatic ducts**, the **cystic duct**, and the **common bile duct** (**CBD**). Bile is transported from the liver via the right and left hepatic ducts and into the cystic duct for storage in the gallbladder. When bile is required in the duodenum for the breakdown of fats, it travels through the cystic duct and into the CBD (the union between the hepatic and cystic ducts), which drains into the duodenum.

Whereas the liver is essential to life, the gallbladder may be surgically removed without too much disruption to body function. After excision of the gallbladder (cholecystectomy), the bile may be stored in the biliary ducts and biliary processes proceed normally.

Memory Key	• The liver

• The liver
  produces bile
  breaks down carbohydrates, fats, and proteins
  stores sugar; vitamins A, D, E, and K; iron; and copper
  detoxifies harmful substances
  synthesizes blood-clotting factors prothrombin and fibrinogen
• The gallbladder stores bile.
• The biliary system consists of the gallbladder, hepatic ducts, cystic ducts, and common bile duct.

THE PANCREAS

The pancreas, illustrated in Figure 15-7, is a long, fish-shaped organ lying behind the stomach. It secretes **pancreatic juice** (enzymes and sodium bicarbonate). The sodium bicarbonate provides the proper environment for the action of enzymes as it neutralizes the acid in chyme. The juice travels along the **pancreatic duct** running the length of the pancreas. The pancreatic duct fuses with the common bile duct from the liver and then empties into the duodenum, where the pancreatic juice is deposited. The **sphincter of Oddi** at the entrance to the duodenum regulates the flow of pancreatic juice and bile into the duodenum. The pancreas also secretes the hormones **insulin** (**IN**-suh-lin) and **glucagon** (**GLOO**-kah-gon), which together regulate the amount of sugar in the bloodstream. See Chapter 11, under pancreas, for details of sugar regulation.

Memory Key	The pancreas secretes pancreatic juice, which runs through the pancreatic duct to the duodenum. The pancreas secretes insulin and glucagon, which regulate blood sugar.

15.8   The Peritoneum

Peritoneum is a membrane lining the abdominopelvic cavity and covering the abdominopelvic organs. The abdominopelvic cavity lies below the diaphragm. The lining of its walls is called **parietal peritoneum** (pah-**RYE**-eh-tal **per**-ih-toh-**NEE**-um) because the term **parietal** means "wall." The covering of the organs is referred to as **visceral** (**VIS**-er-al) **peritoneum**, because visceral means "organ." The space between the parietal and visceral peritoneum is called the **peritoneal** (**per**-ih-toh-**NEE**-al) **cavity**. It is filled with **peritoneal fluid**, a watery fluid that prevents friction between the parietal and visceral layers. Organs such as the kidneys that lie near the posterior abdominal wall but behind the peritoneal cavity are in a **retroperitoneal** (**ret**-roh-**per**-ih-toh-**NEE**-al) position. Figure 15-8 illustrates all of the above.

FIGURE 15-8
Abdominal cavity and peritoneal membranes

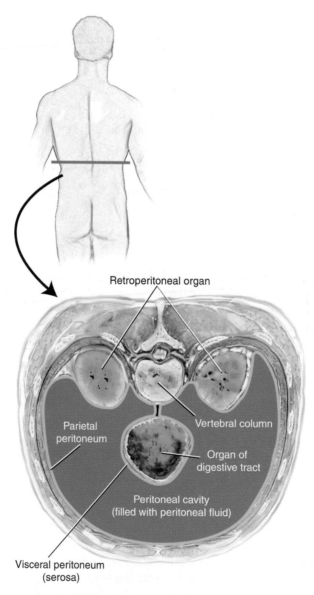

Retroperitoneal organ

Parietal peritoneum

Vertebral column

Organ of digestive tract

Peritoneal cavity
(filled with peritoneal fluid)

Visceral peritoneum
(serosa)

15.9   Additional Word Elements

Use these additional word elements when studying the medical terms in this chapter.

Root	Meaning
chol/e	bile; gall
hiat/o	gape; opening
intestin/o	intestine
umbilic/o	navel

Suffix	Meaning
-clysis	washing; irrigation
-flux	flow
-lytic	pertaining to destruction, separation, or breakdown
-tresia	opening
-tripsy	crushing

Prefix	Meaning
re-	back
retro-	backward; back

15.10   Term Analysis and Definition

	an/o	anus
Term	**Term Analysis**	**Definition**
anorectal (ay-noh-**RECK**-tal)	-al = pertaining to rect/o = rectum	pertaining to the anus and rectum

Term	Term Analysis	Definition
perianal (**peh**-ree-**AY**-nal)	-al = pertaining to peri- = around	pertaining to around the anus

	append/o; appendic/o	**appendix**
appendectomy (**ap**-en-**DECK**-toh-mee)	-ectomy = excision; surgical removal	surgical removal of the appendix
appendicitis (ah-**pen**-dih-**SIGH**-tis)	-itis = inflammation	inflammation of the appendix

	bil/i	**bile**
biliary (**BILL**-ee-air-ee)	-ary = pertaining to	pertaining to bile

	bucc/o	**cheek**
buccal mucosa (**BUK**-ahl myou-**KOH**-sa)	-al = pertaining to mucosa = mucous membrane	pertaining to the mucous membrane of the cheek

	cec/o	**cecum**
cecopexy (**SEE**-koh-**peck**-see)	-pexy = surgical fixation	surgical fixation of the cecum

	cheil/o	**lips**
cheiloplasty (**KYE**-loh-**plas**-tee)	-plasty = surgical reconstruction; surgical repair	surgical repair of the lips
cheilorrhaphy (kye-**LOR**-ah-fee)	-rrhaphy = suture (to sew)	suturing of the lips
cheilosis (kye-**LOH**-sis)	-osis = abnormal condition	abnormal condition of the lips characterized by deep cracklike sores

	cholangi/o	bile duct; bile vessel
Term	**Term Analysis**	**Definition**
cholangiogram (koh-**LAN**-jee-oh-gram)	-gram = record; writing	a record of the bile ducts
cholangiopancreatography (koh-**lan**-jee-oh-**pan**-kree-ah-**TOG**-rah-fee)	-graphy = process of recording **pancreat/o** = pancreas	process of recording the bile ducts and pancreas

	cholecyst/o	gallbladder
cholecystectomy (**koh**-lee-sis-**TECK**-toh-mee)	-ectomy = excision; surgical removal	excision of the gallbladder
cholecystitis (**koh**-lee-sis-**TYE**-tis)	-itis = inflammation	inflammation of the gallbladder

	choledoch/o	common bile duct (CBD)
choledochotomy (**koh**-led-oh-**KOT**-oh-mee)	-tomy = to cut; to cut into; incision	incision into the common bile duct

	col/o; colon/o	colon
colitis (koh-**LYE**-tis)	-itis = inflammation	inflammation of the colon
colocolostomy (**koh**-loh-koh-**LAHS**-toh-mee)	-stomy = new opening	creation of a new opening between two segments of the colon; anastomosis between two segments of the colon. *NOTE:* The surgical joining of two structures that are normally separate is called **anastomosis**. An anastomosis of the colon may be performed after excision of a cancerous portion of colon.
colostomy (koh-**LAHS**-toh-mee)	-stomy = new opening	creation of a new opening between the colon and the abdominal wall (see Figure 15-9)

Memory Key   Be aware when spelling words using **chol/e** and **col/o**. The first syllable is pronounced the same but is spelled differently.

FIGURE 15-9
Ascending colostomy. The transverse, descending, and sigmoid colons are removed. The ascending colon remains and is attached to the abdominal wall.

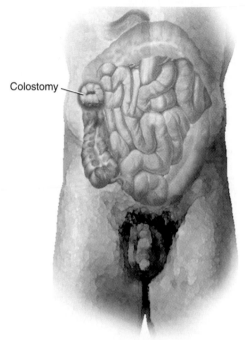

Colostomy

Ascending colostomy

	dent/o; odont/o	tooth
Term	**Term Analysis**	**Definition**
edentulous (ee-**DEN**-tyou-lus)	-ous = pertaining to e- = without	without teeth; having had teeth but lost them
dental caries (**DEN**-tal **KAYR**-eez)	-al = pertaining to caries = decay; cavities	tooth decay
endodontist (**en**-doh-**DON**-tist)	-ist = specialist endo- = within	dentist who specializes in the diagnosis and treatment of diseases within the tooth such as pulp
orthodontist (**or**-thoh-**DON**-tist)	-ist = specialist ortho- = straight	dentist who specializes in the correction of deformed or maloccluded teeth
periodontist (**per**-ee-oh-**DON**-tist)	-ist = specialist peri- = around	specialist in diseases of tissues around the tooth such as the gums and cementum. *NOTE:* The structures around the tooth are collectively known as the periodontium.

	duoden/o	**duodenum**
Term	**Term Analysis**	**Definition**
duodenal (**dew**-oh-**DEE**-nal)	-al = pertaining to	pertaining to the duodenum

	enter/o	**small intestine; intestine**
gastroenteritis (**gas**-troh-en-ter-**EYE**-tis)	-itis = inflammation **gastr/o** = stomach	inflammation of the stomach and intestines
gastroenterology (**gas**-troh-**en**-ter-**OL**-oh-jee)	-logy = study of **gastr/o** = stomach	study of the stomach and intestines including diseases and treatment
gastroenterologist (**gas**-troh-**en**-ter-**OL**-oh-jist)	-ist = specialist **gastr/o** = stomach	specialist in the study of the stomach and intestines including diseases and treatment

	esophag/o	**esophagus**
esophageal atresia (eh-**sof**-ah-**JEE**-al ah-**TREE**-zha)	-eal = pertaining to -tresia = opening a- = no; not	closure of the esophagus
gastroesophageal reflux (GER) (**gas**-troh-eh-**sof**-ah-**JEE**-al **REE**-flucks)	-eal = pertaining to **gastr/o** = stomach re- = back -flux = flow	backward flow of gastric contents into the esophagus

	gastr/o	**stomach**
gastrectomy (gas-**TRECK**-toh-mee)	-ectomy = excision; surgical removal	excision of the stomach
gastrointestinal (**gas**-troh-in-**TES**-tih-nal)	-al = pertaining to **intestin/o** = intestine	pertaining to the stomach and intestine
gastrotomy (gas-**TROT**-oh-mee)	-tomy = to cut; incise process of cutting	to cut into the stomach
nasogastric tube (nay-zoh-**GAS**-trick)	-ic = pertaining to **nas/o** = nose	a tube placed into the nose and extending into the stomach for the insertion or withdrawal of substances

	gingiv/o	gums
Term	**Term Analysis**	**Definition**
gingivobuccal (**jin**-jih-voh-**BUK**-ahl)	-al = pertaining to **bucc/o** = cheek	pertaining to the gums and cheeks
gingivitis (**jin**-jih-**VYE**-tis)	-itis = inflammation	inflamed gums

	gloss/o	tongue
glossectomy (glos-**ECK**-toh-mee)	-ectomy = excision; surgical removal	excision of the tongue

	hepat/o	liver
hepatocellular (**hep**-ah-toh-**SEL**-you-lar)	-ar = pertaining to **cellul/o** = cell	pertaining to liver cells
hepatitis (**hep**-ah-**TYE**-tis)	-itis = inflammation	inflammation of the liver
hepatoma (**hep**-ah-**TOH**-mah)	-oma = tumor; mass	tumor of the liver

	herni/o	**hernia; protrusion or displacement of an organ through a structure that normally contains it**
herniorrhaphy (**her**-nee-**OR**-ah-fee)	-rrhaphy = suture	hernia repair. *NOTE:* This surgical procedure is performed by making an incision over the hernial site. The organ, usually the intestine, is returned back to its normal position and the area secured.
hiatal hernia (high-**AY**-tal **HER**-nee-ah)	-al = pertaining to **hiat/o** = gape; opening	displacement of the stomach above the diaphragm into the thoracic cavity (see Figure 15-10B)
inguinal hernia (**ING**-gwih-nal **HER**-nee-ah)	-al = pertaining to **inguin/o** = groin	displacement of intestines through the inguinal canal, an opening in the groin area; more common in males than females (see Figure 15-10A)

FIGURE 15-10
(A) Inguinal hernia, (B) hiatal hernia

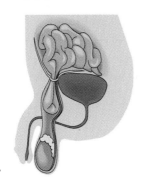

A.

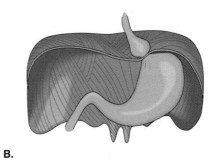

B.

Term	Term Analysis	Definition
femoral hernia (**FEM**-or-al **HER**-nee-ah)	-al = pertaining to **femor/o** = thigh	displacement of intestines through the femoral canal, an opening in the upper thigh area; more common in females than males
umbilical hernia (um-**BILL**-ih-cahl **HER**-nee-ah)	-al = pertaining to **umbilic/o** = navel	displacement of intestines through a weak spot in the abdominal wall near the umbilicus (navel)
	ile/o	**ileum**
ileostomy (**ill**-ee-**OS**-toh-mee)	-stomy = new opening	creation of a new opening between the ileum and the abdominal wall
ileotomy (**ill**-ee-**OT**-oh-mee)	-tomy = to cut; incise, process of cutting	to cut into the ileum
	jejun/o	**jejunum**
gastrojejunostomy (**gas**-troh-**jeh**-jyou-**NOS**-toh-me)	-stomy = new opening **gastr/o** = stomach	new opening between the stomach and jejunum; anastomosis between the stomach and jejunum
jejunal (jeh-**JOO**-nal)	-al = pertaining to	pertaining to the jejunum

	labi/o	lips
Term	Term Analysis	Definition
labial (**LAY**-bee-al)	-al = pertaining to	pertaining to the lips
labioglossopharyngeal (**lay**-bee-oh-**glos**-oh-far-**IN**-jee-al)	-eal = pertaining to **gloss/o** = tongue **pharyng/o** = throat; pharynx	pertaining to the lips, tongue, and throat

	lapar/o	abdomen
laparoscope (**LAP**-ah-roh-skohp)	-scope = instrument used to visually examine	instrument used to visually examine the inside of the abdomen
laparoscopy (**lap**-ah-**ROS**-koh-pee)	-scopy = process of visually examining (a body cavity or organ)	process of visually examining the inside of the abdomen (see Figure 4-1)
laparotomy (**lap**-ah-**ROT**-oh-mee)	-tomy= to cut; incise	incision into the abdominal wall

	lingu/o	tongue
sublingual (sub-**LING**-gwal)	-al = pertaining to sub- = under	pertaining to under the tongue

	lith/o	stone
cholecystolithiasis (**koh**-lee-**sis**-toh-lih-**THIGH**-ah-sis)	-iasis = abnormal condition **cholecyst/o** = gallbladder	condition of stones in the gallbladder (see Figure 15-11)
choledocholithiasis (koh-**led**-uh-koh-lih-**THIGH**-ah-sis)	-iasis = condition **choledoch/o** = common bile duct	condition of stones in the common bile duct (see Figure 15-11)
litholytic agent (**lith**-oh-**LIT**-ick)	-lytic = pertaining to destruction, separation, or breakdown	oral drugs used to break down gallstones, thereby eliminating the need for surgery
lithotripsy (**LITH**-oh-**trip**-see)	-tripsy = crushing	crushing of gallstones into pebbles tiny enough to be discharged from the organ
choledocholithotripsy (koh-**led**-uh-koh-**LITH**-oh-**trip**-see)	-tripsy = crushing **choledoch/o** = common bile duct	crushing of stones in the common bile duct

FIGURE 15-11
Cholelithiasis and choledocholithiasis

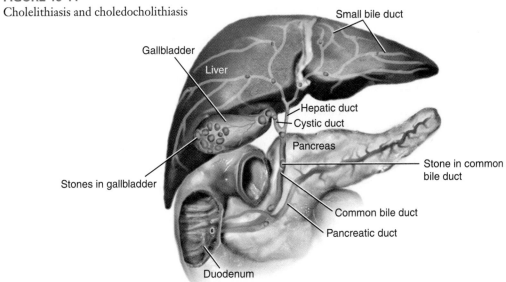

Small bile duct

Gallbladder

Liver

Hepatic duct

Cystic duct

Pancreas

Stones in gallbladder

Stone in common
bile duct

Common bile duct

Pancreatic duct

Duodenum

	orex/i	appetite
Term	**Term Analysis**	**Definition**
anorexia (**an**-oh-**RECK**-see-ah)	-ia = condition a(n)- = no; not; lack of	loss of appetite
	or/o	**mouth**
oral (**OR**-al)	-al = pertaining to	pertaining to the mouth
	pancreat/o	**pancreas**
pancreatitis (**pan**-kree-ah-**TYE**-tis)	-itis = inflammation	inflammation of the pancreas
	peritone/o	**peritoneum**
peritonitis (**per**-ih-toh-**NIGH**-tis)	-itis = inflammation	inflammation of the peritoneum. *NOTE:* A life-threatening condition often due to a ruptured appendix, which releases intestinal bacteria resulting in an inflamed peritoneum.

Term	Term Analysis	Definition
retroperitoneal (**ret**-roh-**per**-ih-toh-**NEE**-al)	-al = pertaining to retro- = behind	behind the peritoneum
ventriculoperitoneal shunt (ven-**trick**-you-loh-**per**-ih-toh-**NEE**-al)	-al = pertaining to **ventricul/o** = ventricles of the brain shunt = a device used to divert the flow of fluid	the use of a shunt to divert cerebrospinal fluid from the ventricles to the peritoneum
	pharyng/o	**throat; pharynx**
pharyngeal (**far**-in-**JEE**-al)	-eal = pertaining to	pertaining to the pharynx
	proct/o	**rectum**
proctologist (prock-**TOL**-oh-jist)	-ist = specialist	specialist in the study of the rectum
proctoclysis (prock-**TOCK**-lih-sis)	-clysis = washing; irrigation	irrigation of the rectum
	pylor/o	**pylorus (distal portion of the stomach); pyloric sphincter**
pyloric stenosis (pie-**LOR**-ick steh-**NOH**-sis)	-ic = pertaining to stenosis = narrowing	narrowing of the pylorus
pylorospasm (pie-**LOR**-oh-spasm)	-spasm = sudden, involuntary contraction	sudden, involuntary contraction of the pylorus
pyloromyotomy (pye-**lor**-oh-my-**OT**-oh-mee)	-tomy = to cut; incise; process of cutting **my/o** = muscle	incision into the pyloric sphincter for pyloric stenosis
	rect/o	**rectum**
rectostenosis (**reck**-toh-sten-**OH**-sis)	-stenosis = narrowing; stricture	narrowing or stricture of the rectum. *NOTE:* -stenosis can be used as a suffix as evident in this example, or it can stand alone as a medical word as in *pyloric stenosis.*

	sial/o	saliva
Term salivary (**SAL**-ih-ver-ee)	**Term Analysis** -ary = pertaining to	**Definition** pertaining to the saliva

	sialaden/o	salivary gland
sialadenitis (**sigh**-al-**ad**-eh-**NIGH**-tis)	-itis = inflammation	inflammation of the salivary gland

	sigmoid/o	sigmoid colon
sigmoidoscopy (**sig**-moi-**DOS**-koh-pee)	-scopy = process of visually examining (a body organ or cavity)	process of visually examining the sigmoid colon

	steat/o	fat
steatorrhea (**stee**-ah-toh-**REE**-ah)	-rrhea = discharge; flow	discharge of fat in the feces

	stomat/o	mouth
stomatitis (**sto**-mah-**TYE**-tis)	-itis = inflammation	inflammation of the mouth

Memory Key   **Stomat/o**, rather than **or/o**, is commonly used in reference to pathology of the mouth.

	viscer/o	internal organs
visceroptosis (**vis**-er-op-**TOH**-sis)	-ptosis = drooping; sagging; prolapse	drooping of the internal organs

SUFFIXES

	-chalasia	relaxation
Term	**Term Analysis**	**Definition**
achalasia (**ack**-ah-**LAY**-zee-ah)	a- = no; not; lack of	inability of the muscles of the digestive tract to relax

	-grade	to step; to go
retrograde (**RET**-roh-grayd)	retro- = backward; back	backward flow of fluid

	-emesis	vomiting
hyperemesis (**high**-per-**EM**-eh-sis)	hyper- = excessive; above normal	excessive vomiting
hematemesis (**hem**-ah-**TEM**-eh-sis)	**hemat/o** = blood	vomiting of blood
melanemesis (**mel**-ah-**NEM**-eh-sis)	**melan/o** = black	black vomit caused by the mixing of blood with intestinal contents. *NOTE:* Melanemesis may be an indication of bleeding ulcers.

	-lith	stone
cholelith (**KOH**-lee-lith)	**chol/e** = bile; gall	gallstones
sialolith (sigh-**AL**-oh-lith)	**sial/o** = saliva	stone in the salivary gland or duct

	-phagia	eating; swallowing
aphagia (ah-**FAY**-jee-ah)	a- = no; not; lack of	no eating
dysphagia (dis-**FAY**-jee-ah)	dys- = difficult; painful; bad	difficulty in eating
polyphagia (**pol**-ee-**FAY**-jee-ah)	poly- = many	excessive eating

	-plakia	patches
Term	**Term Analysis**	**Definition**
leukoplakia (**loo**-koh-**PLAY**-kee-ah)	**leuk/o** = white	white patches on the mucous membrane

	-pepsia	**digestion**
dyspepsia (dis-**PEP**-see-ah)	dys- = difficult; painful; bad	indigestion

	-prandial	**meal**
postprandial (pohst-**PRAN**-dee-al)	post- = after	after a meal

PREFIXES

	endo-	**within**
Term	**Term Analysis**	**Definition**
endoscopy (en-**DOS**-koh-pee)	-scopy = process of visually examining (a body cavity or organ)	process of visually examining the internal body cavities by inserting a tube equipped with a light and lens system; examples are gastroscopy, laparoscopy, and colonoscopy (see Figure 4-1)

15.11 Review of Terms

Define the terms in Tables 15-1 through 15-4 in the space provided.

TABLE 15-1

REVIEW OF ANATOMICAL TERMS

anorectal	biliary	buccal mucosa

continued on page 342

Table 15-1 *continued from page 341*

duodenal	endodontist	gastroenterologist
gastroenterology	gastrointestinal	gingivobuccal
hepatocellular	jejunal	labial
labioglossopharyngeal	oral	orthodontist
perianal	periodontist	pharyngeal
proctologist	retroperitoneal	salivary
sublingual		

TABLE 15-2

REVIEW OF PATHOLOGIC TERMS

achalasia	anorexia	aphagia
appendicitis	cheilosis	cholecystitis
cholecystolithiasis	choledocholithiasis	cholelith
colitis	dental caries	dyspepsia
dysphagia	edentulous	esophageal atresia
femoral hernia	gastroenteritis	gastroesophageal reflux
gingivitis	hematemesis	hepatitis
hepatoma	hiatal hernia	hyperemesis

continued on page 343

Table 15-2 *continued from page 342*

inguinal hernia	leukoplakia	melanemesis
pancreatitis	peritonitis	polyphagia
pyloric stenosis	pylorospasm	rectostenosis
sialadenitis	sialolith	steatorrhea
stomatitis	umbilical hernia	visceroptosis

TABLE 15-3

REVIEW OF DIAGNOSTIC TERMS

cholangiogram	cholangiopancreatography	endoscopy
laparoscopy	laparotomy	retrograde
sigmoidoscopy		

TABLE 15-4

REVIEW OF MEDICAL AND SURGICAL TERMS

appendectomy	cecopexy	cheiloplasty
cheilorrhaphy	cholecystectomy	choledocholithotripsy
choledochotomy	colocolostomy	colostomy
gastrectomy	gastrotomy	glossectomy
herniorrhaphy	ileostomy	ileotomy

continued on page 344

Table 15-4 *continued from page 343*

litholytic agents	lithotripsy	nasogastric tube
postprandial	proctoclysis	pyloromyotomy
ventriculoperitoneal shunt		

15.12 Abbreviations

Abbreviation	Meaning
BE	barium enema (x-ray of the large bowel following the placement of barium into the rectum. Barium is a contrast medium used to highlight the large bowel.)
CBD	common bile duct
ERCP	endoscopic retrograde cholangio-pancreatography (x-ray of the bile ducts and pancreas following injection of a contrasting dye. Because the dye flows against the normal flow of substances, the term *retrograde*, meaning "to flow back," is used.)
GB	gallbladder
GBS	gallbladder series (type of x-ray)
GER	gastroesophageal reflux
GERD	gastroesophageal reflux disorder
GI	gastrointestinal
IVC	intravenous cholangiogram

continued on page 345

continued from page 344

Abbreviation	Meaning
NG	nasogastric
NGT	nasogastric tube
NPO	nothing by mouth
PTC	percutaneous transhepatic cholangiography (after injection of a contrast medium through the skin into the liver's biliary system, an x-ray examination of the bile ducts is performed.)
S&D	stomach and duodenum
TE	tracheoesophageal
UGI	upper gastrointestinal

15.13 Putting It All Together

Exercise 15-1   SHORT ANSWER

1. Name three functions of the digestive tract.

_____

_____

2. Name six major structures of the gastrointestinal tract and four accessory organs.

_____

_____

_____

_____

3. Describe the location of the:

   (a) lower esophageal sphincter

   _____

   (b) pyloric sphincter

   _____

4. Name the sections of the large intestine, in sequence, starting from the ileocecal valve.

   _____

   _____

5. Name the sections of the small intestine, proximal to distal.

   _____

6. Name the three salivary glands.

   _____

7. What is the function of salivary amylase?

   _____

8. List six functions of the liver.

   _____

   _____

   _____

   _____

   _____

   _____

9. Name two hormones secreted by the pancreas. What is their function?

   _____

   _____

10. Define: parietal peritoneum, visceral peritoneum, and peritoneal cavity.

    _____

    _____

    _____

11. Define hepatic duct, cystic duct, and common bile duct.

    _____

    _____

Exercise 15-2   MATCHING

Match the structure in Column A with its function in Column B.

Column A	Column B
_____ 1. uvula	A. mastication
_____ 2. rugae	B. prevents aspiration of food into the trachea
_____ 3. papillae	C. produces bile
_____ 4. villi	D. increase the surface area of the small intestine
_____ 5. large intestine	E. closes off the nasal passages during swallowing
_____ 6. teeth	F. increase the surface area of the stomach
_____ 7. plicae circulares	G. defecation
_____ 8. liver	H. absorption of digested foodstuffs
_____ 9. epiglottis	I. stores bile
_____ 10. gallbladder	J. contain taste buds

Exercise 15-3   DEFINITIONS

Define the following component parts.

1. bucc/o _____

2. cec/o _____

3. cheil/o _____

4. cholangi/o _____

5. cholecyst/o _____

6. choledoch/o _____

7. odont/o _____

8. enter/o _____

9. gingiv/o _____

10. gloss/o _____

11. hepat/o _____

12. ile/o _____

13. jejun/o _____

14. labi/o _____

15. lapar/o _____

16. lingu/o _____

17. lith/o _____

18. orex/i _____

19. proct/o _____

20. sial/o _____

21. sialaden/o _____

22. steat/o _____

23. stomat/o _____

24. or/o _____

25. viscer/o _____

26. -chalasia _____

27. -grade _____

28. -emesis _____

29. -phagia _____

30. -pepsia _____

31. -plakia _____

32. -prandial _____

33. peri- _____

34. -emia _____

Exercise 15-4   TERM DEFINITIONS

Define the following terms.

1. buccal mucosa _____

2. glossectomy _____

3. anorexia _____

4. oral _____

5. rectocele _____

6. sialolith _____

7. steatorrhea _____

8. sigmoidoscopy _____

9. stomatitis _____

10. visceroptosis _____

11. achalasia _____

12. retrograde _____

13. dyspepsia _____

14. postprandial _____

15. endoscopy _____

Exercise 15-5   BUILDING MEDICAL TERMS

Build the medical term.

1. pertaining to the anus and rectum

2. pertaining to around the anus

3. surgical removal of the appendix

4. inflammation of the appendix

5. surgical fixation of the cecum

6. pertaining to the ventricles and peritoneum

7. surgical repair of the lips

8. suturing of the lip

9. abnormal condition of the lips

10. inflammation of the colon

11. hernia repair

12. creation of a new opening between the colon and the abdomen

13. creation of a new opening between two segments of the colon

14. pertaining to liver cells

15. bile stones

16. tumor of the liver

17. displacement of intestines through the inguinal canal

18. excessive vomiting

19. vomiting of blood

20. black vomit

21. no eating

22. difficulty in eating

23. excessive eating

Exercise 15-6   IDENTIFYING SURGICAL AND CLINICAL PROCEDURES

Mark an **X** beside the terms indicating surgical or clinical procedures.

1. perianal   _____

2. cheiloplasty   _____

3. cecopexy   _____

4. cholecystitis   _____

5. edentulous   _____

6. orthodontist   _____

7. gastroesophageal reflux   _____

8. esophageal atresia   _____

9. gastrotomy   _____

10. postprandial   _____

11. choledocholithotripsy   _____

12. proctoclysis   _____

13. dyspepsia   _____

14. visceroptosis   _____

15. endoscopy   _____

Exercise 15-7   ADJECTIVAL FORMS

Mark an **X** beside the adjectival forms found in the list below.

1. anus   _____

2. biliary   _____

3. cecum   _____

4. duodenal   _____

5. colon   _____

6. periodontist   _____

7. esophageal   _____

8. anorexia   _____

9. pylorus   _____

10. salivary   _____

Exercise 15-8   **SPELLING PRACTICE**

Circle any misspelled words in the list below and correctly spell them in the space provided.

1. iliocecal valve   _____

2. melanemesis   _____

3. colecystitis   _____

4. cholitis   _____

5. gingivobuccal   _____

6. chielorhaphy   _____

7. pancreatitis   _____

8. saliviary   _____

9. visceroptosis   _____

10. vomitting   _____

16 CHAPTER

The Urinary and Male Reproductive Systems

CHAPTER ORGANIZATION

This chapter will help you learn about the urinary and male reproductive systems. It is divided into the following sections:

CHAPTER OBJECTIVES

On completion of this chapter, you will be able to do the following:

1. Name and locate the organs of the urinary system

2. Describe the function of the urinary system

3. Describe the structure and functions of the kidney, ureters, bladder, and urethra

4. Describe glomerular filtration, tubular reabsorption, and tubular secretion

5. Name and locate the organs of the male reproductive system

6. Describe the functions of the male reproductive system

7. Analyze, define, pronounce, and spell common terms of the urinary and male reproductive systems

8. Define common abbreviations of the urinary and male reproductive systems

INTRODUCTION

In this chapter, you will learn about the terminology associated with the male and female urinary systems, as well as basic structure and function. Because some structures of the male urinary system also function in the reproductive system, that system is dealt with here as well. The female reproductive system is discussed in Chapter 17.

16.1   Urinary System

The urinary system, as illustrated in Figure 16-1, consists of two **kidneys**, two tubes called **ureters** (you-**REE**-ters), a sac called the **urinary bladder**, and another tube called the **urethra** (you-**REE**-thra). The ureters drain fluid called **urine** from the kidneys into the urinary bladder. From there, the urine travels through the urethra and is excreted from the body. The only difference between male and female systems is that the male has a longer urethra, because it extends through the penis.

Memory Key	The urinary system consists of	
	two kidneys	a urinary bladder
	two ureters	a urethra

FIGURE 16-1
Anterior view of the
urinary system

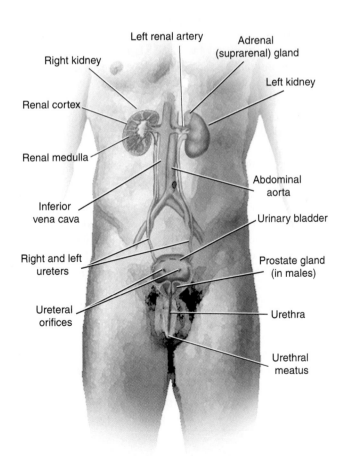

The body's tissue cells are surrounded by fluid called **extracellular fluid**. This fluid contains minerals such as sodium, calcium, and potassium, referred to as **electrolytes** (ee-**LECK**-troh-lights). It also contains nitrogenous waste products such as **urea** (you-**REE**-ah), **uric acid**, and **creatinine** (kree-**AT**-ih-neen). When the level of extracellular fluid is too high, some of the fluid seeps through capillary walls into the blood and lymph systems, carrying with it any excess electrolytes and nitrogenous wastes. The fluid is then transported to the kidneys. There, the fluid and electrolytes are either excreted or reabsorbed if the body now needs them. In this way, the urinary system maintains fluid and electrolyte balance in the body and rids the body of nitrogenous wastes. This is another example of how the body maintains **homeostasis** (hoh-mee-oh-**STAY**-sis). Death comes quickly if fluid and electrolyte homeostasis is not maintained.

> **Memory Key** | The urinary system maintains homeostasis of extracellular fluid by filtering out electrolytes and nitrogenous wastes and excreting them with excess fluid. The excretion is called urine.

THE KIDNEYS

The kidneys are bean-shaped, fist-sized organs lying on each side of the lumbar vertebrae. Their location is **retroperitoneal** (ret-roh-**per**-ih-toh-**NEE**-al), which means they are behind the peritoneal membrane. Each kidney is covered with tissue called the **renal** (**REE**-nal) **capsule** and is encased in a layer of **perirenal** (per-ih-**REE**-nal) **fat**, held in place by a thin membrane called the **renal fascia** (**REE**-nal **FASH**-ee-ah). These coverings prevent movement. The indented medial region of the kidney is called the **hilum** (**HIGH**-lum), the area of entry and exit for nerves, the renal artery, and the renal vein.

> **Memory Key** | • The kidneys lie retroperitoneally on each side of the lumbar area.
> • The outer covering of the kidney is the renal capsule, covered by perirenal fat and the renal fascia.
> • The nerves, renal artery, and renal vein enter and exit at the hilum.

The internal structure of the kidney is illustrated in Figure 16-2. Underlying the renal capsule is a layer called the **cortex** (**KOR**-tecks). Extensions of the cortex called **renal columns** lie between the **renal pyramids**, which are pyramid-shaped structures constituting the next layer, the **renal medulla** (meh-**DULL**-lah). The tip of each renal pyramid is called the **renal papilla** (pah-**PILL**-ah). This structure secretes urine into a small cavity called a **minor calyx** (**KAL**-icks) (pl. **calyces**). From there, the urine drains into larger cavities called **major calyces** (**KAL**-ih-sees), and then into ducts leading to the **renal pelvis**, which is the dilated, proximal portion of the ureter.

> **Memory Key** | • Under the renal capsule is the cortex, which projects inward in columns.
> • Between the columns are the renal pyramids of the renal medulla, tipped with renal papilla, which drain urine into minor calyces.
> • The urine then flows into the major calyces and then drains through ducts into the renal pelvis.

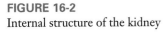

FIGURE 16-2
Internal structure of the kidney

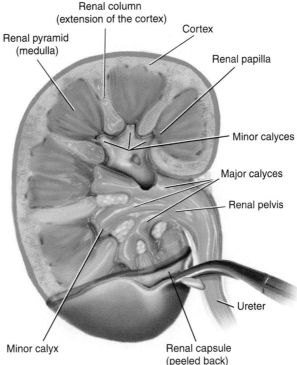

THE URETERS, URINARY BLADDER, AND URETHRA

The ureters are long, narrow tubes connecting the kidney to the bladder. Urine is moved along each ureter by peristalsis (per-ih-**STAL**-sis), the same type of muscle contraction that moves food through the digestive tract. The ureters empty into an expandable sac called the **urinary bladder**, which, along with associated structures, is illustrated in Figure 16-3. Note the **trigone** (**TRI**-gohn) area of the bladder, defined by the triangle formed by the two ureteral openings and the opening into the urethra.

The storage capacity of the bladder allows for occasional rather than constant urination. When sufficient urine has collected, muscle fibers in the wall of the bladder contract, causing the urine to pass into the **urethra**, through which it is voided. This process is called urination or **micturition** (**mick**-too-**RISH**-un), and the reflex action of the external sphincter is called the **micturition reflex**.

Memory Key • Urine empties from the renal pelvis of each kidney into the ureters and is pushed along by peristalsis to the trigone of the urinary bladder.
 • Muscle contraction pushes the urine out of the bladder into the urethra, from which it is voided from the body.

FIGURE 16-3
Ureters, urinary bladder,
and urethra

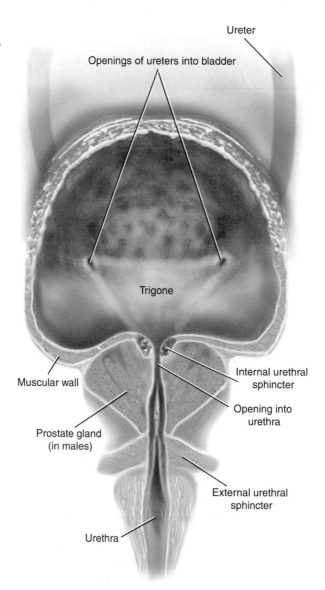

Ureter

Openings of ureters into bladder

Trigone

Muscular wall

Prostate gland
(in males)

Internal urethral
sphincter

Opening into
urethra

External urethral
sphincter

Urethra

URINE PRODUCTION IN THE KIDNEY

Within each kidney are approximately one million nephrons (see Figure 16-4). These tiny structures are responsible for producing urine. In very general terms, they do so by filtering out excess electrolytes and waste products from the blood. Filtration of the blood occurs in a network of capillaries known as glomerular capillaries. Each cluster of glomerular capillaries is called a **glomerulus** (gloh-**MER**-you-lus). The walls of these capillaries allow a mixture of water, electrolytes, and waste products to pass through into the **Bowman's** (glomerular) **capsule**, which surrounds the glomerulus. This mixture, called **filtrate** (**FIL**-trayt), then flows into long twisting tubes, still part of the nephron, called **renal tubules**. As filtrate travels along renal tubules, there is a continuous exchange of substances between

FIGURE 16-4
Anatomy of the kidney: (A) kidneys, ureters, and bladder, posterior view. (B) the nephron includes the glomerulus, Bowman's capsule, and renal tubule, which includes the proximal convoluted tubule, Henle's loop, and distal convoluted tubule. Note the capillary net surrounding the renal tubule.

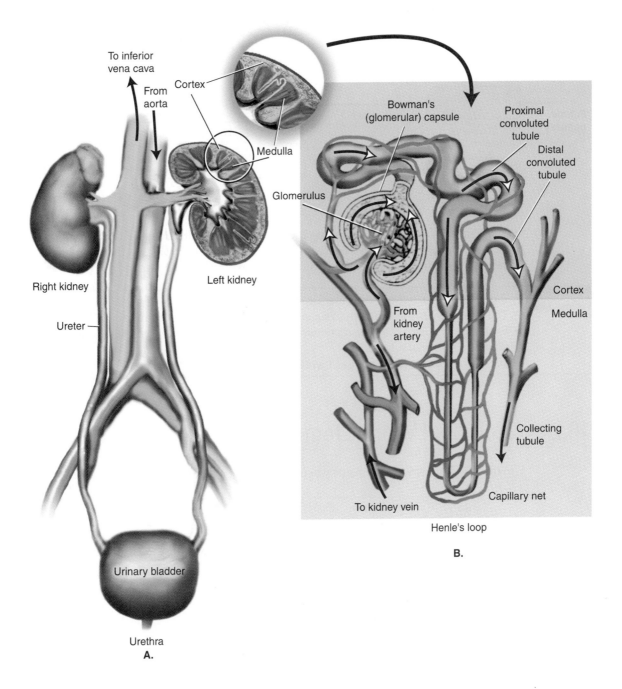

FIGURE 16-5

Exchange of substances between blood and capillaries

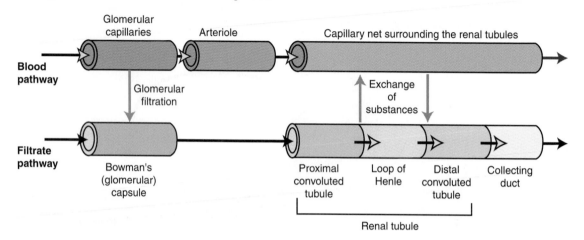

the blood in the capillaries surrounding the tubules and the filtrate inside them (see Figure 16-5). After the filtrate has traveled its entire course, urine is left, which is then excreted out of the nephron into collecting ducts, onto the calyces, and into the ureters.

Memory Key
- Blood is filtered in the glomerular capillaries or glomerulus.
- The filtrate passes into Bowman's capsules and then into renal tubules.
- Exchange of substances occurs between the blood in surrounding capillaries and the filtrate in the renal tubules.
- Urine is left after the filtrate has traveled the entire renal tubule.

16.2   Additional Word Elements

Use these additional word elements when studying the medical terms in this chapter.

Root	Meaning
bacteri/o	bacteria
crypt/o	hidden
noct/o	night
protein/o	protein
spermat/o	sperm

Suffix	Meaning
-cidal	to kill
-continence	to stop

Prefix	Meaning
trans-	through; across

16.3 Term Analysis and Definition Pertaining to the Urinary System

	calic/o; calyc/o	calix; calyx
Term	**Term Analysis**	**Definition**
caliceal (calyceal) (kal-ih-SEE-al)	-eal = pertaining to	pertaining to the calyces (calices)
caliectasis (calyectasis) (kal-ih-ECK-tah-sis)	-ectasis = dilation; stretching	dilation of the calyx
	catheter/o	**something inserted**
catheterization (kath-eh-ter-eye-ZAY-shun)	-ion = process	the process of inserting a flexible tube into a body cavity, such as the urinary tract, for the purpose of removing fluid
	corpor/o	**body**
extracorporeal (ecks-trah-kor-POR-ee-al)	-eal = pertaining to extra- = outside	pertaining to outside the body

	cortic/o	cortex; outer layer
Term cortical (**KOR**-tih-kal)	**Term Analysis** -al = pertaining to	**Definition** pertaining to the cortex or outer layer of the kidney

	cyst/o	bladder
cystitis (sis-**TYE**-tis)	-itis = inflammation	inflammation of the bladder
cystoscope (**SIS**-toh-skope)	-scope = instrument used to visually examine	instrument used to visually examine the bladder
cystoscopy (sis-**TOS**-koh-pee)	-scopy = process of visual examination	process of visually examining the bladder (see Figure 16-6)

	glomerul/o	glomerulus
glomerulonephritis (glow-**mer**-you-low-neh-**FRY**-tis)	-itis = inflammation **nephr/o** = kidney	inflammation of the glomeruli of the kidney

FIGURE 16-6
Cystoscopy

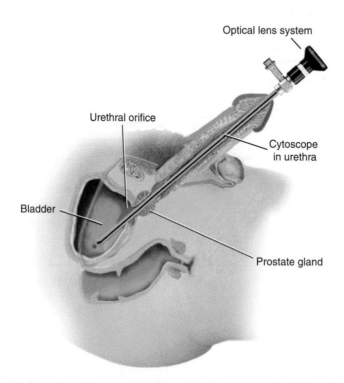

Optical lens system

Urethral orifice

Cytoscope
in urethra

Bladder

Prostate gland

Term	Term Analysis	Definition
glomerulosclerosis (gloh-**mer**-you-loh-skleh-**ROH**-sis)	-sclerosis = hardening	hardening of the glomerulus
	lith/o	**stone**
lithotripsy (**LITH**-oh-**trip**-see)	-tripsy = crushing	surgical crushing of kidney stones using procedures such as **extracorporeal shock wave lithotripsy** (ESWL), which utilizes ultrasound to break up the stones into small pieces, facilitating expulsion from the urinary tract (see Figure 16-7)
	meat/o	**meatus**
meatotomy (**me**-ah-**TOT**-oh-me)	-tomy = process of cutting	process of cutting into the urethral meatus (to widen the meatus (see urethral meatus, Figure 16-1)

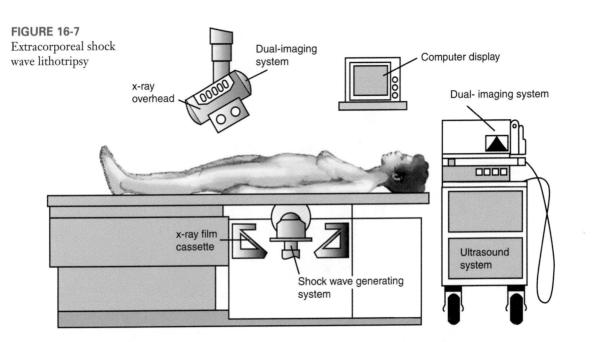

FIGURE 16-7
Extracorporeal shock wave lithotripsy

Dual-imaging system

Computer display

x-ray overhead

Dual- imaging system

x-ray film cassette

Shock wave generating system

Ultrasound system

	medull/o	medulla
Term	**Term Analysis**	**Definition**
medullary (**MED**-you-lar-ee)	-ary = pertaining to	pertaining to the medulla

	nephr/o	kidney
nephrolithiasis (**nef**-roh-lih-**THIGH**-ah-sis)	-iasis = abnormal condition **lith/o** = stones	kidney stones. *NOTE:* The kidney stones can travel, causing urinary obstruction anywhere along the urinary tract (see Figure 16-8).
nephrolithotomy (**nef**-roh-lih-**THOT**-oh-mee)	-tomy = process of cutting **lith/o** = stones	process of removing stones by cutting into the kidney
nephropathy (neh-**FROP**-ah-thee)	-pathy = disease	disease of the kidney
nephropexy (**NEF**-roh-**peck**-see)	-pexy = surgical fixation	surgical fixation of the kidney

FIGURE 16-8
Nephrolithiasis

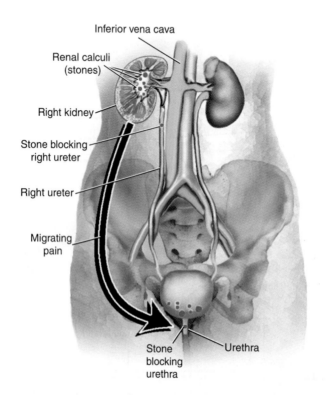

Inferior vena cava

Renal calculi (stones)

Right kidney

Stone blocking right ureter

Right ureter

Migrating pain

Stone blocking urethra

Urethra

Term	Term Analysis	Definition
nephroptosis (**nef**-rop-**TOH**-sis)	-ptosis = drooping; prolapse; sagging	drooping kidney
nephrotomography (**nef**-roh-toh-**MOG**-rah-fee)	-graphy = process of recording; producing images **tom/o** = cut	procedure that utilizes x-rays to show the renal tissue at various depths. *NOTE:* Tomography gives different "cuts" or views of the kidney.
hydronephrosis (high-droh-neh-FROH-sis)	-osis = abnormal condition **hydr/o** = water	accumulation of fluid in the renal pelvis due to the obstruction of the normal urinary pathway (see Figure 16-9)

FIGURE 16-9
Hydronephrosis

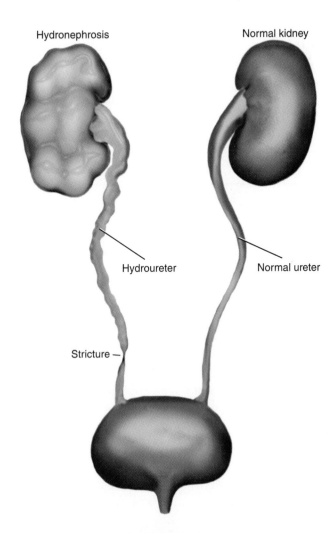

Hydronephrosis

Normal kidney

Hydroureter

Normal ureter

Stricture

Term	Term Analysis	Definition
nephroblastoma (**nef**-roh-blas-**TOH**-mah)	-oma = tumor; mass -blast = immature; a growing thing	malignant tumor of the kidney, usually occurring in children; also known as Wilm's tumor
	pyel/o	**renal pelvis**
pyelogram (**PYE**-eh-loh-gram)	-gram = record	record of the ureter and kidney, particularly the renal pelvis
pyelonephritis (**pye**-eh-loh-neh-**FRY**-tis)	-itis = inflammation **nephr/o** = kidney	inflammation of the kidney pelvis and kidney
	ren/o	**kidney**
renal hypoplasia (**REE**-nal **high**-poh-**PLAY**-zee-ah)	-al = pertaining to -plasia = formation; development hypo- = under; below normal; deficient	underdeveloped kidney
	trigon/o	**trigone**
trigonitis (**trig**-oh-**NIGH**-tis)	-itis = inflammation	inflammation of the trigone
	ureter/o	**ureter**
ureteral (you-**REE**-ter-al)	-al = pertaining to	pertaining to the ureter
ureterectasis (you-**ree**-ter-**ECK**-tah-sis)	-ectasis = dilation; stretching	stretching of the ureters
ureteroileostomy (you-**ree**-ter-oh-**il**-ee-**OS**-toh-mee)	-stomy = new opening **ile/o** = ileum; portion of the small intestine	new opening between the ureter and ileum. *NOTE:* This procedure diverts urine from the ureter to the ileum.
ureterolith (you-**REE**-ter-oh-lith)	-lith = stone	stone in the ureter

Term	Term Analysis	Definition
ureterostenosis (you-**ree**-ter-oh-steh-**NOH**-sis)	-stenosis = narrowing	narrowing of the ureter
ureterostomy (you-**ree**-ter-**OS**-toh-mee)	-stomy = new opening	new opening between the ureter and abdominal wall. *NOTE:* This procedure diverts urine to the exterior of the body
	urethr/o	**urethra**
cystourethrography (**sis**-toh-you-ree-**THROG**-rah-fee)	-graphy = process of recording; producing images **cyst/o** = bladder	process of producing an image of the bladder and urethra using x-rays. If this procedure is performed as the patient is discharging urine, it is called a **voiding** cystourethrography (VCUG).
transurethral (**trans**-you-**REE**-thral)	-al = pertaining to trans- = across or through	performed through the urethra
urethrorrhagia (you-**ree**-throh-**RAY**-jee-ah)	-rrhagia = burst forth; hemorrhage	hemorrhaging from the urethra
urethroplasty (you-**REE**-throh-**plas**-tee)	-plasty = surgical repair; surgical reconstruction	surgical repair of the urethra
	urin/o	**urine**
urinary (**YOU**-rih-**nar**-ee)	-ary = pertaining to	pertaining to urine
	ur/o	**urinary tract; urine; urination**
uremia (you-**REE**-mee-ah)	-emia = blood condition	accumulation of waste products in the blood due to loss of kidney function; azotemia

Term	Term Analysis	Definition
urogram (**YOU**-roh-gram)	-gram = record	record of the urinary tract. *NOTE:* Two types of urograms are (a) **excretory urogram**, an x-ray examination of the urinary tract following injection of a contrast medium into a vein. Also known as intravenous urogram (IVU), or intravenous pyelogram (IVP). (b) **retrograde urogram**, in which a contrast medium is injected into the ureters through a cystoscope and allowed to flow backward, highlighting the urinary structures; also known as retrograde pyelogram. In Figure 16-10, note the kidneys and ureters as seen on an excretory urogram.
urologist (you-**ROL**-oh-jist)	-logist = specialist	specialist in the study of the urinary system in females and the urinary and reproductive systems in males

FIGURE 16-10
Excretory urogram

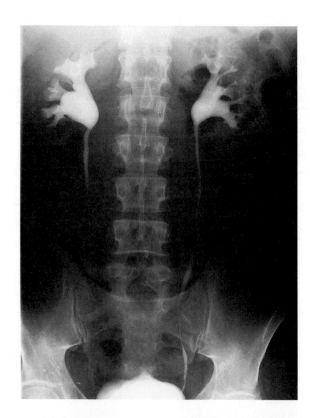

	vesic/o	bladder
Term	**Term Analysis**	**Definition**
vesicosigmoidostomy (**ves**-ih-koh-**sig**-moi-**DOS**-toh-mee)	-stomy = new opening	new opening between bladder and sigmoid colon
vesicoureteral reflux (**ves**-ih-koh-you-**REE**-ter-al **REE**-flucks)	-al = pertaining to **ureter/o** = ureter -flux = flow re- = back	backward flow of urine from bladder to ureter

SUFFIXES

	-lysis	**separate; breakdown; destruction**
Term	**Term Analysis**	**Definition**
dialysis (dye-**AL**-ih-sis)	dia- = through; complete	mechanical replacement of kidney function when the kidney is dysfunctional. *NOTE:* Types include hemodialysis (HD), in which the blood is passed through a kidney machine for waste removal; and peritoneal dialysis (PD), in which fluid is injected into the peritoneal cavity. Wastes flow out of the blood into the fluid, and the fluid is removed (see Figures 16-11 and 16-12).
urinalysis (**you**-rih-**NAL**-ih-sis)	-lysis = breakdown; separate; destruction ana- = apart	laboratory analysis of urine

	-uria	**urine; urination**
anuria (ah-**NEW**-ree-ah)	an- = no; not; lack of	no urine formation; also known as suppression
bacteriuria (back-**tee**-ree-**YOU**-ree-ah)	**bacteri/o** = bacteria	bacteria in the urine
dysuria (dis-**YOU**-ree-ah)	dys- = painful; difficult; bad	painful urination

FIGURE 16-11
Hemodialysis

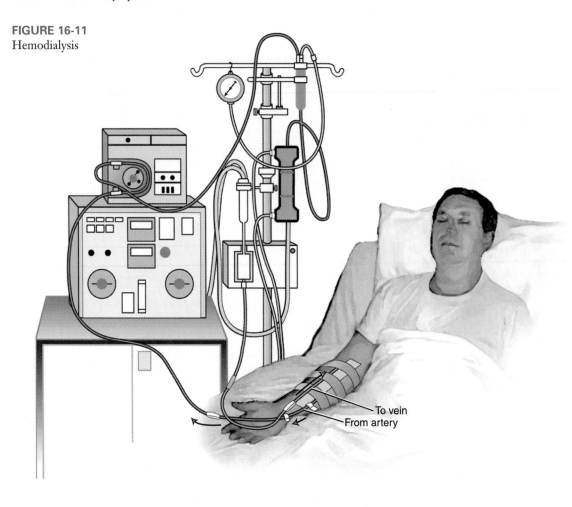

To vein
From artery

Term	Term Analysis	Definition
hematuria (**hem**-ah-**TOO**-ree-ah)	**hemat/o** = blood	blood in the urine
nocturia (nock-**TOO**-ree-ah)	**noct/o** = night	frequent urination at night
oliguria (**ol**-ih-**GOO**-ree-ah)	oligo- = deficient; few; scanty	decreased urination
proteinuria (**pro**-teen-**YOU**-ree-ah)	**protein/o** = protein	excessive amounts of protein in the urine; albuminuria
pyuria (pye-**YOU**-ree-ah)	**py/o** = pus	pus in the urine

FIGURE 16-12
Peritoneal dialysis

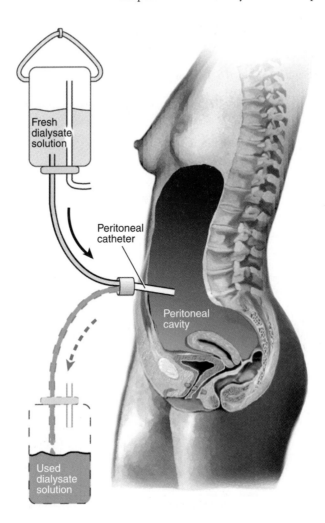

Fresh
dialysate
solution

Peritoneal
catheter

Peritoneal
cavity

Used
dialysate
solution

PREFIXES

	in-	no; not
Term	**Term Analysis**	**Definition**
incontinence (in-**KON**-tih-nens)	-continence = to stop	no control of excretory functions such as urination
	poly-	**many**
polyuria (**pol**-ee-**YOU**-ree-ah)	-uria = urine; urination	excretion of large amounts of urine
polycystic kidneys (**pol**-ee-**SIS**-tick)	-ic = pertaining to **cyst/o** = sac; cysts	kidney with many cysts

16.4   Review of Terms Pertaining to the Urinary System

Define the terms in Tables 16-1 through 16-4 in the space provided.

TABLE 16-1

REVIEW OF ANATOMICAL TERMS

caliceal	cortical	extracorporeal
medullary	transurethral	ureteral
urinary		

TABLE 16-2

REVIEW OF PATHOLOGIC TERMS

anuria	bacteriuria	caliectasis
cystitis	dysuria	glomerulonephritis
glomerulosclerosis	hematuria	hydronephrosis
incontinence	nephroblastoma	nephrolithiasis
nephropathy	nephroptosis	nocturia
oliguria	polycystic kidneys	polyuria
proteinuria	pyelonephritis	pyuria
renal hypoplasia	trigonitis	uremia
ureterectasis	ureterolith	ureterostenosis
urethrorrhagia	vesicoureteral reflux	

TABLE 16-3

REVIEW OF DIAGNOSTIC TERMS

cystourethrography	nephrotomography	pyelogram
urinalysis	urogram	

TABLE 16-4

REVIEW OF CLINICAL AND SURGICAL PROCEDURES

catheterization	cystoscope	cystoscopy
dialysis	lithotripsy	meatotomy
nephrolithotomy	nephropexy	ureteroileostomy
ureterostomy	urethroplasty	vesicosigmoidostomy

16.5   Abbreviations Pertaining to the Urinary System

Abbreviation	Meaning
ARF	acute renal failure
BUN	blood urea nitrogen (test that measures amount of urea nitrogen, a waste product, in the blood; increased amounts indicate glomerular dysfunction)
CAPD	continuous ambulatory peritoneal dialysis
CRF	chronic renal failure
cysto	cystoscopic examination

continued on page 372

continued from page 371

Abbreviation	Meaning
ESWL	extracorporeal shock wave lithotripsy
GU	genitourinary
HD	hemodialysis
IVP	intravenous pyelogram
IVU	intravenous urogram
KKUB	kidney, kidney, ureter, and bladder
KUB	kidney, ureter, and bladder
PD	peritoneal dialysis
PKU	phenylketonuria (a genetic disorder whereby an important digestive enzyme is missing. Lack of this enzyme may result in mental retardation if not treated promptly.)
QNS	quantity not sufficient
RP	retrograde pyelogram
UA	urinalysis
UTI	urinary tract infection
VCUG	voiding cystourethrography

16.6   Male Reproductive System

The kidneys can be thought of as manufacturing centers for the product urine. The urinary tract is the distribution network. The male reproductive system can be viewed in a similar way. The **testes** (**TEST**-tees), or **testicles** (**TEST**-ick-els), are the manufacturing centers for the product **sperm**, and the **reproductive tract** is the distribution network. The other components are the **accessory reproductive organs** and the **external genitalia**, all illustrated in Figure 16-13.

Memory Key	The male reproductive system consists of the
	testes accessory reproductive organs
	reproductive tract external genitalia

FIGURE 16-13
Male reproductive system

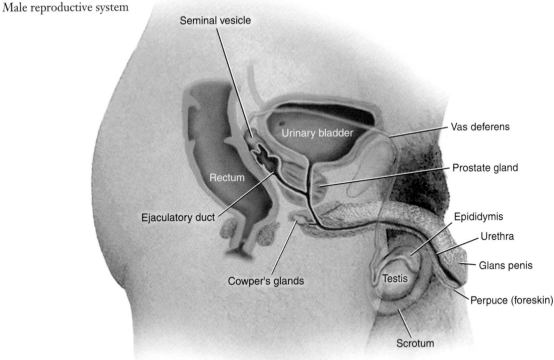

The testes are located in an external skin sac called the **scrotum** (**SKROH**-tum). Sperm production is called **spermatogenesis** (**sper**-mah-toh-jen-**EE**-sis) and takes place within tiny tubes inside the testes called **seminiferous tubules** (see Figure 16-14). Interstitial (Leydig) cells in the testes produce the hormone **testosterone** (tes-**TOS**-ter-own), which is essential for spermatogenesis and the development of secondary male gender characteristics such as facial hair and pubescent voice change.

- The testes lie in the scrotum.
- Sperm production (spermatogenesis) takes place in seminiferous tubules in the testes.
- The sex hormone testosterone is produced in interstitial cells in the testes.

The reproductive tract begins with the **epididymis** (ep-ih-**DID**-ih-mis), a coiled tube on the superior surface of each testicle. The epididymis stores sperm and leads into a duct called the **ductus deferens** or **vas deferens** (vas-**DEF**-er-enz), which circles the urinary bladder and joins a duct from the **seminal vesicle** (**SEM**-ih-nal **VES**-ih-kal) to form the **ejaculatory duct**. This duct leads through the **prostate** (**PROS**-tayt) **gland** and joins the urethra.

Memory Key The reproductive tract starts at the epididymis, then on to the ductus (vas) deferens, joining the seminal vesicle to form the ejaculatory duct, and continuing through the prostate gland to join the urethra.

FIGURE 16-14
Internal structures of the testes. The paths of these structures are indicated by the arrows.

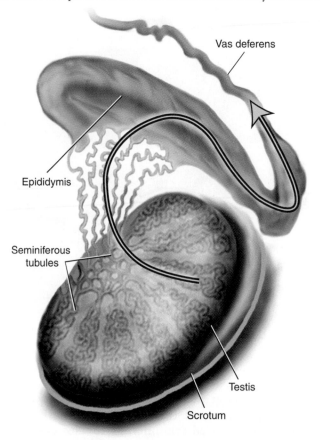

Vas deferens

Epididymis

Seminiferous
tubules

Testis

Scrotum

The accessory organs are the **seminal vesicles**, **prostate**, and **bulbourethral** (**bul**-boh-you-**REE**-thral), or **Cowper's**, **glands**. These glands secrete substances that together form the fluid in which sperm is ejaculated, called **semen**. This substance nourishes and protects sperm.

Memory Key	The accessory organs are the seminal vesicles, prostate, and bulbourethral (Cowper's) glands, which together secrete semen.

The scrotum and the penis are the external genitalia. The tip of the penis is called the **glans penis** (glanz **PEE**-nis), which contains the opening for urination and ejaculation, the **urethral orifice**, also called the urinary **meatus** (me-**AY**-tus). The glans is covered with loose skin called **foreskin** or **prepuce** (**PRE**-pyous), which is often removed by a surgical process called **circumcision** (ser-kum-**SIZH**-un).

Memory Key	• The external genitalia includes the penis and scrotum. • The glans penis is the tip of the penis. • The meatus is the urethral opening. • The prepuce is excess skin covering the glans penis.

16.7   Term Analysis and Definition Pertaining to the Male Reproductive System

	andr/o	male
Term	**Term Analysis**	**Definition**
androgenic (**an**-droh-**JEN**-ick)	-genic = producing	producing masculinizing effects
	balan/o	**glans penis**
balanitis (**bal**-ah-**NIGH**-tis)	-itis = inflammation	inflammation of the glans penis
balanorrhea (**bal**-an-oh-**REE**-ah)	-rrhea = flow; discharge	discharge from the glans penis
	epididym/o	**epididymis**
epididymitis (**ep**-ih-did-ih-**MY**-tis)	-itis = inflammation	inflammation of the epididymis
	orchid/o; orchi/o	**testicle; testis**
cryptorchidism (krip-**TOR**-kih-**diz**-um)	-ism = process **crypt/o** = hidden	undescended testicles. *NOTE:* During fetal development, the testicles fail to descend into the scrotum, remaining instead in the abdominal cavity. This condition can result in sterility if not treated.
orchidopexy (**OR**-kid-oh-**peck**-see)	-pexy = surgical fixation	surgical fixation of the testicle onto the scrotum; treatment for cryptorchidism
orchitis (or-**KYE**-tis)	-itis = inflammation	inflammation of the testicle
	prostat/o	**prostate**
prostatitis (**pros**-tah-**TYE**-tis)	-itis = inflammation	inflammation of the prostate

Term	Term Analysis	Definition
prostatectomy (**pros**-tah-**TECK**-toh-mee)	-ectomy = excision; surgical removal	excision of the prostate
	sperm/o; spermat/o	**spermatozoa; sperm**
aspermatogenesis (ay-**sper**-mah-toh-**JEN**-eh-sis)	-genesis = production; formation a- = no; not; lack of	no production of spermatozoa. *NOTE:* The singular of spermatozoa is spermatozoon.
oligospermia (**ol**-ih-goh-**SPER**-mee-ah)	oligo- = deficient; scanty; few	deficient number of spermatozoa
spermatocidal (**sper**-mah-toh-**SYE**-dal)	-cidal = to kill	to kill or destroy spermatozoa; spermicidal
	testicul/o	**testicle; testis**
testicular (tes-**TICK**-you-lar)	-ar = pertaining to	pertaining to the testicle
	vas/o	**vas deferens**
vasectomy (vah-**SECK**-toh-mee)	-ectomy = excision; surgical removal	excision of the vas deferens or a portion of it (see Figure 16-15)

FIGURE 16-15
Vasectomy

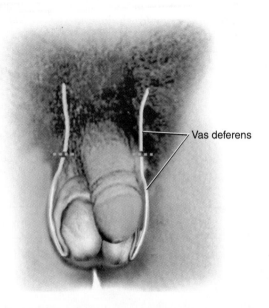

Vas deferens

SUFFIXES

	-cele	hernia
Term	**Term Analysis**	**Definition**
hematocele (**HE**-mah-toh-**seel**)	**hemat/o** = blood	accumulation of blood around the testicles
hydrocele (**HIGH**-droh-seel)	**hydr/o** = water	accumulation of fluid around the testicles (see Figure 16-16)
spermatocele (**SPER**-mah-toh-seel)	**spermat/o** = sperm	accumulation of a milky fluid in the testicles or epididymis
varicocele (**VAR**-ih-koh-**seel**)	**varic/o** = varicose vein; dilated, twisted vein	dilatation of testicular veins inside the scrotum (see Figure 16-17)

FIGURE 16-16
Hydrocele

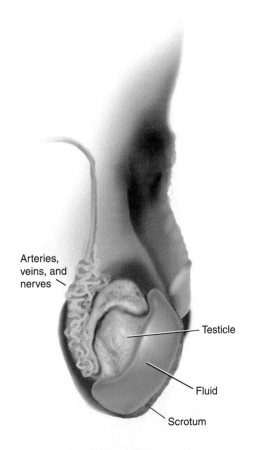

Arteries, veins, and nerves

Testicle

Fluid

Scrotum

FIGURE 16-17
Varicocele

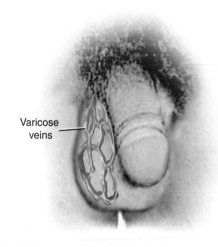

Varicose
veins

	-potence	power
Term	**Term Analysis**	**Definition**
impotence (**IM**-poh-tens)	in(m) = no or not	inability to achieve and maintain an erection

Memory Key   -in changes to -im before word elements starting with *p*.

	-spadias	opening; split
epispadias (**ep**-ih-**SPAY**-dee-as)	epi- = on; upon; above	congenital opening of the meatus on the dorsum (top side) of the penis (see Figure 16-18)
hypospadias (**high**-poh-**SPAY**-dee-as)	hypo- = under	congenital opening of the meatus on the ventral (underside) of the penis (see Figure 16-19)

	-trophy	nourishment
benign prostatic hypertrophy (BPH) (be-**NINE** proh-**STAT**-ick **HIGH**-per-troh-fee)	hyper- = excessive benign = harmless; not malignant prostatic = pertaining to the prostate	benign enlargement of the prostate that squeezes on the urethra, obstructing the passage of urine (see Figure 16-20)

FIGURE 16-18
Epispadias

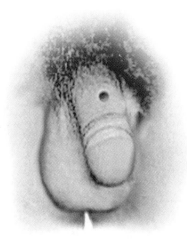

FIGURE 16-19
Hypospadias

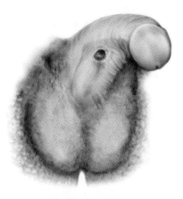

FIGURE 16-20
Benign prostatic hypertrophy

Benign prostatic hypertrophy

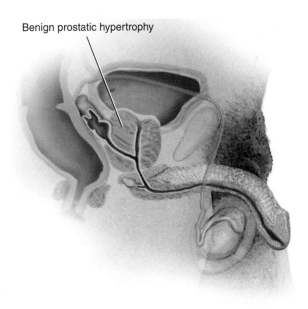

PREFIXES

	circum-	around
Term	**Term Analysis**	**Definition**
circumcision (**ser**-kum-**SIZH**-un)	-ion = process **cis/o** = to cut	removal of the prepuce or foreskin
	re-	**back**
transurethral resection (TUR or TURP) (**trans**-you-**REE**-thral ree-**SECK**-shun)	-ion = process **sect/o** = to cut transurethral = pertaining to across the urethra	excision (to cut back) all or part of the prostate through the urethra (see Figure 16-21). *NOTE:* This procedure is performed for benign prostatic hypertrophy.

FIGURE 16-21
Transurethral resection

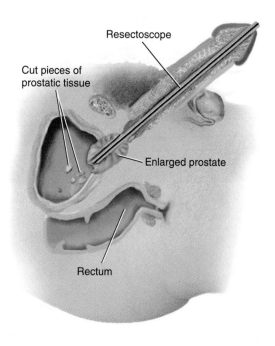

Resectoscope

Cut pieces of prostatic tissue

Enlarged prostate

Rectum

16.8   Abbreviations Pertaining to the Male Reproductive System

Abbreviation	Meaning
BPH	benign prostatic hypertrophy
TUR	transurethral resection
TURP	transurethral resection of the prostate

16.9   Review of Terms Pertaining to the Male Reproductive System

Define the terms in Tables 16-5 through 16-7 in the space provided.

TABLE 16-5

REVIEW OF ANATOMICAL AND PHYSIOLOGICAL TERMS

androgenic	testicular

TABLE 16-6

REVIEW OF PATHOLOGIC TERMS

aspermatogenesis	balanitis	balanorrhea
benign prostatic hypertrophy	cryptorchidism	epididymitis

continued on page 382

Table 16-6 *continued from page 381*

epispadias	hematocele	hydrocele
hypospadias	impotence	oligospermia
orchitis	prostatitis	spermatocele
spermatocidal	varicocele	

TABLE 16-7

REVIEW OF SURGICAL PROCEDURES

circumcision	orchidopexy	prostatectomy
transurethral resection	vasectomy	

16.10 Putting It All Together

Exercise 16-1   MATCHING

Match the term in Column A with its definition in Column B.

Column A	Column B
_____ 1. renal medulla	A. filter blood
_____ 2. renal pelvis	B. triangular area of the bladder
_____ 3. trigone	C. inner layer of the kidney
_____ 4. seminiferous tubules	D. function in spermatogenesis
_____ 5. renal fascia	E. membrane surrounding the kidney
_____ 6. glomeruli	F. dilated, upper portion of the ureter

Exercise 16-2   IDENTIFICATION

Write the suffix; root, and/or prefix for the following:

1. glans penis _____

2. calix _____

3. bladder _____

4. stone _____

5. kidney _____

6. testicle _____

7. kidney pelvis _____

8. vas deferens _____

9. urine _____

10. urinary tract _____

11. hernia _____

12. opening; split _____

13. around _____

14. outside _____

15. hardening _____

16. narrowing _____

17. crushing _____

18. process of cutting _____

19. abnormal condition _____

20. blood condition _____

21. surgical fixation _____

22. drooping _____

23. record _____

24. deficient; scanty _____

25. to kill _____

26. across _____

27. varicose vein _____

28. through; complete _____

29. night _____

30. disease _____

Exercise 16-3   BUILDING MEDICAL TERMS

Build the medical term for the following.

1. pertaining to outside the body _____

2. instrument used to visually examine
   the bladder _____

3. crushing of stones _____

4. accumulation of fluid in the renal pelvis
   due to the obstruction of the normal
   urinary pathway _____

5. undescended testicles _____

6. deficient numbers of spermatozoa _____

7. hemorrhaging from the urethra _____

8. new opening between the bladder and
   sigmoid colon _____

9. new opening between the ureter
   and ileum _____

10. new opening between the ureter and
    abdominal wall _____

11. process of cutting into the urinary meatus _____

12. surgical repair of the urethra _____

Exercise 16-4   BUILDING TERMS

I. Use -cele to build terms for the following definitions.

1. accumulation of blood around
   the testicles _____

2. accumulation of fluid around
   the testicles _____

3. accumulation of a milky fluid in
   the testicles or epididymis _____

4. dilation of testicular veins inside
   the scrotum _____

II. Use -uria to build terms for the following definitions.

  5. no urine formation   _____

  6. bacteria in the urine   _____

  7. painful urination   _____

  8. blood in the urine   _____

  9. frequent urination at night   _____

  10. decreased urination   _____

  11. excessive amounts of protein in
    the urine   _____

  12. pus in the urine   _____

III. Use **nephr/o** to build terms for the following definitions.

  13. kidney stones   _____

  14. process of removing stones by
    cutting into the kidney   _____

  15. disease of the kidney   _____

  16. surgical fixation of the kidney   _____

  17. drooping kidney   _____

  18. procedure that utilizes x-rays to
    show renal tissue at various depths   _____

  19. malignant tumor of the kidney,
    made up of undeveloped material   _____

Exercise 16-5   IDENTIFICATION

Place an **X** beside the terms indicating a surgical or clinical procedure.

  1. androgenic   _____

  2. glomerulosclerosis   _____

  3. lithotripsy   _____

  4. nephrolithiasis   _____

  5. nephrolithotomy   _____

  6. cryptorchidism   _____

  7. orchidopexy   _____

  8. renal hypoplasia   _____

  9. vasectomy   _____

10. cystourethrography _____

11. urinary _____

12. vesicoureteral reflux _____

13. epispadias _____

14. circumcision _____

Exercise 16-6 — DEFINITIONS

Define the following terms.

1. aspermatogenesis _____

2. spermatocidal _____

3. uremia _____

4. vesicoureteral reflux _____

5. dialysis _____

6. urinalysis _____

7. hypospadias _____

8. incontinence _____

9. circumcision _____

10. polycystic kidneys _____

Exercise 16-7 — ADJECTIVES

Write the adjective for the following.

1. body _____

2. cortex _____

3. calyx _____

4. bladder _____

5. glomerulus _____

6. kidney _____

7. testicle _____

8. ureter _____

9. urethra _____

10. urine _____

Exercise 16-8   PLURALS

Write the plural for the following. Use the dictionary if necessary.

1. cortex _____

2. calix; calyx _____

3. epididymis _____

4. glomerulus _____

5. meatus _____

6. testis _____

7. kidney pelvis _____

8. testicle _____

9. spermatozoon _____

10. ureter _____

Exercise 16-9   SPELLING

Circle any misspelled words in the list below and correctly spell them in the space provided.

1. balanorhea _____

2. orchitis _____

3. cysitis _____

4. epididymus _____

5. caliseal _____

6. prostratectomy _____

7. trigonitis _____

8. ureterorrhagia _____

9. incontinance _____

10. extracorporeal _____

17 CHAPTER

The Female Reproductive System and Obstetrics

CHAPTER ORGANIZATION

This chapter will help you learn about the female reproductive system and obstetrics. It is divided into the following sections:

CHAPTER OBJECTIVES

On completion of this chapter, you will be able to do the following:

1. Name, locate, and describe the structures of the female reproductive system

2. Describe the menstrual, ovulatory, and secretory periods

3. Describe the terms related to pregnancy and parturition

4. Analyze, define, pronounce, and spell common terms of the female reproductive system and obstetrics

5. Define common abbreviations of the female reproductive system and obstetrics

INTRODUCTION

The female reproductive system consists of the **ovaries** (**OH**-vah-rees), the **uterus** (**YOU**-ter-us), the **uterine** or **fallopian** (fal-**LOH**-pee-an) **tubes**, the **vagina** (vah-**JIGH**-nah) or **vaginal orifice**, the **external genitalia**, and the **mammary glands**. Figure 17-1 has two illustrations of these structures (except the mammary glands).

Memory Key	The female reproductive system consists of ovaries, uterus, uterine (fallopian) tubes, vagina, external genitalia, and mammary glands.

17.1   Structures of the Female Reproductive System

THE OVARIES

The almond-shaped ovaries are glands. They are located in the pelvic cavity, one on each side of the uterus. They are held in place by ligaments (broad, ovarian, and suspensory) (see Figure 17-1B). Their functions are to discharge the **egg** or **ovum** (pl. ova), and to produce various hormones. The ovaries of a newborn female contain a lifetime supply of immature eggs. Puberty brings on egg release. In approximately 28-day cycles, alternating from ovary to ovary, one egg is released. This process is called **ovulation** (ov-you-**LAY**-shun).

Memory Key	The ovaries are glands that discharge ova and produce sex hormones. The process of egg release is called ovulation.

The ovaries regulate the menstrual cycle (discussed below) by the release of the sex hormones **estrogen** (**ES**-troh-jen) and **progesterone** (pro-**JES**-ter-on). Estrogen is important in the development of secondary female characteristics such as the breasts and pubic hair growth. Progesterone stimulates the growth of blood vessels in the uterus, which will be needed to supply blood if the egg is fertilized. The estrogen stimulates the thickening of the lining of the uterus to prepare for the implantation of a fertilized egg. If no fertilization takes place, this buildup of tissue is sloughed off in a process called **menstruation** (men-stroo-**AY**-shun) or **menses** (**MEN**-seez). Sometime between the ages of 45 and 55, all of the eggs either have been discharged or have degenerated. The reproductive cycle then ceases, and the woman is in **menopause** (**MEN**-oh-pawz), discussed below.

Memory Key	Stimulated by the hormones estrogen and progesterone, the lining of the uterus becomes thicker and more vascular to prepare for implantation of a fertilized egg. Menstruation follows if fertilization does not occur.

THE FALLOPIAN TUBES

The fallopian tubes can be seen in Figure 17-1B. They link the ovaries and the uterus. The distal end of each tube is funnel-shaped and is called the **infundibulum** (in-fun-**DIB**-you-lum). It is equipped with tiny fingerlike projections called **fimbriae** (**FIM**-bree-ee), which sweep back and forth, creating waves in the fluid surrounding the ovary. This action pulls

FIGURE 17-1

Structures of the female reproductive system: (A) female reproductive organs in relation to the urinary and digestive tracts; (B) uterus, ovaries, fallopian tubes, and related structures

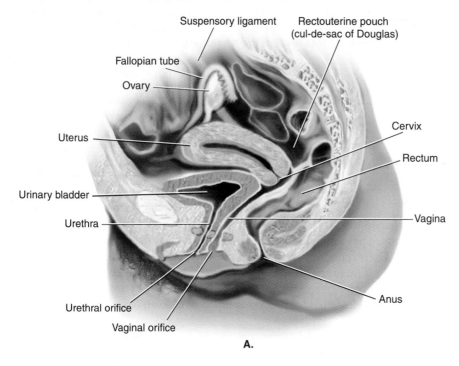

A.

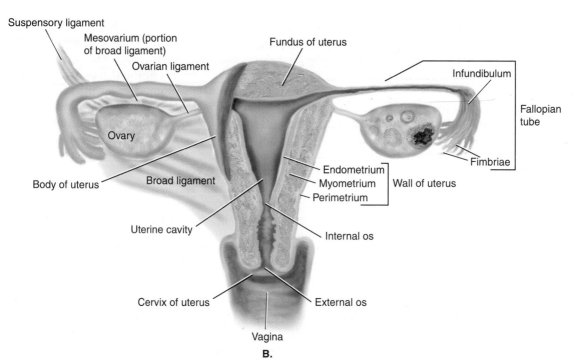

B.

the ovum into the tube for transport to the uterus. If the ovum is fertilized, it begins to grow and is called a **zygote** (**ZYE**-goht). If it is not fertilized, it breaks down within 48 hours.

> **Memory Key**
> - The fallopian tubes link the ovaries and uterus.
> - Fingerlike fimbriae in the funnel-shaped distal end of the tubes create waves that pull the ovum into the tube and down to the uterus.
> - A fertilized egg is called a zygote.

THE UTERUS

The uterus is a muscular, thick-walled organ, hollow and shaped like an inverted pear. It is held in place in the pelvic cavity by ligaments. The superior, rounded portion is called the **fundus** (**FUN**-dus). The middle portion is the **body**. The inferior portion is the **cervix uteri** (**SER**-vicks **YOU**-ter-eye), which projects into the vagina. The superior and inferior openings of the cervix are called the **internal os** and the **external os**, respectively (see Figure 17-1B). Lying between the uterus and the rectum is the lowest point of the abdominal cavity, the **rectouterine** (**reck**-toh-**YOU**-ter-in) **pouch**, also called the **cul-de-sac of Douglas** (see Figure 17-1A). This is a gathering place for microorganisms and is therefore prone to an infection called **pelvic inflammatory disease** (PID).

> **Memory Key**
> - The uterus consists of the
>   fundus
>   body
>   cervix uteri
> - The superior and inferior openings of the cervix are the internal os and the external os.

THE VAGINA

The vagina is a muscular tube leading from the cervix to the exterior. It is approximately 6 inches long and is lined with mucous membrane. The entrance to the vagina, the **introitus** (in-**TRO**-ih-tus) is covered by the hymen (**HIGH**-men), a fold of mucous membrane.

> **Memory Key**   The muscular vagina leads from cervix to the exterior. The opening is the introitus.

THE EXTERNAL GENITALIA

The **external genitalia**, or **vulva** (**VUL**-vah), are illustrated in Figure 17-2. Included are the **clitoris** (**KLIT**-oh-ris), the **labia** (**LAY**-bee-a) **majora**, **labia minora**, **mons pubis**, and **Bartholin's** (**BAR**-toh-linz) **glands**, which secrete lubricant for intercourse. The area from the vulva to the anus is called the **perineum** (per-ih-**NEE**-um).

> **Memory Key**
> - The external genitalia consist of the
>   clitoris   mons pubis
>   labia majora   Bartholin's glands
>   labia minora
> - The area from the vulva to the anus is the perineum.

FIGURE 17-2
External genitalia

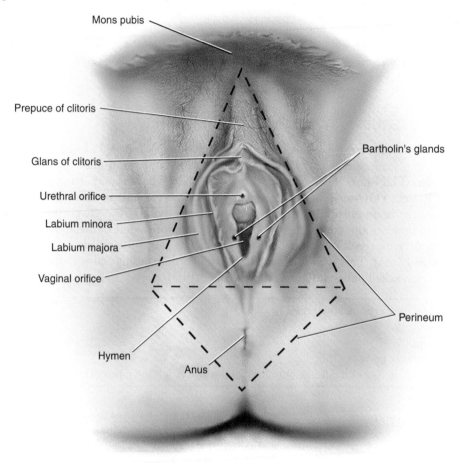

Mons pubis

Prepuce of clitoris

Glans of clitoris

Bartholin's glands

Urethral orifice

Labium minora

Labium majora

Vaginal orifice

Perineum

Hymen

Anus

THE BREASTS

Figure 17-3 illustrates the structures of the **breast** or mammary gland. The **nipple** is surrounded by a darker ring of skin called the **areola**. The **mammary glands** produce milk after childbirth. The milk is stored in **lactiferous** (lack-**TIF**-er-us) **sinuses** and travels through the **lactiferous ducts** to tiny openings in the nipple. Oils produced by glands in the areola help minimize drying out of the skin around the nipple due to breastfeeding.

Memory Key	The breast includes
	nipple
	areola
	lactiferous sinuses
	lactiferous ducts

FIGURE 17-3
Breast

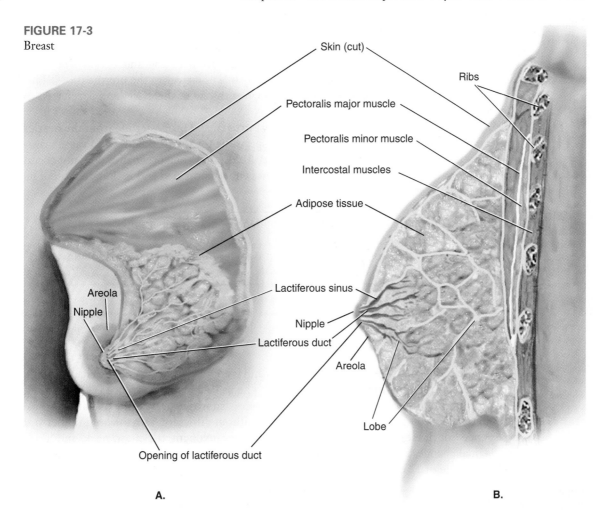

A.

B.

17.2   Menstrual Cycle

The time of life when the **menstrual cycle** first begins (puberty) is called **menarche** (men-**AR**-kee). It is continuous for approximately 40 years except during pregnancy. The average length of the menstrual cycle is 28 days and consists of three periods: the **menstrual period**, the **ovulatory period**, and the **secretory period**.

Memory Key	• Menarche is when the menstrual cycle first begins.
	• The menstrual cycle consists of the menstrual, ovulatory, and secretory periods.

The menstrual period lasts from 3 to 6 days. The endometrium (the inner lining of the uterus) has become thickened and more vascular, preparing itself for housing a fertilized egg.

If pregnancy does not occur, the endometrium is unnecessary and is sloughed off along with blood cells in what is known as a **period**, **menses**, or **menstruation**.

During the ovulatory period, the egg is released from its sac and breaks free from the ovary into the abdominal cavity, where it slowly makes its way to the uterine tubes. This event occurs at midcycle, approximately the fourteenth day of the cycle, and is referred to as **ovulation**.

During the secretory period, the hormones estrogen and progesterone from the ovaries are secreted into the bloodstream. They are responsible for the thickening and vascularization of the endometrium, preparing it for the fertilized egg. When pregnancy does not occur, these hormones decrease, and the endometrium is not maintained and is sloughed off. The menstrual period starts again.

Memory Key	• During the menstrual period the thickened lining of the uterus is sloughed off.
	• During the ovulatory period the egg travels to the uterine tubes.
	• During the secretory period estrogen and progesterone are secreted, stimulating the endometrium to thicken and vascularize.

17.3   Menopause

Menopause is the complete stoppage of menses and is commonly known as the change of life or the **climacteric** (kli-**MACK**-ter-ick) period. The usual age of occurrence is 45–55 years. During this time, there is a decrease of hormones from the ovary, and ovulation stops. Although many women pass through this period without difficulty, a significant number will experience hot flashes (involuntary, sudden heat waves involving the chest, neck, and head) and vaginal changes as estrogen levels fall. A woman is in menopause when menses has been absent for at least 12 consecutive months.

Memory Key	Menopause is the complete stoppage of menses.

17.4   Additional Word Elements

Use these additional word elements when studying the medical terms in this chapter.

Root	Meaning
flex/o	bend
men/o	menstruation; menses; month
tub/o	tube; fallopian tube
versi/o	tilting; turning; tipping

Suffix	Meaning
-an	pertaining to
-ine	pertaining to
-pause	stoppage; cessation

Prefix	Meaning
nulli-	none
oxy-	sharp
primi-	first
secundi-	second

17.5   Term Analysis and Definition Pertaining to the Female Reproductive System

	cervic/o	cervix; neck of uterus; cervix uteri
Term	**Term Analysis**	**Definition**
cervicitis (**ser**-vih-**SIGH**-tis)	-itis = inflammation	inflammation of the cervix
cervical polyp (**SER**-vih-kal **POL**-up)	-al = pertaining to polyp = protruding growth of the mucous membrane	polyp extending from the mucous membrane of the cervix uteri (see Figure 17-12)
	colp/o	vagina
colporrhaphy (kol-**POR**-ah-fee)	-rrhaphy = suture	suture of the vagina
colposcopy (kol-**POS**-koh-pee)	-scopy = process of visually examining	process of visually examining the vagina

		culd/o	cul-de-sac
Term	**Term Analysis**	**Definition**
culdocentesis (**kul**-doh-sen-**TEE**-sis)	-centesis = surgical puncture to remove fluid	surgical puncture to remove fluid from the cul-de-sac of Douglas
culdoscope (**KUL**-doh-skohp)	-scope = instrument used to visually examine	instrument used to visually examine the cul-de-sac of Douglas
	episi/o	**vulva; external genitalia; pudendum**
episiotomy (eh-**piz**-ee-**OT**-oh-mee)	-tomy = process of cutting	process of cutting the vulva. *NOTE:* An episiotomy is used to assist delivery of the fetus.
episiorrhaphy (eh-**piz**-ee-**OR**-ah-fee)	-rrhaphy = suture	suturing the vulva and perineum
	fibr/o	**fibers; fibrous tissue**
uterine fibroid (**YOU**-ter-in **FYE**-broid)	-oid = resembling -ine = pertaining to **uter/o** = uterus	benign, smooth muscle tumor of the uterus; also known as leiomyoma (see Figure 17-12)
	galact/o	**milk**
galactorrhea (gah-**lack**-toh-**REE**-ah)	-rrhea = discharge; flow	discharge of milk from the breast after breastfeeding has stopped
	gynec/o	**woman**
gynecologist (**guy**-neh-**KOL**-oh-jist)	-logist = specialist	specialist in the study of diseases and treatment of the female genital tract
gynecology (**guy**-neh-**KOL**-oh-jee)	-logy = study of	the study of diseases and treatment of the female genital tract

	hyster/o	**uterus**
Term	**Term Analysis**	**Definition**
hysterectomy (**hiss**-ter-**ECK**-toh-mee)	-ectomy = excision; surgical removal	surgical removal of the uterus through the abdomen (abdominal hysterectomy) or the vagina (vaginal hysterectomy). *NOTE:* Types of hysterectomies include total hysterectomy, in which the uterus plus the cervix are removed, and subtotal, in which the cervix is left intact.
hysterotomy (**his**-ter-**OT**-oh-mee)	-tomy = process of cutting	process of cutting into the uterus (usually to remove the fetus)
	labi/o	**lips**
labial (**LAY**-bee-al)	-al = pertaining to	pertaining to the lips
	lact/o	**milk**
lactogenesis (**lack**-toh-**JEN**-ih-sis)	-genesis = production; formation	production and secretion of milk from the breast
	lapar/o	**abdomen**
laparoscopy (**lap**-ar-**OS**-koh-pee)	-scopy = process of visually examining	process of visually examining the contents of the abdominal cavity. *NOTE:* A laser may be used with a laparoscope to remove or destroy tissue without opening the abdominal cavity (see Figure 17-4).
	ligati/o	**binding; tying**
tubal ligation (**TOO**-bal lye-**GAY**-shun)	-ion = process -al = pertaining to **tub/o** = tube; fallopian tube	method of sterilization whereby the lumen of the fallopian tube is blocked by tying the tube with a threadlike material (see Figure 17-5)

FIGURE 17-4
Laparoscopy

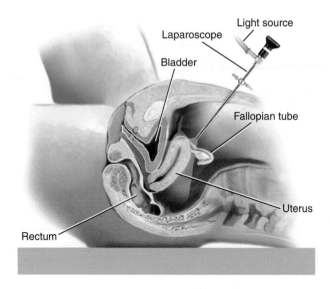

Light source

Laparoscope

Bladder

Fallopian tube

Uterus

Rectum

FIGURE 17-5
Tubal ligation

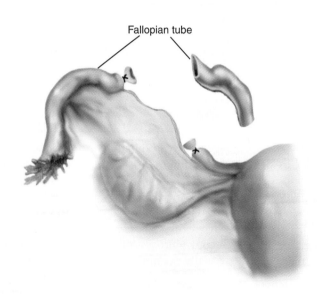

Fallopian tube

	mamm/o; mast/o	breast
Term	**Term Analysis**	**Definition**
mammary (**MAM**-ah-ree)	-ary = pertaining to	pertaining to the breast
mammography (mam-**OG**-rah-fee)	-graphy = process of recording; producing images	x-ray of the breast to diagnose abnormalities that may not show up on a typical physical examination (see Figure 3-4)

Term	Term Analysis	Definition
mammoplasty (**MAM**-oh-**plas**-tee)	-plasty = surgical repair; surgical reconstruction	surgical reconstruction of the breast. *NOTE:* Includes post mastectomy reconstruction and breast enlargement.
mastectomy (mas-**TECK**-toh-mee)	-ectomy = excision; surgical removal	excision of the breast
mastopexy (**MAS**-toh-**peck**-see)	-pexy = surgical fixation	surgical fixation of the breast. *NOTE:* A mastopexy is performed to improve breast shape when the breast is sagging.

	men/o	**menses; menstruation; month**
amenorrhea (ah-**men**-oh-**REE**-ah)	-rrhea = discharge; flow a- = no; not; lack of	no menstruation
dysmenorrhea (**dis**-men-oh-**REE**-ah)	dys- = painful; difficult; bad	painful menstruation
menopause (**MEN**-oh-pawz)	-pause = stoppage; cessation	stoppage of menstruation usually occurring at about 45–55 years of age
menorrhea (**men**-oh-**REE**-ah)	-rrhea = discharge; flow	normal menstruation
menorrhagia (**men**-oh-**RAY**-jee-ah)	-rrhagia = burst forth	excessive uterine bleeding during menstruation
oligomenorrhea (**ol**-ih-goh-**men**-oh-**REE**-ah)	-rrhea = discharge; flow oligo- = diminished; scanty; deficient; few	diminished or infrequent menstruation
menometrorrhagia (**men**-oh-**met**-roh-**RAY**-jee-ah)	-rrhagia = burst forth **metr/o** = uterus	excessive uterine bleeding during menstruation and at variable intervals

	metr/o	**uterus**
endometriosis (**en**-doh-**mee**-tree-**OH**-sis)	-osis = abnormal condition endo- = within	endometrial tissue found at sites other than the uterus (see Figure 17-12)
endometrium (**en**-doh-**MEE**-tree-um)	-ium = structure endo- = within	inner wall of the uterus (see Figure 17-1B)

Term	Term Analysis	Definition
metroptosis (**meh**-troh-**TOH**-sis)	-ptosis = falling	displacement of the uterus through the vaginal canal; uterine prolapse
metrorrhagia (**meh**-troh-**RAY**-jee-ah)	-rrhagia = burst forth	uterine bleeding at times other than at the regular menstrual period
myometrium (**my**-oh-**MEE**-tree-um)	-ium = structure **my/o** = muscle	muscular wall of the uterus (see Figure 17-1B)
parametrium (par-ah-**MEE**-tree-um)	-ium = structure para- = near; beside	structures located beside the uterus such as supporting ligaments
perimetrium (**per**-ih-**MEE**-tree-um)	-ium = structure peri- = around	the outermost wall of the uterus (see Figure 17-1B)
	o/o; ov/o	**egg**
oocyte (**OH**-oh-sight)	-cyte = cell	egg cell; the developing ovum
ovoid (**OH**-void)	-oid = resembling	resembling an egg shape
	oophor/o	**ovary**
oophororrhagia (oh-**of**-oh-**RAY**-jee-ah)	-rrhagia = burst forth	hemorrhaging from the ovary
	ovari/o	**ovary**
ovarian cyst (oh-**VAR**-ree-an **SIST**)	-an = pertaining to cyst = a closed sac or cavity that contains fluid, solid, or semisolid material	cyst formed on an ovary (see Figure 17-12)
	perine/o	**perineum**
colpoperineoplasty (**kol**-poh-**per**-in-**EE**-oh-**plas**-tee)	-plasty = surgical reconstruction; surgical repair **colp/o** = vagina	surgical reconstruction of the vagina and perineum

Term	Term Analysis	Definition
perineorrhaphy (**per**-ih-nee-**OR**-ah-fee)	-rrhaphy = suture	suture of the perineum
	salping/o	**fallopian tube; uterine tube**
hysterosalpingectomy (**his**-ter-oh-**sal**-pin-**JECK**-toh-mee)	-ectomy = excision; surgical removal **hyster/o** = uterus	excision of the uterus and fallopian tubes
hysterosalpingogram (HSG) (**his**-ter-oh-sal-**PING**-oh-gram)	-gram = record **hyster/o** = uterus	record of the uterus and fallopian tubes by the use of x-rays after injection of a contrast medium
salpingopexy (sal-**PING**-oh-**peck**-see)	-pexy = surgical fixation	surgical fixation of the fallopian tubes
salpingo-oophorectomy (sal-**ping**-goh-**oh**-of-oh-**RECK**-toh-mee)	-ectomy = excision; surgical removal **oophor/o** = ovary	excision of the fallopian tubes and ovaries; may be bilateral or unilateral
	thel/o	**nipple**
polythelia (**pol**-ee-**THEE**-lee-ah)	-ia = condition poly- = many	more than one nipple present on the breast
thelitis (thee-**LYE**-tis)	-itis = inflammation	inflammation of the nipple
	uter/o	**uterus**
intrauterine (**in**-trah-**YOU**-ter-in)	-ine = pertaining to intra- = within	pertaining to within the uterus
rectouterine (**reck**-toh-**YOU**-ter-in)	-ine = pertaining to **rect/o** = rectum	pertaining to the rectum and uterus
uterovesical (**you**-ter-oh-**VES**-ih-kal)	-al = pertaining to **uter/o** = uterus	pertaining to the uterus and bladder
	vagin/o	**vagina**
vaginitis (**vag**-ih-**NIGH**-tis)	-itis = inflammation	inflammation of the vagina

Term	Term Analysis	Definition
vaginomycosis (**vag**-in-oh-mye-**KOH**-sis)	-osis = abnormal condition **myc/o** = fungus	fungal infection of the vagina
	vulv/o	**vulva; external genitalia; pudendum**
vulvectomy (vul-**VECK**-toh-mee)	-ectomy = excision; surgical removal	excision of the vagina
vulvorectal (**vul**-voh-**RECK**-tal)	-al = pertaining to **rect/o** = rectum	pertaining to the vulva and rectum

SUFFIXES

	-arche	beginning
	-arche	**beginning**

Term	Term Analysis	Definition
menarche (men-**AR**-kee)	**men/o** = menses; menstruation; month	beginning of the regular menstrual cycle occurring at approximately 13 years of age
	-cele	**hernia (protrusion of an organ from the structure that normally contains it)**
cystocele (**SIS**-toh-seel)	**cyst/o** = bladder	hernia of bladder against the vaginal wall (see Figure 3-1)
rectocele (**RECK**-toh-seel)	**rect/o** = rectum	hernia of the rectum against the vaginal wall (see Figure 3-2)
	-logy	**the study of**
cytology (sigh-**TOL**-oh-jee)	**cyt/o** = cells	the study of cells. A cytology commonly performed is the **Papanicolaou (pap-ah-nick-oh-LAY-ooh) smear**, or **Pap smear**, which differentiates normal cells from precancerous and cancerous cells of the cervix uteri.

	-opsy	to view
Term	**Term Analysis**	**Definition**
biopsy (**BYE**-op-see)	**bi/o** = life	living tissue is excised from the body and viewed under a microscope. *NOTE:* Common biopsies on the cervix uteri are **conization** (kon-ih-**ZAY**-shun), in which a piece of cervix, shaped like a cone, is surgically removed for the purposes of microscopic examination; and **punch biopsy**, which removes a circular piece of tissue.

	-salpinx	**fallopian tube; uterine tube**
hematosalpinx (**hem**-ah-toh-**SAL**-pinks)	**hemat/o** = blood	accumulation of blood in the fallopian tube
hydrosalpinx (**high**-dro-**SAL**-pinks)	**hydr/o** = water	accumulation of a watery fluid in the fallopian tube
pyosalpinx (**pye**-oh-**SAL**-pinks)	**py/o** = pus	accumulation of pus in the fallopian tube

PREFIXES

	ante-	**before**
Term	**Term Analysis**	**Definition**
anteflexion (**an**-tee-**FLECK**-shun)	-ion = process **flex/o** = bending	bending forward of a part of an organ. *NOTE:* Anteflexion describes the position of the uterus as it bends forward over the bladder (see Figure 17-6).
anteversion (**an**-tee-**VER**-shun)	-ion = process **versi/o** = turning; tilting; tipping	tilting forward of an organ. *NOTE:* Anteversion describes the position of the uterus as it tilts over the bladder. Considered a malposition of the uterus (see Figure 17-7).

FIGURE 17-6
Anteflexion

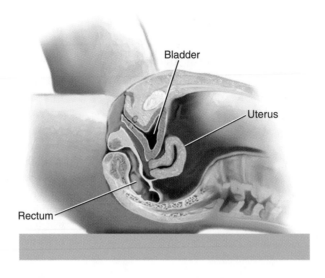

FIGURE 17-7
Anteversion

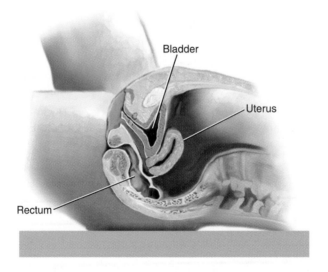

	retro-	**back; behind**
Term	**Term Analysis**	**Definition**
retroflexion (**ret**-roh-**FLECK**-shun)	-ion = process **flex/o** = bending	bending back of a part of an organ. *NOTE:* Retroflexion describes the malpositioned uterus as it bends backward toward the rectum (see Figure 17-8).

FIGURE 17-8
Retroflexion

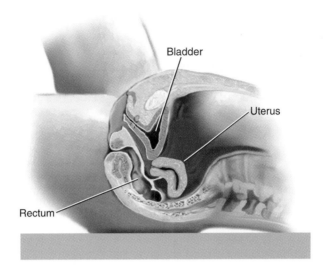

Term	Term Analysis	Definition
retroversion (**ret**-roh-**VER**-shun)	-ion = process **versi/o** = turning; tilting; tipping	tilting backward of an organ. *NOTE:* Retroversion describes a malpositioned uterus as it tilts backward toward the rectum (see Figure 17-9).

FIGURE 17-9
Retroversion

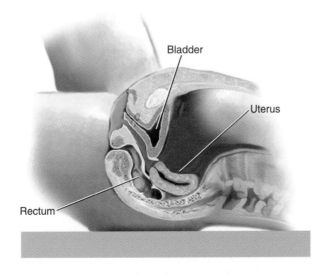

17.6   Review of Terms Pertaining to the Female Reproductive System

Define the terms in Tables 17-1 through 17-4 in the space provided.

TABLE 17-1

REVIEW OF ANATOMICAL AND PHYSIOLOGICAL TERMS OF THE FEMALE REPRODUCTIVE SYSTEM

endometrium	gynecologist	gynecology
intrauterine	labial	lactogenesis
mammary	menarche	menopause
menorrhea	myometrium	oocyte
ovoid	parametrium	perimetrium
rectouterine	uterovesical	vulvorectal

TABLE 17-2

REVIEW OF PATHOLOGIC TERMS PERTAINING TO THE FEMALE REPRODUCTIVE SYSTEM

amenorrhea	anteflexion	anteversion
cervical polyp	cervicitis	cystocele
dysmenorrhea	endometriosis	galactorrhea
hematosalpinx	hydrosalpinx	menometrorrhagia
menorrhagia	metroptosis	metrorrhagia

continued on page 407

Table 17-2 *continued from 406*

oligomenorrhea	oophororrhagia	ovarian cyst
polythelia	pyosalpinx	rectocele
retroflexion	retroversion	thelitis
uterine fibroids	vaginitis	vaginomycosis

TABLE 17-3

REVIEW OF DIAGNOSTIC TERMS OF THE FEMALE REPRODUCTIVE SYSTEM

cytology	hysterosalpingogram	mammography
Pap smear (Papanicolaou)		

TABLE 17-4

REVIEW OF CLINICAL PROCEDURES AND SURGICAL INSTRUMENTS OF THE FEMALE REPRODUCTIVE SYSTEM

colpoperineoplasty	colporrhaphy	colposcopy
conization biopsy	culdocentesis	culdoscope
episiorrhaphy	episiotomy	hysterectomy
hysterosalpingectomy	hysterotomy	laparoscopy
mammoplasty	mastectomy	mastopexy
perineorrhaphy	punch biopsy	salpingo-oophorectomy
salpingopexy	tubal ligation	vulvectomy

17.7   Abbreviations Pertaining to the Female Reproductive System

Abbreviation	Meaning
BSO	bilateral salpingo-oophorectomy
D&C	dilation and curettage (a type of operation in which the uterus is dilated and the surface of the endometrium is scraped, or curetted)
Gyn; Gyne	gynecology
HRT	hormone replacement therapy
HSG	hysterosalpingogram
IUD	intrauterine device (a type of contraceptive device)
LMP	last menstrual period
Pap smear	Papanicolaou smear
PID	pelvic inflammatory disease
TAH	total abdominal hysterectomy
STD	sexually transmitted disease
VD	venereal disease

17.8   Obstetrics

PREGNANCY

If fertilization does occur in the uterine tube, the fertilized egg (the zygote) travels to the uterus and implants in the uterine wall. The uterus begins to enlarge. The zygote is referred to as the **embryo** (**EM**-bree-oh) from the second to the eighth week of pregnancy. For the remainder of the **gestation** period the name **fetus** (**FEE**-tus) is used. Gestation is the length of time from conception (fertilization) to birth, on the average, 40 weeks.

Memory Key   The zygote becomes the embryo, which becomes the fetus.

At the beginning of pregnancy, the placenta develops and attaches to the uterine wall. The placenta is the organ that allows for the exchange of nutrients and waste products between the developing embryo and the mother. The placenta is made up of embryonic tissue: the **chorion**, the outermost layer surrounding the embryo, and the **amnion**, the innermost layer (see Figure 17-10). The amnion forms the amniotic cavity, which holds the embryo floating in **amniotic fluid**. Thus, the embryo develops in a protective environment, the amniotic fluid, which acts as a shock absorber for the embryo. Near the time of birth, the amnion ruptures, releasing its fluid, and signaling the onset of labor. After delivery, the placenta detaches from the uterus, hence the term **afterbirth**.

During placental development, fingerlike projections called chorionic villi form and extend from the chorion into the endometrial tissue of the mother. This arrangement allows the vessels of the embryo (chorionic villi) to lie side by side with the mother's blood vessels. At no time during gestation does the fetal blood mix with the maternal blood, yet nutrients and waste products are exchanged.

Materials that are exchanged must be transported to and from the embryo. This transport is made possible by the **umbilical** (um-**BILL**-ih-cahl) **cord**. The umbilical cord contains two arteries and one vein, which become the lifelines between the mother and the baby, carrying nutrients and waste products to and from the developing embryo.

The placenta secretes **human chorionic gonadotropin (HCG) hormone**. This hormone confirms pregnancy when tested for in women who suspect they are pregnant. HCG stimulates the releases of estrogen and progesterone. These hormones maintain the uterine wall—an important contribution to fetal development. Low levels of these hormones can lead to a spontaneous abortion, or miscarriage.

Detection of fetal abnormalities can be determined by two diagnostic procedures: **amniocentesis** and **chorionic villus sampling** (**CVS**) as seen in Figure 17-11. Amniocentesis withdraws amniotic fluid from the amniotic sac for laboratory analysis at 15 to 18 weeks' gestation. Chorionic villus sampling removes placental tissue for chemical and microscopic examination at 9 to 11 weeks' gestation.

FIGURE 17-10
The amniotic sac

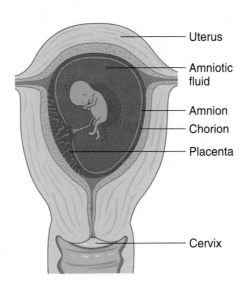

- Uterus
- Amniotic fluid
- Amnion
- Chorion
- Placenta
- Cervix

FIGURE 17-11

(A) Chorionic villi sampling (9–11 weeks), (B) amniocentesis (15–18 weeks)

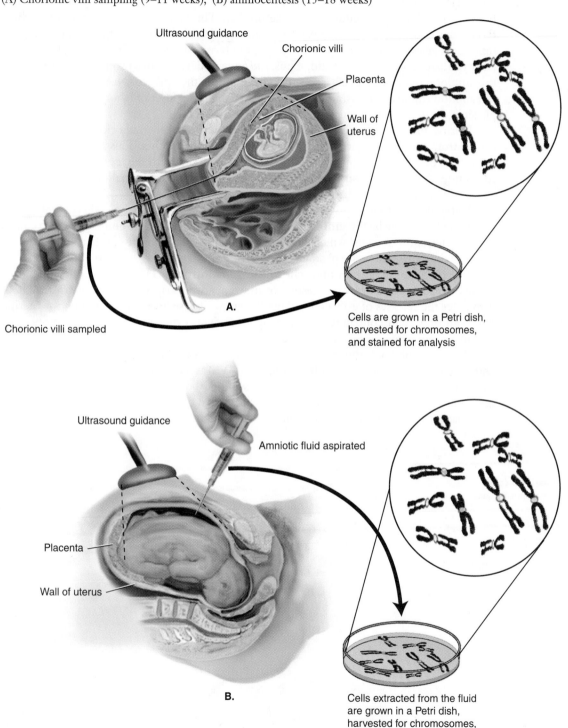

A.

Ultrasound guidance

Chorionic villi

Placenta

Wall of uterus

Chorionic villi sampled

Cells are grown in a Petri dish, harvested for chromosomes, and stained for analysis

B.

Ultrasound guidance

Amniotic fluid aspirated

Placenta

Wall of uterus

Cells extracted from the fluid are grown in a Petri dish, harvested for chromosomes, and stained for analysis

PARTURITION

The birth process is known as **parturition** (**par**-tyou-**RISH**-un). At about 9 months, the uterine muscles begin to contract. This marks the beginning of labor, which has three stages: **cervical dilatation** (dil-ah-**TAY**-shun), **fetal delivery**, and **placental delivery**. During cervical dilatation, the cervix begins to dilate, ultimately reaching approximately 4 inches (10.2 cm) in diameter. During fetal delivery, uterine contractions move the infant through the cervix and vagina to the outside world. The umbilical cord connecting the infant to the placenta is severed once the baby is out. The placenta is expelled from the uterus during placental delivery.

Memory Key	The birth process is parturition. The stages of labor are cervical dilatation, fetal delivery, and placental delivery.

The fetus is delivered head first. If the buttocks presents first, it is in a **breech** position. In such cases, or when the fetus is too large for vaginal delivery, a surgical procedure known as **cesarean** (see-**SAY**-ree-an) **section** (**CS**) may be used. This involves removal of the fetus through an incision in the abdomen and uterus.

Memory Key	If the fetus is too large or in breech position, delivery may be by cesarean section.

The condition of the newborn is evaluated within one minute of birth and again 15 minutes later. A numerical rating called an **Apgar score** is obtained by evaluating each of the following on a 2-point scale, 2 being the highest: heart rate, respiration, muscle tone, reflex response, and color. The highest rating is therefore 10.

Memory Key	• Apgar scoring rates heart rate, respiration, muscle tone, reflex response, and color, each out of a highest possible score of 2. • The best possible score is 10.

The 6 to 8 weeks following parturition are known as the **postpartum period**. During this period, the uterus returns to normal size, a process known as **involution**, and the mammary glands are stimulated to produce milk; the production of milk is called lactation. During the first few days, the mammary glands produce **colostrum** (kuh-**LOS**-trum), which is a highly nourishing fluid containing antibodies to protect the infant.

Memory Key	Colostrum is produced by the mammary glands during the first few days of the postpartum period.

The terms **gravida** (**GRAV**-ih-dah) and **para** are used to describe a woman's obstetrical history. *Gravida* refers to the number of times she has been pregnant, whereas *para* refers to the number of times a pregnancy has resulted in viable offspring, regardless of whether the child was alive at birth. So, for example, a woman who is **primigravida** (pregnant for the first time) is described as gravida I, para 0 before the birth. If a viable child is born, the woman is then described as gravida I, para I, whether she has a single child, twins, or triplets, because *para* refers only to the number of occasions a woman has given birth to a viable child and not to the number of children born on any of those occasions. During her next pregnancy, this same woman would be described as gravida II, para I. If she gives birth to viable offspring, she is gravida II, para II. If she does not, she will remain gravida ll, para l.

Memory Key	• *Gravida* refers to the number of times a woman has been pregnant. • *Para* refers to the number of times she has given viable births.

17.9   Term Analysis and Definition Pertaining to Obstetrics

	amni/o	amnion; sac in which the fetus lies in the uterus
Term	**Term Analysis**	**Definition**
amniocentesis (**am**-nee-oh-sen-**TEE**-sis)	-centesis = surgical puncture	surgical puncture to withdraw or aspirate fluid from the amniotic sac for analysis
	nat/o	birth
antenatal (**an**-tee-**NAY**-tal)	-al = pertaining to ante- = before	pertaining to before birth
postnatal period (pohst-**NAY**-tal)	-al = pertaining to post- = after	pertaining to the period after birth (referring to the newborn)
prenatal (pre-**NAY**-tal)	-al = pertaining to pre- = before	pertaining to before birth, referring to the fetus
	top/o	place
ectopic pregnancy (eck-**TOP**-ick **PREG**-nan-see)	-ic = pertaining to ec- = out	pregnancy occurring in a place other than the uterus, such as in the fallopian tube (see Figure 17-12)

FIGURE 17-12
Ectopic pregnancy, endometriosis, leiomyoma, ovarian cyst, cervical polyp

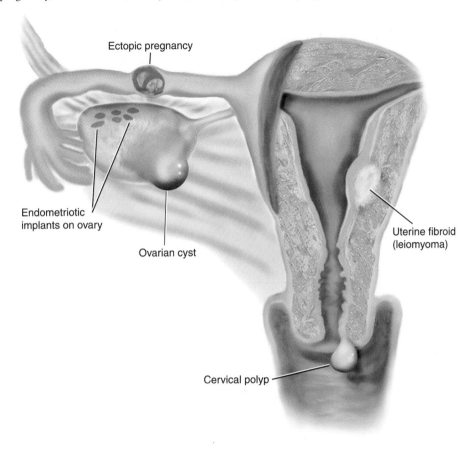

SUFFIXES

	-cyesis	pregnancy
Term	**Term Analysis**	**Definition**
pseudocyesis (**soo**-doh-sigh-**EE**-sis)	pseudo- = false	false pregnancy

	-emesis	vomit
hyperemesis gravidarum (**high**-per-**EM**-eh-sis **grav**-ih-**DAR**-um)	hyper- = excessive; above normal gravidarum = pregnancy	excessive vomiting during pregnancy

	-gravida	pregnancy
Term	**Term Analysis**	**Definition**
multigravida (**mul**-tih-**GRAV**-ih-dah)	multi- = multiple	a woman who has been pregnant two or more times (written gravida II, gravida III, gravida IV, etc., or as GII, GIII, GIV, etc.)
nulligravida (**nul**-ih-**GRAV**-ih-dah)	nulli- = none	a woman who has never been pregnant
primigravida (**prih**-mih-**GRAV**-ih-dah)	primi- = first	a woman who is pregnant for the first time (written gravida I or GI)
secundigravida (see-**kun**-dih-**GRAV**-ih-dah)	secundi- = second	a woman pregnant for the second time (written gravida II or GII)
	-metry	**process of measuring**
pelvimetry (pel-**VIM**-eh-tree)	**pelv/i** = pelvis	process of measuring the dimensions of the mother's pelvis to determine if its dimensions will allow the passage of the fetus through the birth canal
	-para	**to bear; give birth; part with child**
multipara (mul-**TIP**-ah-rah)	multi- = multiple	a woman who has given birth to viable offspring two or more times (written as para II, para III, para IV, etc., or as PII, PIII, PIV, etc.)
nullipara (nul-**LIP**-ah-rah)	nulli- = none	a woman who has never given birth to viable offspring
primipara (prye-**MIP**-ah-rah)	primi- = first	a woman who has given birth to viable offspring for the first time (written para I or PI)
secundipara (see-kun-**DIP**-ah-rah)	secundi- = second	a woman who has given birth to viable offspring twice (written para II or PII)

	-partum	**labor; delivery; childbirth**
Term	**Term Analysis**	**Definition**
antepartum (an-tee-**PAR**-tum)	ante- = before	before birth (referring to the mother)
postpartum (pohst-**PAR**-tum)	post- = after	after birth (referring to the mother)

	-tocia; -tocin	**labor**
dystocia (dis-**TOH**-see-ah)	dys- = painful; difficult; bad	difficult labor
oxytocin (**ock**-see-**TOH**-sin)	oxy- = sharp	hormone secreted from the posterior pituitary that initiates uterine contractions, starting childbirth

PREFIXES

	ultra-	**excess; beyond**
Term	**Term Analysis**	**Definition**
pelvic ultrasonography (**PEL**-vick **ul**-trah-son-**OG**-rah-fee)	-graphy = process of recording **son/o** = sound pelvic = pertaining to the pelvis	process of recording high-frequency sound waves as they bounce off organs in the pelvic area. *NOTE:* This procedure may be used to determine fetal size and position.

17.10 Review of Obstetrical Terms

Define the terms in Tables 17-5 and 17-6 in the space provided.

TABLE 17-5

REVIEW OF OBSTETRICAL TERMS

antenatal	antepartum	dystocia

continued on page 416

Table 17-5 *continued from page 415*

ectopic pregnancy	hyperemesis gravidarum	multigravida
multipara	nulligravida	nullipara
oxytocin	prenatal	postnatal
postpartum	primigravida	primipara
pseudocyesis	secundigravida	secundipara

TABLE 17-6

REVIEW OF DIAGNOSTIC TERMS PERTAINING TO OBSTETRICS

amniocentesis	pelvimetry	ultrasonography

17.11 Abbreviations Pertaining to Obstetrics

Abbreviation	Meaning
AB	abortion (termination of the pregnancy before the embryo or fetus is outside the uterus)
CPD	cephalopelvic disproportion
CS; C-section	cesarean section (incision into the uterus to remove the fetus)
CVS	chorionic villus sampling
DOB	date of birth
EDC	expected date of confinement

continued on page 417

continued from page 416

Abbreviation	Meaning
FHS	fetal heart sound
G	gravida
HCG	human chorionic gonadotrophin (hormone secreted by the placenta)
NB	newborn
Ob; OB	obstetrics
P	para
UC	uterine contractions

17.12 Putting It All Together

Exercise 17-1   MATCHING

Match the word in Column A with its definition in Column B.

Column A

_____ 1. estrogen

_____ 2. fundus

_____ 3. parturition

_____ 4. progesterone

_____ 5. introitus

_____ 6. fimbriae

_____ 7. Bartholin's glands

_____ 8. lactiferous sinuses

_____ 9. placenta

_____ 10. colostrum

Column B

A. fingerlike projections at the distal ends of the fallopian tubes

B. secrete lubricant for intercourse

C. store milk produced by mammary glands

D. birth process

E. provides fetus with nourishment

F. stimulates development of secondary female characteristics

G. entrance to the vagina

H. fluid secreted from the mammary gland containing antibodies

I. superior rounded portion of the uterus

J. stimulates the growth of blood vessels in the uterus

Exercise 17-2   IDENTIFICATION

Write the suffix, root, or prefix for the medical term for each of the following.

1. vagina _____

2. vulva _____

3. woman _____

4. milk _____

5. breast _____

6. menstruation _____

7. birth _____

8. ovary _____

9. fallopian tube _____

10. place _____

11. beginning _____

12. pregnancy _____

13. to bear; give birth _____

14. labor _____

15. before _____

Exercise 17-3   BUILDING MEDICAL TERMS

Build the medical term for each of the following definitions.

1. inflammation of the neck of the uterus _____

2. suturing the vulva _____

3. surgical puncture to remove fluid from the cul-de-sac of Douglas _____

4. specialist in the study of diseases and treatment of the female genital tract _____

5. surgical removal of the uterus _____

6. pertaining to the breast _____

7. excision of the breast _____

8. resembling an egg shape _____

9. excision of the fallopian tubes and ovaries _____

10. more than one nipple present on the breast _____

11. pregnancy occurring in a place other than the uterus _____

12. fungal infection of the vagina _____

13. hernia of the bladder against the vaginal wall _____

14. false pregnancy _____

15. after birth, referring to the mother   _____

16. accumulation of pus in the fallopian tube   _____

17. difficult labor   _____

18. bending back of an organ   _____

Exercise 17-4   ADJECTIVES

Write the adjective for each of the following. Use the dictionary if necessary.

1. cervix   _____

2. breast   _____

3. uterus   _____

4. birth   _____

5. ovary   _____

6. perineum   _____

7. vagina   _____

Exercise 17-5   BUILDING TERMS

I. Use **men/o** to build terms for the following definitions.

1. no menstruation   _____

2. painful menstruation   _____

3. stoppage of menstruation at about
   45 to 55 years of age   _____

4. normal menstruation   _____

5. excessive uterine bleeding at time
   of menstruation   _____

6. diminished or infrequent
   menstruation   _____

7. excessive uterine bleeding during
   menstruation and at variable intervals   _____

II. Use **metr/o** to build terms for the following definitions.

8. uterine prolapse   _____

9. uterine bleeding at times other than
   at the regular menstrual period   _____

10. muscular wall of the uterus   _____

11. outermost wall of the uterus   _____

12. innermost wall of the uterus   _____

III. Use -gravida to build terms for the following definitions.

13. a woman who has been pregnant
    two or more times   _____

14. a woman who has never been
    pregnant   _____

IV. Use -para to build terms for the following definitions.

15. a woman who has given birth for
    the first time   _____

16. a woman who has given birth to
    viable offspring twice   _____

Exercise 17-6   DEFINITIONS

Define the following terms.

1. endometriosis   _____

2. galactorrhea   _____

3. rectouterine   _____

4. menarche   _____

5. menopause   _____

6. parturition   _____

7. zygote   _____

8. slough   _____

9. embryo   _____

10. hyperemesis
    gravidarum   _____

Exercise 17-7   IDENTIFICATION

Place an **X** beside the terms indicating a surgical or clinical procedure.

1. lactogenesis   _____

2. menarche   _____

3. colporrhaphy   _____

4. oophororrhagia   _____

Exercise 17-8   PLURALS

Write the plural for each of the following. Use the dictionary if necessary.

1. uterus _____

2. ovary _____

Exercise 17-9   SPELLING

Circle any misspelled words in the list below and correctly spell them in the space provided.

1. cervixitis _____

2. mamography _____

3. oligomenorrhea _____

4. perimetrium _____

5. dismenorrhea _____

6. ocyte _____

7. colpoperineoplasty _____

8. salpingo-oophorectomy _____

9. polythilea _____

10. extopic _____

11. vulvoectomy _____

12. pseudocyesis _____

13. secundigravida _____

14. retroflextion _____

15. episiotomy _____

APPENDIX

Answers to Exercises

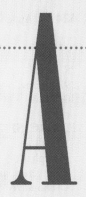

CHAPTER 1

EXERCISE 1-1
1. prefix, root, and suffix
2. suffix
3. suffix, and then define the beginning of the word
4. arthr
5. the combining form is the name given to a root, which is followed by a combining vowel. The combining vowel is used to attach the root to a suffix or another root. It is usually an *o*, but sometimes *e* or *i*

EXERCISE 1-2
1. T
2. F
3. T
4. F
5. T

EXERCISE 1-3
1. thoraces
2. neuroses
3. ganglions; ganglia
4. viruses
5. phalanges
6. fibromas; fibromata
7. varices
8. diverticula
9. scapulae
10. emboli

EXERCISE 1-4
1. larynx
2. carcinoma
3. calyx; calix
4. acetabulum

5. sclera
6. bronchus
7. diagnosis
8. sinus
9. septum
10. index

CHAPTER 2

EXERCISE 2-1
1. joint
2. ear
3. bladder
4. rectum
5. brain
6. stomach
7. bronchus
8. vessel
9. blood
10. fat
11. bone
12. heart
13. kidney
14. cell
15. eyelid
16. hair
17. nose
18. spleen
19. artery
20. disease
21. nerve
22. abdomen
23. tonsil
24. bone marrow; spinal cord
25. life
26. trachea; windpipe

27. eye
28. liver
29. internal organs
30. head

EXERCISE 2-2

1. axill/o
2. cephal/o
3. onych/o; ungu/o
4. chondr/o
5. crani/o
6. tend/o; tendin/o
7. ophthalm/o; ocul/o
8. enter/o
9. col/o
10. gloss/o; lingu/o
11. vas/o
12. thyroid/o
13. ven/o; phleb/o
14. pneum/o; pneumon/o; pulmon/o
15. thorac/o
16. lymphangi/o
17. vulv/o
18. orchid/o; test/o
19. epididym/o
20. ovari/o; oophor/o

EXERCISE 2-3

1. Anatomy is the study of structure. Physiology is the study of function.
2. See Figures 2-2 to 2-13 for a list of the body systems and their organs.

CHAPTER 3

EXERCISE 3-1

Suffixes indicating pathologic conditions
1. pain
2. pain
3. vomiting
4. abnormal condition; abnormal increase
5. hernia
6. softening
7. tumor; mass
8. deficiency; decrease
9. blood condition
10. drooping; sagging; prolapse; downward displacement
11. bursting forth
12. rupture
13. narrowing; stricture

Suffixes indicating diagnostic and surgical procedures
14. excision; surgical removal
15. record; writing
16. instrument used to record
17. to view
18. surgical reconstruction; surgical repair
19. instrument used to visually examine (a body cavity or organ)
20. stoppage; stopping; controlling
21. instrument used to cut

GENERAL SUFFIXES
22. cell
23. specialist; one who specializes; specialist in the study of
24. process of
25. study of
26. production; manufacture; formation

ADJECTIVAL SUFFIXES
27. produced by; producing
28. resembling
29. small
30. pertaining to

EXERCISE 3-2
1. -cele
2. -meter
3. -emia
4. -itis
5. -lysis
6. -megaly
7. -osis
8. -phobia
9. -ptosis
10. -ptysis
11. -rrhea
12. -sclerosis
13. -y
14. -desis
15. -graphy
16. -metry
17. -pexy
18. -rrhaphy
19. -scopy
20. -stasis
21. -tome
22. -cyte
23. -logy
24. -plasia; -poiesis
25. -oid

EXERCISE 3-3
The following suffixes mean pertaining to:
-al, -ous, -eal, -ary, -ic, -ac

EXERCISE 3-4
The following suffixes indicate a diagnostic or surgical procedure:
-ectomy, -stomy, -pexy, -rrhaphy

EXERCISE 3-5
1. breast pain
2. vomiting of blood
3. inflammation of the small intestine
4. softening of the brain
5. abnormal condition of the kidney
6. drooping eyelid
7. discharge from the ear
8. narrowing of a vein
9. process of recording the breast
10. surgical reconstruction of the testicle
11. cutting of the tendon
12. process of visually examining the bronchus
13. tissue cell
14. specialist licensed to prepare and dispense drugs
15. cartilage formation

EXERCISE 3-6
1. renal
2. mammary
3. pharyngeal
4. gastric
5. venous

EXERCISE 3-7
The following terms were misspelled:
1. oophorectomy
2. inflammation
4. pelvimetry
6. splenorrhexis
8. orchidoplasty
10. practitioner

CHAPTER 4

EXERCISE 4-1
1. circum-   around
2. epi-   upon; on; above
3. hyper-   excessive; above
4. infra-   below; beneath
5. meta-   beyond; change
6. post-   after
7. retro-   behind
8. trans-   across
9. contra-   against
10. hemi-   half
11. tri-   three
12. macro-   large
13. neo-   new
14. syn-   together; joined; with
15. tachy-   fast

EXERCISE 4-2
1. D
2. J
3. F
4. H
5. A
6. I
7. C
8. E
9. B
10. G

EXERCISE 4-3
1. ad-
2. post-
3. hypo-; infra-; sub-
4. ecto-; ex-; exo-; extra-; e-
5. tachy-
6. macro-
7. ana-
8. infra-; hypo-; sub-

EXERCISE 4-4
1. abduction
2. prenatal
3. excision
4. incision
5. prodrome
6. transection
7. indigestible
8. unilateral
9. polyadenoma
10. tachycardia

EXERCISE 4-5
1. mal-; dys-
2. sub-; infra-; hypo-
3. hyper-; epi-; supra-
4. anti-; contra-
5. pre-; pro-; ante-
6. circum-; peri-

CHAPTER 5

EXERCISE 5-1
1. T
2. F
3. T
4. F
5. F
6. F
7. T
8. F
9. T
10. T

EXERCISE 5-2
1. F
2. C
3. D
4. A
5. G
6. H
7. B
8. E

EXERCISE 5-3
1. gastr   pertaining to below the stomach
2. ili   pertaining to the hip
3. dors   pertaining to the back
4. inguin   pertaining to the groin
5. viscer   pertaining to the internal organs
6. crani   pertaining to the skull
7. phren   pertaining to the diaphragm
8. anter   pertaining to the front
9. super   pertaining to a structure or organ situated either above another or toward the head
10. thorac   pertaining to the chest
11. caud   pertaining to the lower end of the body or tail

CHAPTER 6

EXERCISE 6-1
1. epidermis and dermis
2. integumentum
3. nerves and blood vessels
4. connective
5. protection
6. hair follicle
7. sebaceous glands secrete sebum; sweat glands or sudoriferous glands secrete sweat; ceruminous glands secrete a wax called cerumen

EXERCISE 6-2
1. cutane   pertaining to under the skin
2. cyano   pertaining to a bluish discoloration of skin
3. derm   pertaining to under the skin
4. epitheli   pertaining to the epithelium
5. erythemat   pertaining to a redness of skin
6. hidr   excessive secretion of sweat
7. leuko   lack of pigmentation of skin showing up as white patches
8. necro   pertaining to death (of tissue)
9. onych   inflammation of tissue around the nail
10. sebo   increased discharge of sebum from the sebaceous glands
11. steat   fatty tumor of the sebaceous glands
12. rhytid   removal of wrinkles
13. xero   dry skin
14. melano   tumor arising from the melanocytes
15. albin   lack of pigment in the skin, hair, and eyes

EXERCISE 6-3
1. tumor
2. pertaining to
3. skin
4. flow; discharge
5. producing
6. condition; state of
7. structure
8. abnormal condition
9. cell
10. process
11. pertaining to
12. study of

EXERCISE 6-4
1. rhytidectomy
2. cyanotic
3. dermatologist
4. anhidrosis
5. melanocyte
6. dermatomycosis
7. onychomycosis
8. scleroderma
9. carcinoma
10. melanoma

EXERCISE 6-5
1. D
2. F
3. B

4. C
5. G
6. A
7. J
8. H
9. E
10. I

EXERCISE 6-6

1. E
2. F
3. G
4. D
5. C
6. I
7. J
8. H
9. A
10. B

EXERCISE 6-7

1. cyanotic
3. diaphoresis
4. epithelial
5. erythema
10. anhidrosis

CHAPTER 7

EXERCISE 7-1

1. cranium
2. protection, support, production of blood cells, movement, storage of minerals
3. calcium and phosphorus
4. Osteoclasts break down and reabsorb bone. Osteocytes are mature bone cells. Osteoblasts are immature bone cells.

EXERCISE 7-2

1. axial
2. appendicular
3. axial
4. appendicular
5. axial
6. appendicular
7. appendicular

EXERCISE 7-3

1. d	2. e	3. h	4. e, h
5. a	6. b	7. e	8. g
9. a	10. h	11. b	12. e

13. h	14. d	15. g	16. c
17. h	18. d	19. g	20. c
21. h	22. e	23. b	24. h
25. e	26. f		

EXERCISE 7-4

1. myeloma
2. osteomyelitis
3. osteoarthritis
4. osteoblast
5. osteochondritis
6. osteocyte
7. osteogenesis; ossification
8. osteoma
9. osteosarcoma
10. craniotomy
11. cranioplasty
12. craniofacial
13. chondrocyte
14. chondroma
15. chondrosarcoma
16. costochondral
17. costovertebral
18. subcostal
19. arthralgia
20. arthritis
21. arthropathy
22. arthroplasty
23. arthroscopy

EXERCISE 7-5

1. chest
2. collarbone
3. wrist
4. upper arm
5. elbow
6. hip
7. heel
8. thighbone
9. shin bone

EXERCISE 7-6

The following are surgical procedures: osteoclasis, arthrodesis, cranioplasty.

EXERCISE 7-7

The following terms were incorrectly spelled:
1. calcaneus
2. tibia
4. myeloma
5. temporomandibular
6. iliosacral

7. osteogenesis
9. malleolus
10. coccyx
11. humerus
14. arthrodesis

EXERCISE 7-8
1. cranial
2. facial
3. ethmoidal
4. mandibular
5. maxillary
6. zygomatic
7. sternal
8. coccygeal
9. malleolar
10. sacral
11. vertebral
12. thoracic
13. clavicular
14. scapular
15. olecranal
16. radial
17. acetabular
18. ischial
19. calcaneal
20. fibular

EXERCISE 7-9
1. inadequate cartilage formation, resulting in a type of dwarfism
2. benign tumor of cartilage
3. malignant tumor of cartilage
4. lower back pain
5. inflammation of the vertebrae
6. inflammation of bone
7. inflammation of bones and joints
8. softening of bone
9. exaggerated posterior curvature of the thoracic spine; humpback
10. exaggerated anterior curvature of the lumbar spine; swayback
11. abnormal lateral curvature of the spine
12. loss of bone density resulting in open spaces within bony substance
13. lumbar pain
14. softening of cartilage
15. benign tumor of bone marrow
16. inflammation of bone and bone marrow
17. inflammation of bone and cartilage
18. benign tumor of bone
19. malignant tumor of bone

EXERCISE 7-10
1. process of visually examining a joint cavity with an arthroscope
2. surgical puncture of a joint to remove fluid; aspiration of a joint cavity

EXERCISE 7-11
1. incision into the skull
2. surgical repair of the skull
3. excision of a carpal (wrist) bone
4. surgical repair of the hip socket
5. surgical fixation of the knee
6. surgical repair of a joint
7. instrument used to cut bone
8. process of cutting bone
9. surgical fracture or refracture of a bone
10. surgical fusion of a joint

EXERCISE 7-12
1. pertaining to the arm and head
2. cartilaginous material found at both ends of a long bone
3. pertaining to the neck
4. pertaining to the cranium and face
5. pertaining to the ribs and cartilage
6. resembling a wedge; refers to the sphenoid bone
7. pertaining to the ribs and vertebrae
8. surgical specialty dealing with the correction of deformities and dysfunctions of the skeletal system
9. pertaining to the heel
10. pertaining to the upper jaw

CHAPTER 8

EXERCISE 8-1
(a) Voluntary muscles perform movement on command. Involuntary muscles move automatically without conscious control.
(b) Skeletal muscles lie on top of bone. Cardiac muscle is found in the heart. Visceral muscles are found in internal organs.
(c) Origin is an attachment of the muscle that remains stable when a muscle contracts. Insertion is the attachment of the muscle that undergoes the greatest movement when a muscle contracts.
(d) Ligaments connect bone to bone. Tendons connect muscle to bone.

EXERCISE 8-2
1. electromyogram
2. myalgia

3. myositis
4. myopathy
5. polymyositis
6. bradykinesia
7. dyskinesia
8. hyperkinesia
9. atrophy
10. dystrophy
11. hypertrophy

EXERCISE 8-3

1. muscle that moves a part toward the midline
2. muscle that moves a part away from the midline
3. pertaining to the fascia (a band of tissue surrounding a muscle)
4. pertaining to a tendon
5. abnormal muscle tone or tension
6. benign tumor of smooth muscle
7. malignant tumor of striated muscle
8. inflammation of a tendon
9. muscle weakness
10. record of the electrical characteristics of a muscle
11. instrument used to measure movement
12. heat applied to deep tissue
13. suturing of fascia
14. surgical fixation of tendon

EXERCISE 8-4

1. masseter
2. sternocleidomastoid
6. trapezius
7. latissimus dorsi
8. teres major
9. rhomboideus
10. Achilles

EXERCISE 8-5

1. adduction
2. flexion
3. dorsiflexion
4. pronation

CHAPTER 9

EXERCISE 9-1

1. The pons
2. Sensory neurons sense internal and external environmental influences and carry these messages to the brain. Motor neurons carry response messages called motor impulses back to the part of the body that has to react.

3. Dura mater, arachnoid mater, and pia mater
4. Eight pairs are cervical, twelve pairs are thoracic, five pairs are lumbar, five pairs are sacral, one pair is coccygeal
5. Surrounds the cerebrum

EXERCISE 9-2

1. C
2. E
3. F
4. G
5. H
6. A
7. D
8. B

EXERCISE 9-3

1. neuralgia
2. neurologist
3. neurolysis
4. polyneuritis
5. electroencephalogram
6. meningocele
7. myelomeningocele
8. anesthesia
9. hypoesthesia
10. hyperesthesia
11. dysesthesia
12. paresthesia
13. diplegia
14. hemiplegia
15. monoplegia
16. paraplegia
17. quadriplegia
18. encephalitis
19. encephalomalacia
20. encephalopathy

EXERCISE 9-4

1. cerebellar
2. cerebral
3. cortical
4. neural
5. dural

EXERCISE 9-5

1. accumulation of water in the brain
2. inflammation of the spinal cord and nerve roots
3. instrument used to record the electrical activity of the brain
4. arteries of the brain are visualized after injection of a contrast medium

5. process of producing an image of the brain using ultrasound
6. accumulation of blood in an organ or space due to a break in a blood vessel
7. lack of myelin sheath
8. inflammation of the pachymeninges (dura mater)

EXERCISE 9-6

1. thalamus
2. medulla
4. encephalomalacia
5. cerebellum
6. epidural space
7. myeloschisis
8. ventriculostomy
9. dysphasia
10. quadriplegia

CHAPTER 10

EXERCISE 10-1

1. I
2. F
3. E
4. J
5. A
6. C
7. B
8. G
9. H
10. D

EXERCISE 10-2

1. gonioscopy
   -scopy = process of visually examining
   goni/o = angle (of the anterior chamber)
   process of visually examining the angle of the
       anterior chamber with the aid of a gonioscope
2. anisocoria
   -ia = condition
   an- = no; not; lack of
   is/o = equal
   core/o = pupil
   inequality in the size of the pupil
3. miosis
   -osis = abnormal condition
   mi/o = contraction; less
   abnormal contraction of the pupil
4. mydriatic
   -tic = pertaining to

   mydri/o = wide; dilation
   pertaining to a drug used to dilate the pupil
5. optician
   -ician = specialist; one who specializes; expert
   opt/o = vision; sight
   expert who fills prescriptions for eyeglasses and
       contact lenses
6. tonometry
   -metry = process of measuring
   ton/o = tension
   measurement of intraocular pressure
7. retinoschisis
   -schisis = splitting; cleft
   retin/o = retina
   splitting of the retina
8. hyperopia
   -opia = visual condition; vision
   hyper- = above; beyond
   light rays focus behind the retina; farsightedness
9. presbyopia
   -opia = visual condition; vision
   presby- = old age
   impaired vision due to advanced age
10. entropion
    -tropion = turning
    en- = inward
    inward turning of the eyelid
11. electrocochleography
    -graphy = process of recording
    electr/o = electric
    cochle/o = cochlea
    process of recording the electrical activity of the
        cochlea
12. presbycusis
    -cusis = hearing
    presby- = old age
    diminished hearing due to advanced age
13. otitis media
    -itis = inflammation
    ot/o = ear
    media = middle
    inflammation of the middle ear
14. audiometry
    -metry = process of measuring
    audi/o = hearing
    measurement of a patient's hearing ability
15. aural
    -al = pertaining to
    aur/o = ear
    pertaining to the ear

EXERCISE 10-3
1. blepharopexy
2. blepharoptosis
3. blepharospasm
4. symblepharon
5. iridocyclitis
6. iridectomy
7. keratoconjunctivitis
8. keratoconus
9. keratomycosis
10. keratoplasty
11. otalgia
12. otorrhea
13. myringoplasty; tympanoplasty
14. myringotomy; tympanotomy
15. stapedectomy

EXERCISE 10-4
1. amblyopia = dimness of vision; diplopia = double vision
2. esotropia = turning inward of the eyeball; exotropia = turning outward of the eyeball
3. presbyopia = impaired vision due to advanced age; emmetropia = normal vision; presbycusis = diminished hearing due to advanced age
4. hypertropia = upward turning of the eyeball; hypotropia = downward turning of the eyeball
5. ectropion = outward turning of the eyelid; entropion = inward turning of the eyelid
6. optician = expert who fills prescriptions for eyeglasses and contact lenses; optometrist = specialist in the testing of visual function and in the diagnosis and nonsurgical treatment of eye conditions; ophthalmologist = specialist in the study of diagnosis and medical and surgical treatment of eye disorders
7. vertigo = dizziness; tinnitus = ringing in the ears

EXERCISE 10-5
1. corneal
2. lacrimal
3. ocular; ophthalmic
4. optic
5. palpebral; blepharal
6. retinal
7. pupillary
8. aural; otic
9. auditory
10. cochlear

EXERCISE 10-6
1. symblepharon
2. gonioscopy
4. exophthalmia
6. retinoschisis

EXERCISE 10-7
1. irides
2. palpebrae
3. retinae
4. sclerae

CHAPTER 11

EXERCISE 11-1
1. somatotrophin/somatotrophic hormone
2. thyrotrophin/thyrotrophic hormone
3. gonadotrophin/gonadotrophic hormone
4. gonadotrophin/gonadotrophic hormone
5. cortisol
6. epinephrine

EXERCISE 11-2
I.
1. A, C, G, K
2. D, I
3. B
4. L
5. F, M
6. N
7. E
8. H, J

II.
1. E
2. A
3. G
4. H
5. B
6. I
7. C
8. J
9. D
10. F

EXERCISE 11-3
1. adrenocorticotrophic
2. gonadotrophic
3. somatotrophic
4. thyrotrophic
5. hyperglycemia
6 hypoglycemia
7. hyperkalemia
8. hyponatremia

9. hypercalcemia
10. hypergonadism
11. hypoinsulinism
12. hyperparathyroidism
13. panhypopituitarism
14. hyperthyroidism

EXERCISE 11-4

1. enlargement of many skeletal structures including the extremities, nose, forehead, and jaw
2. substance producing male characteristics
3. female sex hormones
4. a balanced, yet sometimes varying, state
5. produced by the pancreas
6. the study of the endocrine system including diagnosis and treatment of endocrine disorders
7. excessive thirst
8. posterior pituitary gland
9. glands that secrete substances into ducts that deliver secretions directly to a site
10. glands that secrete hormones into the bloodstream

EXERCISE 11-5

1. pancreas
4. endocrine
5. luteinizing
7. hypothalamus
10. hypercalcemia

CHAPTER 12

EXERCISE 12-1

1. Right atrium, tricuspid valve, right ventricle, pulmonary valve, pulmonary artery, lungs, pulmonary veins, left atrium, bicuspid (mitral) valve, left ventricle, aortic valve, aorta, arteries, arterioles, capillaries, venules, veins, superior and inferior venae cavae
2. Pericardium: sac in which the heart lies. Myocardium: heart muscle; middle wall of the heart. Endocardium: inner wall of the heart. Epicardium: outer wall of the heart. The epicardium is the same as the visceral pericardium.
3. Initiates the heartbeat; spreads the electrical impulses throughout the heart; and causes the heart to contract.
   Structures include: sinoatrial node (SA node), atrioventricular node (AV node), atrioventricular bundle (AV bundle, bundle of His), right and left bundle branches, Purkinje fibers.
   The SA node is the pacemaker because it sets the rhythm of the heart.

4. Systolic pressure: pressure against the walls of the artery during ventricular contraction
   Diastolic pressure: pressure against the walls of the artery during ventricular relaxation
   Sphygmomanometer: instrument used to record blood pressure
   P wave: registers atrial contraction.
   P-R interval: length of time it takes for impulses to travel from the SA to the AV node
5. Arteries and veins are named according to the structure through which they pass.

EXERCISE 12-2

1. vasoconstriction
2. hypotension
3. tachycardia
4. systole

EXERCISE 12-3

1. **arteri/o**; removal of the inner lining of the arterial wall
2. **atri/o**; pertaining to between the atria
3. **cardi/o**; inflammation of all the walls of the heart
4. **ech/o**; **cardi/o**; record of the heart using sound waves
5. **phleb/o**; **thromb/o**; abnormal condition of clots in a vein
6. **cerebr/o**; **vascul/o**; disturbance in the flow of blood to one or more parts of the brain
7. **ather/o**; fatty mass or debris

EXERCISE 12-4

1. angiectasis
2. angiography
3. angioplasty
4. angiospasm
5. arteriography
6. arterioles
7. arteriosclerosis
8. venous
9. venule
10. cardiologist

EXERCISE 12-5

1. Accumulation of fatty debris on the inner arterial wall. A type of arteriosclerosis.
2. A holdback of blood to the heart muscle.
3. Inflammation of a vein with clot formation.
4. Escape of fluid into the surrounding tissue.
5. Record of the electrical activity of the heart.

EXERCISE 12-6

1. pericardium
2. ventricle
4. myocardium
7. sphygmomanometer
8. extravasation
9. bicuspid

EXERCISE 12-7

1. vascular
2. aortic
3. arterial
4. atrial
5. cardiac
6. valvular
7. venous; vasal
8. ventricular

CHAPTER 13

EXERCISE 13-1

1. Albumin, globulin, and fibrinogen
2. (a) Plasma: the liquid portion of the blood; serum: plasma minus fibrinogen, the blood-clotting agent
   (b) Eosinophils: release chemicals into the bloodstream that can neutralize toxic substances. basophils: release histamine, a natural toxin that dilates blood vessels, starting the inflammatory process.
   neutrophils: ingest bacteria and other harmful matter.
   (c) Type A blood: has A antigens attached to the surface of the red blood cell.
   Type B blood: has B antigens attached to the surface of the red blood cell.
   Type AB blood: has both A and B antigens attached to the surface of the red blood cell.
   Type O blood: has neither A nor B antigens attached to the surface of the red blood cell.
3. Drains fluid away from body tissues into the bloodstream; carries nutrients, hormones, and oxygen to body tissues, and transports lipids from the digestive system; defends the body against infection.
4. (a) Phagocytes: white blood cells that consume bacteria.
   (b) Thymosin: a hormone that stimulates red bone marrow to produce T cells.
   (c) Pharyngeal tonsils: another name for adenoids, located in the nasopharynx.

(d) T lymphocytes: white blood cells that are produced in the red bone marrow but mature in the thymus gland. T lymphocytes have the ability to recognize when one of the body's cells has been invaded by a virus. T lymphocytes kill that particular virus.
(e) B lymphocytes: white blood cells that develop and mature in the bone marrow. B lymphocytes produce antibodies called immunoglobulins, which attach to foreign cells, labeling them for destruction.

5. cervical, submandibular, axillary, and inguinal lymph nodes

EXERCISE 13-2

1. color
2. network
3. immunity; safe
4. lymph glands
5. lymph vessels
6. clot
7. separate
8. transmission; carrying
9. production; manufacture; formation
10. stopping; controlling

EXERCISE 13-3

1. erythrocytopenia
2. leukocytopenia
3. thrombocytopenia
4. pancytopenia
5. anisocytosis
6. leukocytosis
7. poikilocytosis
8. anemia
9. erythremia
10. hyperbilirubinemia
11. hypercholesterolemia
12. hyperlipidemia

EXERCISE 13-4

1. hyperchromia
2. lymphangiography
3. lymphedema
4. myeloid
5. splenorrhaphy
6. thrombosis
7. erythropoiesis
8. hemostasis
9. autommune
10. myelogenous

EXERCISE 13-5

1. underpigmented red blood cells
2. study of blood and blood disorders
3. inadequate immune response to foreign substances
4. disease (particularly enlargement) of the lymph nodes
5. laboratory test that determines the percentage of erythrocytes in a blood sample
6. a protein that contains iron and has the ability to bind with oxygen and carbon dioxide. Hgb carries oxygen to the tissues and carbon dioxide away from the tissues.
7. laboratory test that separates substances in a mixture (usually protein) by the application of an electrical current
8. hormone that stimulates the production of red blood cells

CHAPTER 14

EXERCISE 14-1

1. Inhalation occurs when oxygen is inhaled into the lungs. Exhalation is when carbon dioxide moves from the blood to the lungs and is exhaled into the air.
2. Nose and nasal cavities: function in the inhalation and exhalation of air; filter out dust particles; warm and moisten air; smell. Pharynx is for the passage of food and air. The larynx is the voice box and also functions for the passage of air. The trachea is lined with cilia, which filter air. The trachea allows for the passage of air. Bronchi are for the passage of air. Lungs are for the exchange of gases.
3. Adam's apple: cartilaginous structure of the larynx that acts as a shield protecting inner structures
   Epiglottis: cartilaginous structure of the larynx that acts as a lid, covering the opening of the larynx during swallowing
   Cilia: hairs throughout the respiratory tract that filter air
   Bronchial tree: the branching and rebranching of the bronchi into smaller bronchi to resemble an inverted tree
   Paranasal sinuses: cavities within the cranial bones, lighten skull bones, and moisten air
4. Root: attaches the lungs to the body
   Hilum: area in the lung through which blood vessels, nerves, bronchi, and lymph vessels enter
   Apex: top of each lung
   Base: bottom of each lung
   Lobes: divisions of the lung. The right lung has three lobes, the superior, middle, and inferior lobe. The left lung has two lobes, the superior and inferior lobes.
   Alveoli: tiny sacs for the exchange of oxygen and carbon dioxide

EXERCISE 14-2

1. alveolar
2. bronchial
3. lobar
4. nasal
5. pharyngeal
6. laryngeal
7. diaphragmatic
8. pleural
9. pulmonary
10. thoracic; pectoral

EXERCISE 14-3

bronchodilator; lobectomy; mucolytic; phrenotomy; thoracocentesis; thoracoplasty

EXERCISE 14-4

1. apnea
2. bradypnea
3. dyspnea
4. eupnea
5. hyperpnea
6. oligopnea
7. orthopnea
8. tachypnea
9. hypercapnia
10. hypocapnia
11. hemothorax
12. hydrothorax
13. pneumothorax
14. pyothorax
15. stethoscope

EXERCISE 14-5

1. inflammation of the alveoli
2. pertaining to the nose and lacrimal apparatus
3. lack of oxygen
4. pertaining to the throat and tongue
5. pain in the pleura
6. inflammation of the lung
7. bleeding from the lungs
8. inflammation of all the sinuses
9. instrument used to cut the tonsils
10. inflammation of the voice box (larynx), windpipe (trachea), and bronchus

EXERCISE 14-6

1. pleurocentesis; thoracentesis, thoracocentesis
2. croup

EXERCISE 14-7

1. alveoli
2. bronchi
3. larynges
4. tonsils
5. tracheae

EXERCISE 14-8

1. alveolar
5. diaphragm
6. pneumoconiosis
7. pneumopleuritis
8. spirometer
10. dyspnea
13. bronchiectasis
14. tonsillar

CHAPTER 15

EXERCISE 15-1

1. Digestion, absorption, and defecation
2. Major structures: oral cavity or mouth; pharynx or throat; esophagus; stomach; small intestine; large intestine. Accessory organs: salivary glands, pancreas, liver, and gallbladder.
3. Lower esophageal sphincter: at the junction between the esophagus and the stomach. Pyloric sphincter: at the junction between the stomach and the duodenum.
4. cecum, ascending colon, transverse colon, descending colon, sigmoid colon, rectum, and anus
5. duodenum, jejunum, and ileum
6. parotid, submandibular, and sublingual
7. begins digestion of carbohydrates
8. 1. Production of bile. 2. Breakdown of carbo-hydrates, fats, and proteins so that they can be absorbed or stored for later use. 3. Storage of excess sugar as glycogen. 4. Storage of vitamins A, D, E, and K; iron; and copper. 5. Detoxification of harmful substances by the action of phagocytic cells called Kupffer's cells. 6. Production of blood proteins such as prothrombin and fibrinogen.
9. Insulin and glucagon regulate the amount of sugar in the bloodstream.
10. Parietal peritoneum: membrane lining the abdominopelvic wall. Visceral peritoneum: membrane covering the abdominopelvic organs. Peritoneal cavity: space between the parietal and visceral pleura
11. The hepatic duct drains bile from the liver. The cystic duct carries bile to and from the gallbladder. The common bile duct is the union of the hepatic, cystic, and pancreatic ducts.

EXERCISE 15-2

1. E
2. F
3. J
4. H
5. G
6. A
7. D
8. C
9. B
10. I

EXERCISE 15-3

1. cheek
2. cecum
3. lips
4. bile duct; bile vessel
5. gallbladder
6. common bile duct
7. tooth
8. small intestine; intestine
9. gums
10. tongue
11. liver
12. ileum (portion of the small intestine)
13. jejunum
14. lips
15. abdomen
16. tongue
17. stone
18. appetite
19. rectum
20. saliva
21. salivary gland
22. fat
23. mouth
24. mouth
25. internal organs
26. relaxation
27. to step; to go
28. vomiting
29. eating; swallowing
30. digestion
31. patches

32. meal
33. around
34. blood condition

EXERCISE 15-4

1. pertaining to the mucous membrane of the cheek
2. excision of the tongue
3. loss of appetite
4. pertaining to the mouth
5. hernia of the rectum with the rectum pushing onto the vaginal wall
6. stone in the salivary gland or duct
7. discharge of fat in the feces
8. process of visually examining the sigmoid colon
9. inflammation of the mouth
10. drooping of the internal organs
11. inability of the muscles of the digestive tract to relax
12. backward flow of fluid
13. indigestion
14. after a meal
15. process of visually examining the internal body cavities

EXERCISE 15-5

1. anorectal
2. perianal
3. appendectomy
4. appendicitis
5. cecopexy
6. ventriculoperitoneal
7. cheiloplasty
8. cheilorrhaphy
9. cheilosis
10. colitis
11. herniorrhaphy
12. colostomy
;13. colocolostomy
14. hepatocellular
15. cholelith
16. hepatoma
17. inguinal hernia
18. hyperemesis
19. hematemesis
20. melanemesis
21. aphagia
22. dysphagia
23. polyphagia

EXERCISE 15-6

cheiloplasty; cecopexy; gastrotomy; choledocholithotripsy; proctoclysis; endoscopy

EXERCISE 15-7

biliary; duodenal; esophageal; salivary

EXERCISE 15-8

1. ileocecal valve
3. cholecystitis
4. colitis
6. cheilorrhaphy
8. salivary
10. vomiting

CHAPTER 16

EXERCISE 16-1

1. C
2. F
3. B
4. D
5. E
6. A

EXERCISE 16-2

1. balan/o
2. calic/o; calyc/o
3. cyst/o; vesic/o
4. lith/o
5. ren/o; nephr/o
6. testicul/o; orchid/o; orchi/o
7. pyel/o
8. vas/o
9. urin/o; ur/o; -uria
10. ur/o
11. -cele
12. -spadias
13. circum-
14. extra-
15. -sclerosis
16. -stenosis
17. -tripsy
18. -tomy
19. -osis; -iasis
20. -emia
21. -pexy
22. -ptosis
23. -gram
24. oligo-
25. -cidal
26. trans-
27. varic/o
28. dia-
29. noct/o
30. -pathy

EXERCISE 16-3

1. extracorporeal
2. cystoscope
3. lithotripsy
4. hydronephrosis
5. cryptorchidism
6. oligospermia
7. urethrorrhagia
8. vesicosigmoidostomy
9. ureteroileostomy
10. ureterostomy
11. meatotomy
12. urethroplasty

EXERCISE 16-4

1. hematocele
2. hydrocele
3. spermatocele
4. varicocele
5. anuria
6. bacteriuria
7. dysuria
8. hematuria
9. nocturia
10. oliguria
11. proteinuria; albuminuria
12. pyuria
13. nephrolithiasis
14. nephrolithotomy
15. nephropathy
16. nephropexy
17. nephroptosis
18. nephrotomography
19. nephroblastoma

EXERCISE 16-5

lithotripsy; nephrolithotomy; orchidopexy; vasectomy;
cystourethrography; circumcision

EXERCISE 16-6

1. no production of spermatozoa
2. to kill or destroy spermatozoa
3. accumulation of waste products in the blood due
   to loss of kidney function
4. backward flow of urine from the bladder to the
   ureter
5. mechanical replacement of kidney function when
   the kidney is dysfunctional
6. laboratory analysis of urine
7. congenital opening of the meatus on the ventral
   (underside) of the penis
8. no control of excretory functions such as urination

9. removal of the prepuce or foreskin
10. pertaining to many cysts on the kidney

EXERCISE 16-7

1. corporeal
2. cortical
3. caliceal; calyceal
4. vesical; cystic
5. glomerular
6. renal; nephric
7. testicular
8. ureteral
9. urethral
10. urinary

EXERCISE 16-8

1. cortices
2. calices; calyces
3. epididymides
4. glomeruli
5. meati
6. testes
7. kidney pelves
8. testicles
9. spermatozoa
10. ureters

EXERCISE 16-9

1. balanorrhea
3. cystitis
4. epididymis
5. caliceal
6. prostatectomy
9. incontinence

CHAPTER 17

EXERCISE 17-1

1. F
2. I
3. D
4. J
5. G
6. A
7. B
8. C
9. E
10. H

EXERCISE 17-2

1. vagin/o; colp/o
2. vulv/o; episi/o

3. gynec/o
4. lact/o; galact/o
5. mamm/o; mast/o
6. men/o
7. nat/o; -partum; -para
8. oophor/o; ovari/o
9. salping/o; salpinx
10. top/o
11. -arche
12. -gravida; -cyesis
13. -para
14. -tocia; tocin; -partum
15. ante-

EXERCISE 17-3
1. cervicitis
2. episiorrhaphy
3. culdocentesis
4. gynecologist
5. hysterectomy
6. mammary
7. mastectomy
8. ovoid
9. salpingo-oophorectomy
10. polythelia
11. ectopic pregnancy
12. vaginomycosis
13. cystocele
14. pseudocyesis
15. postpartum
16. pyosalpinx
17. dystocia
18. retroflexion

EXERCISE 17-4
1. cervical
2. mammary
3. uterine
4. natal
5. ovarian
6. perineal
7. vaginal

EXERCISE 17-5
1. amenorrhea
2. dysmenorrhea
3. menopause
4. menorrhea

5. menorrhagia
6. oligomenorrhea
7. menometrorrhagia
8. metroptosis
9. metrorrhagia
10. myometrium
11. perimetrium
12. endometrium
13. multigravida
14. nulligravida
15. primipara
16. secundipara

EXERCISE 17-6
1. endometrial tissue found at sites other than the uterus
2. discharge of milk from the breast after breastfeeding has stopped
3. pertaining to the rectum and uterus
4. beginning of the regular menstrual cycle, usually occurring at around 13 years of age
5. stoppage of menstruation, usually at about 45–55 years of age
6. birth process
7. fertilized ovum from conception to second week of gestation
8. to shed
9. name given to a developing human between the second and eighth week of gestation
10. excessive vomiting during pregnancy

EXERCISE 17-7
colporrhaphy

EXERCISE 17-8
1. uteri
2. ovaries; ovaria

EXERCISE 17-9
1. cervicitis
2. mammography
5. dysmenorrhea
6. oocyte
9. polythelia
10. ectopic
11. vulvectomy
14. retroflexion

Word Element to Definition

WORD ELEMENT	DEFINITION
a(n)-	inadequate; no; not; lack of
ab-	away from
abdomin/o	abdomen
-ac	pertaining to
acetabul/o	acetabulum; hip socket
acr/o	extremity; top
acromi/o	acromion
ad-	toward
aden/o	gland
adenoid/o	adenoids
adip/o	fat
adren/o	adrenal gland
adrenal/o	adrenal gland
-al	pertaining to
albin/o	white
albumin/o	albumin (a blood protein)
-algia	pain
alveol/o	air sacs; alveolus
ambly/o	dull; dim
amni/o	amnion; sac in which the fetus lies in the uterus
an/o	anus
ana-	apart; up
andr/o	male; man
angi/o	vessel
anis/o	unequal size
ankyl/o	fusion of parts; bent; crooked
ante-	before
anter/o	front
anti-	against
aort/o	aorta
append/o	appendix
aque/o	water
-ar	pertaining to
-arche	beginning

WORD ELEMENT	DEFINITION
arteri/o	artery
arthr/o	joint
articul/o	joint
-ary	pertaining to
-assay	analysis of a mixture to identify its contents
-asthenia	no strength
ather/o	fatty debris; fatty plaque
atri/o	atrium (upper chambers of the heart)
audi/o	hearing
audit/o	hearing
aur/o	ear
auto-	self
axill/o	armpit
bacteri/o	bacteria
balan/o	glans penis (tip of the penis)
bi/o	life
bil/i	bile
bilirubin/o	bilirubin (a bile pigment)
-blast	immature, growing thing
blephar/o	eyelid
brachi/o	arm
brady-	slow
bronch/o	bronchus
bronchi/o	bronchus
bronchiol/o	bronchioles; little bronchi; small bronchial tubes
bucc/o	cheek
burs/o	bursa (sac filled with synovial fluid located around joints)
calc/o	calcium
calcane/o	heel

WORD ELEMENT	DEFINITION
calic/o; calyc/o	calix; calyx
-capnia	carbon dioxide
capsul/o	capsule
carcin/o	cancer; cancerous
cardi/o	heart
carp/o	wrist
cartilagin/o	cartilage
catheter/o	something inserted
caud/o	tail
cec/o	cecum
-cele	hernia (protrusion of an organ from the structure that normally contains it)
cellul/o	cell
-centesis	surgical puncture to remove fluid
cephal/o	head
cerebell/o	cerebellum
cerebr/o	brain
cervic/o	cervix; neck; neck of uterus; cervix uteri
-chalasia	relaxation
cheil/o	lips
chol/e	bile; gall
cholangi/o	bile ducts
cholecyst/o	gallbladder
choledoch/o	common bile duct
cholesterol/o	cholesterol
chondr/o	cartilage
chori/o	choroid
chrom/o	color
-cidal	to kill
cili/o	hair
-clasis	surgical fracture or refracture
-clast	breakdown
clavicul/o	clavicle; collarbone
-clonus	turmoil
-clysis	washing; irrigation
coagulati/o	to condense; to clot
coccyg/o	coccyx; tailbone
cochle/o	cochlea
col/o	colon; large intestine
colon/o	colon
colp/o	vagina
coni/o	dust
conjunctiv/o	conjunctiva
constrict/o	to draw together
-continence	to stop
-conus	cone-shaped
core/o	pupil
corne/o	cornea

WORD ELEMENT	DEFINITION
coron/o	crown
corpor/o	body
cortic/o	cortex; outer covering; outer layer
cost/o	ribs
crani/o	skull
crin/o	to secrete
-crine	to secrete
-crit	separate
cry/o	cold
crypt/o	hidden
culd/o	cul-de-sac
-cusis	hearing
cutane/o	skin
cycl/o	ciliary body
-cyesis	pregnancy
cyst/o	bladder; sac
cyt/o	cell
-cyte	cell
-cytosis	increase in the number of cells
dacry/o	tears; lacrimal duct
de-	lack of; removal
dent/o	tooth
derm/o	skin
-derma	skin
dermat/o	skin
-dermis	skin
-desis	surgical binding; surgical fusion
di-	two
dia-	complete; through
diaphor/e	profuse sweating
dilat/o	dilation; dilatation; to expand; widen
dipl/o	double
-dipsia	thirst
don/o	donates
dors/o	back
dorsi-	back
duct/o	to draw
duoden/o	duodenum (proximal portion of small intestine)
dur/o	dura mater (outermost membrane surrounding the brain)
-dynia	pain
dys-	bad; difficult; painful; poor
e-	out; outside; outward; without
-eal	pertaining to
-ear	pertaining to

WORD ELEMENT	DEFINITION
ec-	out
ech/o	sound
-ectasis	dilation; dilatation; stretching
-ectomy	excision; surgical removal
-edema	accumulation of fluid
electr/o	electric
-emesis	vomit; vomiting
-emia	blood condition
emmetr/o	in proper measure
en-	inward
encephal/o	brain
endo-	with; within
enter/o	small intestine
epi-	above; on; upon
epididym/o	epididymis
episi/o	vulva; external genitalia; pudendum
epitheli/o	covering
-er	specialist; one who specializes; specialist in the study of
erythemat/o	red
erythr/o	red
eso-	inward
esophag/o	esophagus
-esthesia	sensation
estr/o	female
ethm/o	ethmoid bone; sieve
eu-	normal; good
ex-	out; outside; outward
exo-	out; outside; outward
extra-	out; outside; outward
faci/o	face
fasci/o	fascia
femor/o	femur; thigh bone
fibr/o	fibers; fibrous tissue
fibul/o	fibula
flex/o	bending
-flux	flow
front/o	frontal bone
galact/o	milk
gastr/o	stomach
-gen	producing
-genesis	development; production
-genic	producing; produced by
gingiv/o	gums
glen/o	socket; pit; glenoid cavity
gli/o	glue
glomerul/o	glomerulus
gloss/o	tongue

WORD ELEMENT	DEFINITION
gluc/o	sugar
glycogen/o	glycogen (storage form of sugar)
gonad/o	gonads; sex glands
goni/o	angle (of the anterior chamber)
-grade	to step; to go
-gram	record; writing
granul/o	granules
-graph	instrument used to record
-graphy	process of recording; producing images
-gravida	pregnancy
gynec/o	female; woman
hem/o	blood
hemat/o	blood
hemi-	half
hepat/o	liver
herni/o	hernia
hiat/o	hiatus, opening
hidr/o	sweat
hist/o	tissue
histi/o	tissue
home/o	same
humer/o	humerus; upper arm
hydr/o	water
hyper-	abnormal increase; above; above normal; excessive
hypo-	abnormal decrease; below; below normal; under
hyster/o	uterus
-ia	condition; state of
-iasis	abnormal condition; process
-ic	pertaining to
-ician	specialist; one who specializes; expert
ile/o	ileum (distal portion of the small intestine)
ili/o	hip
immun/o	immunity; safe
in-	no; not
-ine	pertaining to
infer/o	below; downward
infra-	within
inguin/o	groin
insulin/o	insulin
inter-	between
intestin/o	intestine
intra-	within
-ion	process

WORD ELEMENT	DEFINITION
-ior	pertaining to
ir/o	iris
irid/o	iris
is/o	equal
isch/o	hold back
ischi/o	ischium (posterior portion of the hip bone)
-ism	condition; process; state of
-ist	specialist; one who specializes; specialist in the study of
-itis	inflammation (the redness, swelling, heat, and pain that occur when the body protects itself from injury)
-ium	structure
jejun/o	jejunum (medial portion of small intestine)
kal/o	potassium
kerat/o	cornea; hard; hornlike
keratin/o	hard; hornlike
kinesi/o	movement
-kinesia	movement; motion
-kinesis	movement; motion
kyph/o	humpback
labi/o	lips
labyrinth/o	inner ear; labyrinth
lacrim/o	lacrimal apparatus; tears
lact/o	milk
lapar/o	abdominal wall; abdomen
laryng/o	larynx; voice box
lei/o	smooth
leuk/o	white
ligati/o	binding; tying
lingu/o	tongue
lip/o	fat
lipid/o	fat
-lith	calculus; stone
lith/o	stone
lob/o	lobe
-logist	specialist; one who specializes; specialist in the study of
-logy	study of; process of study
lord/o	swayback
lumb/o	lower back; loins
lymph/o	lymph (clear, watery fluid)
lymphaden/o	lymph glands; lymph nodes
lymphangi/o	lymph vessels

WORD ELEMENT	DEFINITION
-lysis	breakdown; destruction; separate; separation
-lytic	pertaining to destruction, separation, or breakdown
magnet/o	magnet
-malacia	softening
malleol/o	malleolus (bony projection on the distal aspects of the tibia and fibula)
mamm/o	breast
mandibul/o	mandible; lower jaw
mast/o	breast
maxill/o	maxilla; upper jaw
meat/o	meatus
medi/o	middle
medull/o	marrow; medulla; inner portion of an organ
-megaly	enlargement
melan/o	black
men/o	menses; menstruation; month
mening/o	membrane; meninges
metacarp/o	metacarpals (bones of the hand)
metatars/o	metatarsals (bones of the foot)
-meter	instrument used to measure
metr/o	uterus
-metrist	specialist in the measurement of
-metry	process of measuring; to measure; measurement
mi/o	contraction; less
mono-	one
muc/o	mucus (a bodily secretion, of the mucous membrane, sometimes sticky and frequently thick)
multi-	multiple
muscul/o	muscle
my/o	muscle
myc/o	fungus
mydri/o	dilation (dilatation); wide
-myein	to shut
myel/o	bone marrow; spinal cord
myelin/o	myelin sheath
myos/o	muscle
myring/o	tympanic membrane; eardrum
nas/o	nose
nat/i	birth
natr/o	sodium
necr/o	death
neo-	new

WORD ELEMENT	DEFINITION
nephr/o	kidney
neur/o	nerve
noct/o	night
norm/o	normal
nulli-	none
o/o	egg
occipit/o	occiput (back part of the head)
ocul/o	eye
odont/o	teeth; tooth
-oid	resembling
-ole	small
olecran/o	elbow; olecranon
oligo-	deficient; few; scanty
-oma	mass; tumor
onych/o	nail
oophor/o	ovary
ophthalm/o	eye
-opia	visual condition; vision
-opsia	visual condition; vision
-opsy	to view
-opt/o	vision; sight
-or	one who; person or thing that does something
or/o	mouth
orchi/o	testicle; testis
orchid/o	testicle; testis
orex/i	appetite
ortho-	straight
-ory	pertaining to
-ose	pertaining to
-osis	abnormal condition
oste/o	bone
ot/o	ear
-ous	pertaining to
ov/o	egg
ovari/o	ovary
ox/o	oxygen
oxy-	quick; sharp
palpebr/o	eyelid
pan-	all
pancreat/o	pancreas
papill/o	optic disc; nipple-like
para-	abnormal; beside; near
-para	give birth; near; part with child; to part with
parathyroid/o	parathyroid gland
pariet/o	parietal bone; wall
-partum	labor; delivery; childbirth

WORD ELEMENT	DEFINITION
patell/a	patella; kneecap
patell/o	patella; kneecap
path/o	disease
-pathy	disease
-pause	stoppage; cessation
pector/o	chest
ped/o	child
pelv/i	pelvis
pelv/o	pelvis
-penia	decrease; deficiency
-pepsia	digestion
peri-	around
perine/o	perineum
peritone/o	peritoneum
-pexy	surgical fixation
phac/o	lens
-phagia	swallow; to eat
phalang/o	phalanx (one of the bones making up the fingers or toes)
phall/o	penis
pharmac/o	drug
pharyng/o	pharynx; throat
-phasia	speech
phleb/o	vein
-phobia	fear; irrational fear
-phonia	voice
-phoresis	transmission; carry
phot/o	light
phren/o	diaphragm
physi/o	nature
-physis	to grow
pil/o	hair
pine/o	pineal gland
pituitar/o	pituitary gland
-plakia	patches
-plasia	development; formation
-plasty	surgical repair or reconstruction
-plegia	paralysis (loss or impairment of motor function)
pleur/a	pleura; pleural cavity
pleur/o	pleura; pleural cavity
-pnea	breathing
pneum/o	air; respiration; lungs
pneumat/o	air; respiration; lungs
pneumon/o	lungs
-poiesis	production; manufacture; formation
-poietin	a hormone that stimulates the production of blood cells
poikil/o	variation; irregular
polio-	gray

WORD ELEMENT	DEFINITION
poly-	many
-porosis	porous
post-	after
poster/o	back
practition/o	practice
-prandial	meal
presby-	old age
primi-	first
proct/o	rectum
pronati/o	pronation
prostat/o	prostate; prostate gland
proxim/o	near; close
pseudo-	false
-ptosis	downward displacement; drooping; falling; prolapse; sagging
-ptysis	spitting
pub/o	pubis (a portion of the hip bone)
pulmon/o	lungs
pupill/o	pupil
py/o	pus
pyel/o	renal pelvis (upper dilated portion of the ureter)
pylor/o	pylorus (distal portion of the stomach); pyloric sphincter
quadri-	four
radi/o	radius (one of the bones of the lower arm)
radicul/o	nerve roots
re-	back
rect/o	rectum
ren/o	kidney
reticul/o	network
retin/o	retina
retro-	backward; back; behind
rhabd/o	rod-shaped; striped; striated
rhin/o	nose
rhythm/o	rhythm
-rrhage	bursting forth
-rrhagia	bursting forth
-rrhaphy	suture; sew
-rrhea	flow; discharge
-rrhexis	rupture
sacr/o	sacrum
salping/o	eustachian tube; fallopian tubes; uterine tubes
-salpinx	fallopian tube; uterine tube
-sarcoma	malignant tumor of connective tissue

WORD ELEMENT	DEFINITION
scapul/o	scapula
-schisis	cleft; splitting
-sclerosis	hardening
scoli/o	curved
-scope	instrument used to visually examine (a body cavity or organ)
-scopy	process of visually examining (a body cavity or organ)
seb/o	sebum
sect/o	to cut
secundi-	second
sial/o	saliva
sialaden/o	salivary glands
sigmoid/o	sigmoid colon
sinus/o	sinuses
-sis	state of; condition
skelet/o	skeleton
somat/o	body
son/o	sound
-spadias	opening; split
-spasm	sudden, involuntary contraction
sperm/o	spermatozoa; sperm
spermat/o	spermatozoa; sperm
sphen/o	sphenoid bone; wedge
spin/o	spine; spinal column; backbone
splen/o	spleen
spondyl/o	vertebra
staped/o	stapes
-stasis	standing; stable; stoppage; stopping; controlling
steat/o	fat
-stenosis	narrowing; stricture
stern/o	sternum; breastbone
steth/o	chest
stomat/o	mouth
-stomy	new opening
sub-	tongue; under
super/o	above; toward the head
supinati/o	supination
supra-	above; beyond; excessive
sym-	together; with
synovi/o	synovium (synovial membrane)
tachy-	fast
-taxia	order
tempor/o	temporal bone
ten/o	tendon
tend/o	tendon
tendin/o	tendon
tenosynovi/o	tendon sheath (covering of a tendon)

WORD ELEMENT	DEFINITION
tens/o	stretch
tensi/o	tension
test/o	testicle; testis
testicul/o	testicle; testis
thalam/o	thalamus
thel/o	nipple
-therapy	treatment
-thermy	heat
thorac/o	chest; thorax
-thorax	chest
thromb/o	clot
thym/o	thymus; thymus gland
thyr/o	thyroid gland; shield
thyroid/o	thyroid gland; shield
tibi/o	tibia; shin
-tic	pertaining to
-tocia	labor
-tocin	labor
tom/o	to cut
-tome	instrument used to cut
-tomy	to cut; incise; process of cutting; incision
ton/o	tension
tonsill/o	tonsils
top/o	place
trabecul/o	trabecula (strands of connective tissue)
trache/o	trachea; windpipe
trans-	across
trigon/o	trigone
-tripsy	crushing
-trophic; -tropic	pertaining to nutrition or nourishment
-trophy	development; growth; nutrition
-tropia	turning
-tropion	turning
tub/o	fallopian tube
tympan/o	tympanic membrane; eardrum
-ule	small

WORD ELEMENT	DEFINITION
uln/o	ulnar (one of the bones of the lower arm)
ultra-	excess; beyond
-um	structure
ungu/o	nail
ur/o	urinary tract; urine; urination
ure/o	urea (end product of protein breakdown and is found in urine)
ureter/o	ureters
urethr/o	urethra
-uria	urine; urination
urin/o	urine
-us	condition; thing
uter/o	uterus
uve/o	uvea (includes the choroid, ciliary body, and iris)
vagin/o	vagina
valvul/o	valve
varic/o	varicose vein; dilated, twisted vein
vas/o	vas deferens; vessel
vascul/o	vessel
ven/o	vein
ventr/o	front
ventricul/o	ventricle (lower chambers of the heart)
versi/o	turning; tilting; tipping
vertebr/o	vertebra
vesic/o	bladder
viscer/o	internal organs
vitre/o	glasslike; gel-like
vulv/o	vulva; external genitalia; pudendum
xer/o	dry
xiph/o	sword
-y	process
zygomat/o	cheekbone

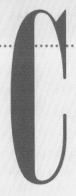
Definition to Word Element

DEFINITION	WORD ELEMENT
abdomen	abdomin/o; lapar/o
abdominal wall	lapar/o
abnormal	para-
abnormal condition	-iasis; -osis
abnormal increase	hyper-
above	epi-; hyper-; super/o; supra-
accumulation of a fluid	-edema
acetabulum	acetabul/o
acromion	acromi/o
across	trans-
adenoids	adenoid/o
adrenal gland	adren/o; adrenal/o
after	post-
against	anti-
air	pneum/o; pneumat/o
air sacs	alveol/o
albumin (a blood protein)	albumin/o
all	pan-
alveolus	alveol/o
amnion	amni/o
analysis of a mixture to identify its contents	-assay
angle (of the anterior chamber)	goni/o
anus	an/o
aorta	aort/o
apart	ana-
appendix	append/o
appetite	orex/i
arm	brachi/o
armpit	axill/o
around	circum-; peri-
artery	arteri/o
aspiration	-centesis
atrium	atri/o

DEFINITION	WORD ELEMENT
away from	ab-
back	dorsi-; dors/o; poster/o; re-; retro-
back part of the head (occiput)	occipit/o
backbone	spin/o
backward	retro-
bacteria	bacteri/o
bad	dys-
bear (to)	-para
before	ante-
beginning	-arche
behind	retro-
below	hypo-; infer/o; sub-
below normal	hypo-
bending	flex/o
bent	ankyl/o
beside	para-
between	inter-
beyond	supra-; ultra-
bile	bil/i; chol/e
bile vessel	cholangi/o
bilirubin (a bile pigment)	bilirubin/o
binding	ligati/o
birth	nat/o
black	melan/o
bladder	cyst/o; vesic/o
blood	hem/o; hemat/o
blood condition	-emia
body	corpor/o; somat/o
bone	osse/o; oste/o
bone marrow	myel/o
bony projection on the distal aspects of the tibia and fibula	malleol/o

DEFINITION	WORD ELEMENT	DEFINITION	WORD ELEMENT
brain	cerebr/o; encephal/o	cone-shaped	-conus
breakdown	-clast; -lysis	contraction	mi/o
breast	mamm/o; mast/o	controlling	-stasis
breastbone	stern/o	cornea	corne/o; kerat/o
breathing	-pnea	cortex	cortic/o
bronchioles	bronchiol/o	covering	epitheli/o
bronchus	bronchi/o; bronch/o	covering of a tendon	tenosynovi/o
bursa	burs/o	crooked	ankyl/o
bursting forth	-rrhage; -rrhagia	crown	coron/o
		crushing	-tripsy
calcium	calc/o	cul-de-sac	culd/o
calculus	-lith	curved	scoli/o
calix	calic/o; calyc/o	cut (to)	cis/o; sect/o; tom/o;
calyx	calic/o; calyc/o		-tomy
cancer	carcin/o		
cancerous	carcin/o	death	necr/o
capsule	capsul/o	decrease	hypo-; -penia
carbon dioxide	-capnia	deficiency	-penia
carry	-phoresis	deficient	oligo-
cartilage	cartilagin/o; chondr/o	delivery	-partum
cecum	cec/o	destruction	-lysis
cell	cellul/o; cyt/o; -cyte	development	-plasia; -trophy; -genesis
cerebellum	cerebell/o	diaphragm	phren/o
cervix	cervic/o	difficult	dys-
cervix uteri	cervic/o	digestion	-pepsia
cessation	-pause	dilated, twisted vein	varic/o
cheek	bucc/o	dilation (dilatation)	dilat/o; -ectasis; mydri/o
cheekbone	zygomat/o	dim	ambly/o
chest	pector/o; steth/o;	discharge	-rrhea
	thorac/o; -thorax	disease	path/o; -pathy
child	ped/o	donates	don/o
childbirth	-partum	double	dipl/o
cholesterol	cholesterol/o	downward	infer/o
choroid	chori/o	downward displacement	-ptosis
ciliary body	cycl/o	draw (to)	duct/o
clavicle	clavicul/o	draw together (to)	constrict/o
clear, watery fluid	lymph/o	drooping	-ptosis
cleft	-schisis	drug	pharmac/o
close	proxim/o	dry	xer/o
clot	thromb/o	dull	ambly/o
clot (to)	coagulati/o	duodenum (proximal	duoden/o
coccyx	coccyg/o	portion of small	
cochlea	cochle/o	intestine)	
cold	cry/o	dura mater (outermost	dur/o
collarbone	clavicul/o	membrane surrounding	
colon	col/o; colon/o	the brain)	
color	chrom/o		
common bile duct	choledoch/o	ear	aur/o; ot/o
complete	dia-	eardrum	myring/o; tympan/o
condense (to)	coagulati/o	eat (to)	-phagia
condition	-ia; -ism; -sis	egg	o/o; ov/o

DEFINITION	WORD ELEMENT	DEFINITION	WORD ELEMENT
elbow	olecran/o	glans penis (tip of penis)	balan/o
electric	electr/o	glasslike	vitre/o
enlargement	-megaly	glenoid cavity	glen/o
epididymis	epididym/o	glomerulus	glomerul/o
equal	is/o	glycogen (storage form of sugar)	glycogen/o
esophagus	esophag/o	go (to)	-grade
ethmoid bone	ethm/o	gonads	gonad/o
eustachian tube	salping/o	good	eu-
excess	ultra-	granules	granul/o
excessive	hyper-; supra-	gray	polio-
excision	-ectomy	groin	inguin/o
expand (to)	dilat/o	grow (to)	-physis
expert	-ician	growing thing	-blast
external genitalia	episi/o; vulv/o	growth	-trophy
extremity	acr/o	gums	gingiv/o
eye	ocul/o; ophthalm/o		
eyelid	blephar/o; palpebr/o	hair	cili/o; pil/o
		half	hemi-
face	faci/o	hard	kerat/o; keratin/o
falling	-ptosis	hardening	-sclerosis; scler/o
fallopian tube	salping/o; -salpinx; tub/o	head	cephal/o
false	pseudo-	hearing	audi/o; -cusis
fascia (band of tissue surrounding a muscle)	fasci/o	heart	cardi/o
		heat	-thermy
fast	tachy-	heel	calcane/o
fat	adip/o; lip/o; lipid/o; steat/o	hernia (protrusion of an organ from the structure that normally contains it)	-cele; herni/o
fatty debris	ather/o		
fatty plaque	ather/o		
fear	-phobia	hiatus	hiat/o
female	estr/o; gynec/o	hidden	crypt/o
femur	femor/o	hip	ili/o
few	oligo-	hip socket	acetabul/o
fibers	fibr/o	hold back	isch/o
fibrous tissue	fibr/o	hormone that stimulates the production of blood cells	-poietin
fibula	fibul/o		
first	primi-		
flow	-flux; -rrhea	hornlike	kerat/o; keratin/o
formation	-plasia; -poiesis	humerus	humer/o
formed in	-genic	humpback	kyph/o
four	quadri-		
front	anter/o; ventr/o	ileum (distal portion of the small intestine)	ile/o
frontal bone	front/o		
fungus	myc/o	immature	-blast
fusion of parts	ankyl/o	immunity	immun/o
		in proper measure	emmetr/o
gall	chol/e	inadequate	a(n)-
gallbladder	cholecyst/o	inadequate formation	-plasia
gel-like	vitre/o	incise	-tomy
give birth	-para		
gland	aden/o		

DEFINITION	WORD ELEMENT	DEFINITION	WORD ELEMENT
incision	-tomy	loss or impairment of motor function	-plegia
increase in the number of cells	-cytosis	lower back	lumb/o
inflammation (redness, swelling, heat, and pain that occur when the body protects itself from injury)	-itis	lower jaw	mandibul/o
		lungs	pneum/o; pneumat/o; pneumon/o; pulmon/o
		lymph (clear, watery fluid)	lymph/o
		lymph glands	lymphaden/o
inner ear	labyrinth/o	lymph node	lymphaden/o
instrument used to cut	-tome	lymph vessels	lymphangi/o
instrument used to measure	-meter		
		magnet	magnet/o
instrument used to record	-graph	male	andr/o
instrument used to visually examine (a body cavity or organ)	-scope	malignant tumor of connective tissue	-sarcoma
		malleolus	malleol/o
insulin	insulin/o	man	andr/o
internal organ	viscer/o	mandible	mandibul/o
intestine	ile/o; intestin/o	manufacture	-poiesis
inward	en-; eso-	many	poly-
iris	irid/o; ir/o	marrow	medull/o
irrational fear	-phobia	mass	-oma
irregular	poikil/o	maxilla	maxill/o
irrigation	-clysis	meal	-prandial
ischium	ischi/o	measure (to)	-metry
		meatus	meat/o
		medulla	medull/o
jejunum (medial portion of small intestine)	jejun/o	membrane	chori/o; mening/o
		meninges	mening/o
joint	arthr/o; articul/o	menses	men/o
		menstruation	men/o
		metacarpals (bones of the hand)	metacarp/o
kidney	nephr/o; ren/o		
kill (to)	-cidal	metatarsals (bones of the foot)	metatars/o
kneecap	patell/a; patell/o		
		middle	medi/o
labor	-partum; -tocia; -tocin	milk	galact/o; lact/o
labyrinth	labyrinth/o	month	men/o
lack of	de-	motion	-kinesia; -kinesis
lacrimal apparatus	lacrim/o	mouth	or/o; stomat/o
lacrimal duct	dacry/o	movement	-kinesia; -kinesis
large intestine	col/o	mucus (a bodily secretion, of the mucous membrane, sometimes sticky and frequently thick)	muc/o
larynx	laryng/o		
lens	phac/o; phak/o		
less	mi/o		
life	bi/o		
light	phot/o	multiple	multi-
lips	cheil/o; labi/o	muscle	muscul/o; myos/o
little bronchi	bronchiol/o	myelin sheath	myelin/o
liver	hepat/o		
lobe	lob/o	nail	onych/o; ungu/o
loins	lumb/o	narrowing	-stenosis

DEFINITION	WORD ELEMENT	DEFINITION	WORD ELEMENT
nature	physi/o	perineum	perine/o
near	proxim/o; para-	peritoneum	peritone/o
neck	cervic/o	person or thing that	-or
neck of uterus	cervic/o	does something	
nerve	neur/o	pertaining to	-ac; -al; -ar; -ary; -eal;
nerve roots	radicul/o		-ear; -ic; ine; -ior; -or;
network	reticul/o		-ory; -ose; -ous; -tic
new opening	-stomy	pertaining to destruction,	-lytic
night	noct/o	separation, or breakdown	
nipple	thel/o	pertaining to nutrition	-trophic; tropic
nipple-like	papill/o	or nourishment	
no	a(n)-; in-	phalanges (one of the	phalang/o
no strength	-asthenia	bones making up	
none	nulli-	the fingers or toes)	
normal	eu-; norm/o	pharynx	pharyng/o
nose	nas/o; rhin/o	pineal gland	pine/o
not	a(n)-; -in	pit	glen/o
nourishment	-trophy	pituitary gland	pituitar/o
nutrition	-trophy	place	top/o
		pleura	pleur/a; pleur/o
		pleural cavity	pleur/a; pleur/o
occiput (back part	occipit/o	poor	dys-
of the head)		porous	-porosis
old age	presby-	posterior portion of	ischi/o
olecranon	olecran/o	the hip bone	
on	epi-	potassium	kal/o
one	mono-	practice	practition/o
one who	-or	pregnancy	-cyesis; -gravida
one who specializes;	-er; -or; -ician; -ist;	process	-iasis; -ion; -ism; -y
specialist	-logist	process of cutting	-tomy
opening	-spadias; hiat/o	process of measuring	-metry
optic disc	papill/o	process of producing	-graphy
order	-taxia	images	
out	e-; ec-; ex-; exo-; extra-	process of recording	-graphy
outer layer	cortic/o	process of study	-logy
outside	e-; ec-; ex-; exo-; extra-	process of visually	-scopy
outward	e-; ec-; ex-; exo-; extra-	examining (a body	
ovary	oophor/o; ovari/o	cavity or organ)	
oxygen	ox/o	produced by	-genic
		producing	-gen; -genic
		producing images	-graphy
pain	-algia; -dynia	production	genesis; -poiesis
painful	dys-	profuse sweating	diaphor/e
pancreas	pancreat/o	prolapse	-ptosis
paralysis	-plegia	pronation	pronati/o
parathyroid gland	parathyroid/o	prostate	prostat/o
parietal bone	pariet/o	protrusion	-cele
part with child	-para	pubis (a portion of	pub/o
patches	-plakia	the hip bone)	
patella	patell/a; patell/o	pudendum	episi/o; vulv/o
pelvis	pelv/i; pelv/o	pupil	core/o; pupill/o
penis	phall/o		

DEFINITION	WORD ELEMENT	DEFINITION	WORD ELEMENT
pus	py/o	skin	cutane/o; derm/o; -derma; dermat/o; -dermis
pyloric sphincter	pylor/o		
pylorus	pylor/o		
quick	oxy-	skull	crani/o
		small	-ole; -ule
radius (bone of lower arm)	radi/o	small bronchial tubes	bronchiol/o
		small intestine	enter/o
reconstruction	-plasty	smooth	lei/o
record	-gram	socket	glen/o
rectum	proct/o; rect/o	sodium	natr/o
red	erythemat/o; erythr/o	softening	-malacia
relaxation	-chalasis	something inserted	catheter/o
removal	de-	sound	ech/o; son/o
renal pelvis	pyel/o	specialist	-ician; -logist
resembling	-oid	specialist in the measurement of	-metrist
respiration	pneumat/o; pneum/o		
retina	retin/o	specialist in the study of; one who specializes; specialist	-er; -or; -ician; -ist; -logist
rhythm	rhythm/o		
ribs	cost/o		
rod-shaped	rhabd/o	speech	-phasia
rupture	-rrhexis	spermatozoa (sperm)	sperm/o; spermat/o
		sphenoid bone	sphen/o
sac	cyst/o	spinal column	spin/o
sac filled with synovial fluid located around joints	burs/o	spinal cord	myel/o
		spine	spin/o
		spitting	-ptysis
sac in which the fetus lies in the uterus	amni/o	spleen	splen/o
		split	-spadias
sagging	-ptosis	splitting	-schisis
saliva	sial/o	stable	-stasis
salivary gland	sialaden/o	standing	-stasis
same	home/o	stapes	staped/o
scanty	oligo-	state of	-ia; -ism; -sis
scapula	scapul/o	step (to)	-grade
sebum	seb/o	sternum	stern/o
second	secundi-	stomach	gastr/o
secrete (to)	crin/o; -crine	stone	-lith; lith/o
self	auto-	stop (to)	-continence
sensation	-esthesia	stoppage	-pause; -stasis
separate	-crit; -lysis	straight	ortho-
sew	-rrhaphy	stretching	-ectasis
sex glands	gonad/o	striated	rhabd/o
sharp	oxy-	stricture	-stenosis
shield	thyr/o; thyroid/o	striped	rhabd/o
shin	tibi/o	structure	-ium; -um
shut (to)	-myein	study of	-logy
sieve	ethm/o	sudden, involuntary contraction	-spasm
sight	opt/o		
sigmoid colon	sigmoid/o	sugar	gluc/o
sinuses	sinus/o	supination	supinati/o
skeleton	skelet/o	surgical binding	-desis

DEFINITION	WORD ELEMENT	DEFINITION	WORD ELEMENT
surgical fixation	-pexy	trachea	trache/o
surgical fracture	-clasis	transmission	-phoresis
surgical fusion	-desis	treatment	-therapy
surgical puncture to remove fluid	-centesis	trigone	trigon/o
		tube	tub/o
surgical reconstruction	-plasty	tumor	-oma
surgical refracture	-clasis	turmoil	-clonus
surgical removal	-ectomy	turning	-tropia; -tropion; versi/o
surgical repair	-plasty	two	di-
suture (to sew)	-rrhaphy	tying	ligati/o
swallow	-phagia	tympanic membrane	tympan/o; myring/o
swayback	lord/o		
sweat	hidr/o	ulna (bone of lower arm)	uln/o
sword	xiph/o	umbilicus	umbilic/o
synovium	synovi/o	under	hypo-; sub-
		unequal size	anis/o
tail	caud/o	up	-ana
tailbone	coccyg/o	upon	epi-
tears	dacry/o; lacrim/o	upper arm	humer/o
teeth	odont/o	upper dilated portion of the ureter	pyel/o
temporal bone	tempor/o		
tendon	tend/o; tendin/o	upper jaw	maxill/o
tendon sheath	tenosynovi/o	urea (end product of protein breakdown and is found in urine)	ure/o
tension	tensi/o; ton/o		
testicle	orchi/o; orchid/o; test/o; testicul/o		
		ureter	ureter/o
testis	orchi/o; orchid/o; test/o; testicul/o	urethra	urethr/o
		urinary tract	ur/o
thalamus	thalam/o	urination	ur/o; -uria
thigh bone	femor/o	urine	ur/o; -uria; urin/o
thing	-us	uterine tube	salping/o; -salpinx
thirst	-dipsia	uterus	uter/o; hyster/o; metr/o
thorax	thorac/o		
throat	pharyng/o	uvea	uve/o
thymus gland	thym/o		
thyroid gland	thyr/o; thyroid/o	vagina	colp/o; vagin/o
tibia	tibi/o	valve	valvul/o
tilting	versi/o	variation	poikil/o
tip of penis	balan/o	varicose vein	varic/o
tipping	versi/o	vas deferens	vas/o
tissue	hist/o; histi/o	vein	phleb/o; ven/o
together	sym-	ventricle (lower chambers of the heart)	ventricul/o
tone	ton/o		
tongue	gloss/o; lingu/o	vertebra	vertebr/o; spondyl/o
tonsils	tonsill/o	vessel	angi/o; vas/o; vascul/o
tooth	dent/o; odont/o	view (to)	-opsy
top	acr/o	vision	-opia; -opsia; opt/o
toward	ad-	visual condition	-opia; -opsia
toward the head	super/o	voice	-phonia
trabecula (strands of connective tissue)	trabecul/o	voice box	laryng/o
		vomit	-emesis

DEFINITION	WORD ELEMENT	DEFINITION	WORD ELEMENT
vulva	episi/o; vulv/o	windpipe	trache/o
wall	pariet/o	with	endo-; sym-
washing	-clysis	within	endo-; infra-; intra-
water	aque/o; hydr/o	without	e-
wedge	sphen/o	woman	gynec/o
white	albin/o; leuk/o	wrist	carp/o
wide	mydri/o	writing	-gram
widen	dilat/o		

Index

NOTE: Page numbers followed by "F" refer to figures. Page numbers followed by "T" refer to tables.